HANDBOOK OF

Cancer Emergencies

Mark A. Marinella, MD, FACP, CNSP

Associate Clinical Professor of Internal Medicine
Department of Internal Medicine
Wright State University School of Medicine
Hematology/Oncology
Dayton Physicians, LLC
Dayton, OH

JONES AND BARTLETT PUBLISHERS
Sudbury, Massachusetts
BOSTON   TORONTO   LONDON   SINGAPORE

World Headquarters

Jones and Bartlett Publishers
40 Tall Pine Drive
Sudbury, MA 01776
978-443-5000
info@jbpub.com
www.jbpub.com

Jones and Bartlett Publishers
Canada
6339 Ormindale Way
Mississauga, Ontario L5V 1J2
Canada

Jones and Bartlett Publishers
International
Barb House, Barb Mews
London W6 7PA
United Kingdom

Jones and Bartlett's books and products are available through most bookstores and online book-sellers. To contact Jones and Bartlett Publishers directly, call 800-832-0034, fax 978-443-8000, or visit our website, www.jbpub.com.

Substantial discounts on bulk quantities of Jones and Bartlett's publications are available to corporations, professional associations, and other qualified organizations. For details and specific discount information, contact the special sales department at Jones and Bartlett via the above contact information or send an email to specialsales@jbpub.com.

The authors, editor, and publisher have made every effort to provide accurate information. However, they are not responsible for errors, omissions, or for any outcomes related to the use of the contents of this book and take no responsibility for the use of the products and procedures described. Treatments and side effects described in this book may not be applicable to all people; likewise, some people may require a dose or experience a side effect that is not described herein. Drugs and medical devices are discussed that may have limited availability controlled by the Food and Drug Administration (FDA) for use only in a research study or clinical trial. Research, clini-cal practice, and government regulations often change the accepted standard in this field. When consideration is being given to use of any drug in the clinical setting, the healthcare provider or reader is responsible for determining FDA status of the drug, reading the package insert, and re-viewing prescribing information for the most up-to-date recommendations on dose, precautions, and contraindications, and determining the appropriate usage for the product. This is especially important in the case of drugs that are new or seldom used.

Production Credits
Executive Publisher: Christopher Davis
Sr. Editorial Assistant: Jessica Acox
Production Director: Amy Rose
Production Editor: Daniel Stone
Marketing Manager: Ilana Goddess
V.P., Manufacturing and Inventory Control: Therese Connell
Composition: Auburn Associates, Inc.
Cover Design: Scott Moden
Cover Image: © Victoria Field/ShutterStock, Inc.
Printing and Binding: Malloy, Inc.
Cover Printing: Malloy, Inc.

Library of Congress Cataloging-in-Publication Data
Marinella, Mark A., 1967-
 Handbook of cancer emergencies / Mark A. Marinella.
    p. ; cm.
 Includes bibliographical references and index.
 ISBN-13: 978-0-7637-6989-5 (alk. paper)
 ISBN-10: 0-7637-6989-4 (alk. paper)
 1. Cancer—Complications—Handbooks, manuals, etc. 2. Medical
emergencies--Handbooks, manuals, etc. I. Title.
 [DNLM: 1. Emergencies—Handbooks. 2.
Neoplasms--complications—Handbooks. QZ 39 M338h 2010]
 RC270.9.M37 2010
 616.99'4025--dc22
                              2009012143
6048

Printed in the United States of America
13 12 11 10 09   10 9 8 7 6 5 4 3 2 1

Dedication

This book is dedicated to my friend and colleague Robert Barker, MD, who not only gave me my start in medicine but also extended constant mentoring, expert medical advice, unlimited opportunities to grow professionally, and numerous second chances, especially early in my career.

Table of Contents

Section I

Section II

Section III

Section IV

Section V

Section VI

Section IX

Foreword

The clinical manifestations of malignant diseases and their treatment arguably involve the broadest spectrum of acute medical problems of any subspecialty. There has previously not been a single source in which these diverse problems have been collected and presented in a manner that is both comprehensive and succinct. If someone had presented me with the idea of preparing such a text, I would have considered the task formidable and probably impossible to do in such a manner that the result would be something that I would find a useful addition to my library. I would have been wrong.

The utility of this text results from careful thought to the organization of each clinical problem, grouped by organ system affected, beginning with a concise definition and progressing through clinical setting, pathogenesis, etiology, symptoms and signs, diagnostic studies, treatment, and prognosis. The descriptions of pathogenesis are particularly elegant as very few sentences are used to relate relevant, basic, and clinical science information to clinical presentation. What has been accomplished is an improbable marriage of bare bones pocket guide to comprehensive, authoritative text, producing an offspring that is more readable and more quickly useful and informative than either parent.

This text deserves its small-footprint place in the library of any who provide medical care to cancer patients.

Michael A. Baumann, MD
Professor of Medicine
Chief, Division of Hematology/Oncology
Boonshoft School of Medicine
Wright State University
Dayton, OH

Preface

Although much of oncologic care is provided in the outpatient arena to compensated patients, significant numbers of individuals with cancer are at-risk for developing disease-specific, as well as treatment-related, acute complications, some of which can be life-threatening. Most clinicians providing anticancer therapies, or those involved with supportive or more peripheral care of the cancer patient, are aware of the "classic" oncologic emergencies such as cardiac tamponade, spinal cord compression, and hypercalcemia. While these emergent problems are not uncommonly encountered in a busy clinical setting, many other common and not-so-common true oncologic emergencies and acute, less emergent complications unique to the cancer population may invoke significant morbidity and mortality. Since cancer is a leading cause of hospitalization and death in the Western World, clinicians of all specialties are touched by this disease almost daily in their professional endeavors. As such, any physician, nurse, or physician extender involved in cancer care should be at least familiar with the unique presentations and manifestations of various acute complications that afflict patients with malignancy—especially those with advanced disease or who are undergoing systemic therapy. To this end, this text is intended to foster interest in the acute care of the cancer patient by presenting a succinct overview of a spectrum of not only traditional oncologic emergencies, but also acute medical disorders and treatment-related complications that can occur with a variety of malignancies. In addition to oncologists/hematologists and radiation oncologists, I hope this book will prove helpful for physicians of other specialties such as internal medicine, emergency medicine, surgical disciplines, family practice, and a host of other subspecialties who regularly treat patients with cancer. Other clinicians such as nurse practioners, physicians' assistants, and bedside nurses may also find this book useful in providing day-to-day patient care. This work is in no way intended to serve as a substitute for major oncology texts or treatment manuals. Rather, it is meant as a starting point for appreciating the broad spectrum of acute pathologic processes that may complicate malignancy and provide a succinct review of the pathogenesis and approach to diagnosis and management of these various disorders.

Mark A. Marinella, MD, FACP, CNSP

Acknowledgments

I wish to extend my appreciaton to Michael Baumann, MD, and Steven Burdette, MD, for their time and expertise in reviewing the manuscript.

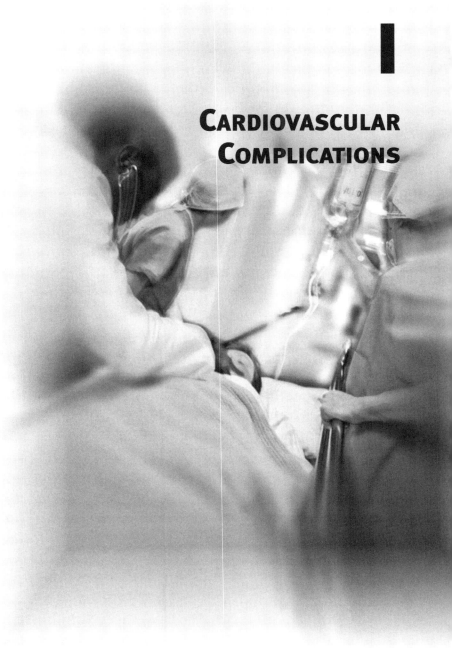

I

CARDIOVASCULAR COMPLICATIONS

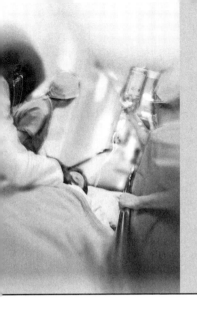

1

Cardiac Tamponade

DEFINITION

Cardiac tamponade is a form of obstructive shock in which increased pericardial pressure from accumulation of blood or fluid within the pericardial space results in impaired cardiac filling, decreased cardiac output, and hemodynamic compromise.

CLINICAL SETTING

Malignancy is the most common cause of cardiac tamponade in medical patients and typically occurs in the setting of known metastastic cancers, most commonly breast and lung cancer.

PATHOGENESIS

Cardiac tamponade occurs when malignant fluid or blood accumulates in the pericardial space impairing ventricular diastolic filling, which results in decreased cardiac output and, eventually, hemodynamic collapse. The pericardium is comprised of a visceral and parietal layer that is separated by a potential space normally containing 10 to 20 milliliters of fluid, a transudate of plasma. Pericardial fluid formation may exceed resorption due to disruption of lymphatic drainage in cases of pericardial inflammation or neoplastic invasion. Pericardial effusions complicating cancer tend to be large due to the slow accumulation of fluid which allows the pericardium to stretch, thereby increasing compliance. However, an acute increase in pericardial fluid, as occurs with hemopericardium, can cause tamponade with only small amounts of fluid (<100 cc) since pericardial compliance is limited.

Hemopericardium occurring in the cancer population may result from disseminated intravascular coagulation (DIC), thrombocytopenia, or anticoagulant drugs.

The three pathogenic mechanisms of cardiac tamponade involve elevation of intracardiac pressures, impaired cardiac diastolic filling, and decreased cardiac output. Impaired cardiac filling results in a decline of cardiac output and, eventually, cardiogenic shock. Increases in central venous pressure are also present. These hemodynamic derangements are responsible for the characteristic clinical manifestations of cardiac tamponade, namely hypotension, elevated jugular venous pressure, and the presence of a pulsus paradoxus. A pulsus paradoxus is defined as a greater than 10 mmHg decline in systolic blood pressure during inspiration. With inspiration during cardiac tamponade, right ventricular enlargement and leftward interventricular shift result in diminished left ventricular cavity volume, which contributes to the decline in cardiac output. As such, during tamponade, the normal inspiratory augmentation of right ventricle volume causes an exaggerated reciprocal decline in left ventricular volume. Since cardiac output is the product of heart rate and stroke volume, this decline in ventricular volume results in decreased stroke volume and, as a result, diminished cardiac output. Eventually, impaired perfusion of vital organs results, culminating in cardiogenic shock and multiple organ failure and, if untreated, death.

ETIOLOGY

Overall, metastatic breast and lung cancer account for the majority of cases of cardiac tamponade in cancer patients. Other tumors, conditions, and drugs unique to the cancer patient may be involved in some patients:

- Malignant pericardial effusion
  - Breast cancer
  - Lung cancer
  - Melanoma
  - Leukemia
  - Lymphoma
- Non-malignant pericardial effusion
  - Congestive heart failure/cardiomyopathy
    - Ischemic heart disease due to prior left-sided chest wall radiation
    - Anthracycline cardiomyopathy
    - Traztuzumab cardiomyopathy
  - Uremia
    - Obstructive uropathy due to prostate or cervical cancer
    - Myeloma kidney
    - Chemotherapy: cisplatinum
  - Chemotherapeutic agents
    - All-trans retinoic acid, busulfan
  - Radiation pericarditis

- ○ Nephrotic syndrome
  - ▪ Multiple myeloma, amyloidosis, paraneoplastic (lymphoma, solid tumors)
- ○ Hemopericardium
  - ▪ Coagulopathy, thrombocytopenia, trauma

Symptoms and Signs

Pericardial effusions may be asymptomatic in the absence of hemodynamic compromise. However, with the development of cardiac tamponade patients are usually symptomatic; common clinical manifestations include:

- Anxiety or "sense of doom"
- Dyspnea
- Orthopnea
- Chest pain
- Fatigue
- Edema
- Tachycardia
- Tachypnea
- Pulsus paradoxus
- Elevated neck veins
- Hypotension
- Quiet heart sounds
- Ewart's sign
  - ○ Area of dullness underneath the angle of the left scapula in the presence of a large pericardial effusion causing compressive atelectasis
- Kussmaul's sign (failure of neck veins to collapse with inspiration)
- Beck's triad: elevated neck veins, quiet heart sounds, and hypotension—present in 10% to 40% of cases

Diagnostic Studies

Diagnosis of cardiac tamponade requires a high index of suspicion. In fact, the diagnosis of cardiac tamponade should be considered in any patient with known cancer who develops dyspnea, chest pain, neck vein distention, or hypotension and the diagnosis pursued with the following:

- Chest radiography
  - ○ May reveal enlarged cardiac silhouette—the so-called "water-bottle" heart
- Computed tomography
  - ○ More sensitive for detection of pericardial fluid than chest radiography, but does not provide information on hemodynamic changes
- Electrocardiogram
  - ○ Sinus tachycardia and low-voltage QRS complexes common
  - ○ Electrical alternans. That is, alternating QRS amplitude resulting from heart "swinging" in pericardial fluid

- Right-sided heart catheterization
  - Invasive, but may provide diagnosis if pulmonary artery catheter already inserted
  - Elevation and equalization of right atrial, pulmonary artery diastolic, and pulmonary capillary wedge pressures
  - Right atrial pressure exceeding 20 mmHg indicates impending hemodynamic collapse
- Echocardiography
  - An echo-free space surrounding the heart
  - Altered mitral and tricuspid inflow
  - Diastolic chamber collapse
    - Right atrium followed by right ventricle and left ventricle collapse

TREATMENT

If the patient is hemodynamically unstable, emergent treatment is required and includes volume infusion with crystalloids via large vein access. Some patients may require vasopressors until definitive pericardial decompression can be performed. In an emergent situation, a percutaneous pericardiocentesis can be performed with a spinal needle and is best performed via echocardiographic guidance. Definitive drainage is typically performed via subxiphoid pericardiostomy (pericardial window), which has a high success rate and is associated with low surgical morbidity. Pericardial sclerosis after drainage may benefit select patients with malignant pericardial disease.

PROGNOSIS

Untreated, cardiac tamponade results in refractory hypotension, shock, and death. Relief of elevated pericardial pressure restores cardiac function. However, even in patients with resolution of cardiac tamponade, the prognosis depends on the stage and response to therapy of the underlying malignancy. However, most patients have a poor prognosis with survival of less than 1 year and median survival of 2 months.

ADDITIONAL READING

Ben-Horin S, Bank I, Guetta V, et al. Large symptomatic pericardial effusion as the presentation of unrecognized cancer: a study of 173 consecutive patients undergoing pericardiocentesis. *Medicine (Baltimore)* 2006;85:49–53.

Keefe DL. Cardiovascular emergencies in the cancer patient. *Semin Oncol* 2000; 27:244–255.

Laham RJ, Cohen DJ, Kuntz RE, et al. Pericardial effusion in patients with cancer: outcome with contemporary management strategies. *Heart* 1996;75:67–71.

Larrea L, De La Rubia J, Jimenez C, et al. Cardiac tamponade and cardiogenic shock as a manifestation of all-trans retinoic acid syndrome: an association not previously reported. *Haematologica* 1997;82:463–464.

Marinella MA. Cardiac tamponade. In: *Recognizing Clinical Patterns: Clues to a Timely Diagnosis.* Philadelphia: Hanley and Belfus, 2002.

Spodick DH. Acute cardiac tamponade. *N Engl J Med* 2003;349:684–690.

Yeh ETH, Tong AT, Lenihan DJ, et al. Cardiovascular complications of cancer therapy: diagnosis, pathogenesis, and management. *Circulation* 2004; 109:3122–3131.

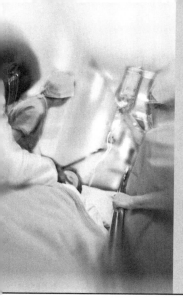

2

Anthracycline Cardiomyopathy

DEFINITION

Anthracycline cardiomyopathy is a dose-dependent form of chronic left ventricular dysfunction characterized by irreversible global systolic impairment following administration of any anthracycline but especially with doxorubicin.

CLINICAL SETTING

Anthracycline cardiomyopathy generally occurs months to years after treatment with an anthracycline, most commonly doxorubicin in cumulative doses exceeding 450 mg/m^2.

PATHOGENESIS

Anthracycline antibiotics are widely utilized cytotoxic agents utilized in the treatment of a variety of neoplasms, such as breast cancer, acute myeloid leukemia, and Hodgkin's and non-Hodgkin's lymphoma. These agents intercalate between strands of DNA causing interruption of DNA synthesis which leads to cell death. Anthracycline cardiomyopathy is most commonly dose-related and is postulated to result from the generation of iron-containing free radicals that induce myocardial inflammation and fibrosis. One theory is that enzymatic reduction of the anthracycline ring results in oxidation of cell membrane phospholipids which causes cell membrane damage. Free-radical damage to intracellular organelles such as mitochondria may contribute to cell damage and death, resulting in fibrosis. Due to fibrosis, the left ventricle typically is normal-sized, without dilatation, which is a characteristic feature of anthracycline cardiomyopathy. Additionally, anthracyclines may lead to intracellular deposition of calcium, which damages cardiomyocytes, impairing systolic function. Development of heart failure symptoms usually occurs within 1 year of treatment, although onset may occur decades later. Gradual development of symptomatic left ventricular dysfunction is most common, but biventricular systolic heart failure and restrictive cardiomyopathy have been reported. As left ventricular function and cardiac output decline, typical physiologic adaptions of systolic cardiomyopathy occur such as neurohumoral activation of the symphatic and renal-angiotensin-aldosterone axes which leads to the various phenotypic changes characteristic of chronic heart failure. Concurrent administration of thoracic radiotherapy, taxanes, traztuzumab, or uncontrolled hypertension increase the risk of cardiac damage. Cyclophosphamide, an alkylating agent that may cause hemorrhagic myonecrosis, may potentiate the cardiotoxic risk of anthracyclines. Doxorubicin doses of greater than 450-550 mg/m^2 are associated with significantly increased risk and should be avoided. Prolonged infusions of doxorubicin and administration of the iron-chelating free-radical scavenger, dexrazoxane, may decrease the risk of anthracycline cardiomyopathy in high-risk patients.

ETIOLOGY

Any of the following anthracyclines can induce cardiomyopathy:

- Doxorubicin
  - Most commonly implicated anthracycline
- Daunorubicin
- Idarubicin
- Epirubicin
- Mitoxantrone
  - An anthracenedione agent that lacks the amino group present on the anthracyclines, which may impart less cardiotoxicity

SYMPTOMS AND SIGNS

Cardiotoxicity from anthracyclines should be considered in any patient who is receiving or has received an anthracycline and develops the following:

- Progressive dyspnea
- Orthopnea
- Edema
- Palpitations
- Tachycardia
- Ventricular gallop
- Elevated jugular venous pressure
- Pulmonary rales

DIAGNOSTIC STUDIES

Diagnosis of anthracycline cardiomyopathy requires judicious use of radiographic and laboratory testing. Some of the most clinically useful tests and findings include:

- Electrocardiogram
  - Sinus tachycardia, low QRS voltage, non-specific ST-T wave changes, and poor R-wave progression across the precordial leads
- Chest radiograph
  - Normal cardiac silhouette size, pleural effusions, venous encouragement, pulmonary edema
- B-natriuretic peptide
  - Sensitive biomarker for impaired left ventricular function, but not specific for anthracycline toxicity
- Myocardial biopsy
  - Invasive and infrequently utilized with improved imaging techniques to assess ventricular function
  - Cytoplasmic changes within cardiomyocytes and fibrosis as assessed by Billingham score may predict risk of cardiomyopathy
- Nuclear stress testing
  - Fall in ejection fraction with stress may indicate limited myocardial reserve which may preclude further anthracycline use in subsequent cycles
- Echocardiography
  - Test of choice: typically reveals septal dyskinesis, mitral regurgitation with a characteristic posteriorly-directed jet, decreased left ventricular compliance and ejection fraction with normal left ventricular mass

TREATMENT

The treatment of patients presenting with symptoms of acute congestive heart failure due to anthracyclines is similar to patients with any type of systolic heart failure. However, a caveat in treating these patients is that the limited left ventricular volume results in a smaller stroke volume and cardiac output than patients with other types of cardiomyopathy. Because of this, avoiding rapid and profound decreases in heart rate is necessary to avoid decompensation. Optimal treatment of traditional cardiac risk factors such as hypertension, hyperlipidemia, diabetes mellitus, and smoking cessation are important. Drug treatment hinges upon beta-antagonists (e.g., carvedilol, metoprolol), angiotensin converting enzyme inhibitors, digoxin, and loop diuretics.

PROGNOSIS

If patients are diagnosed before severe ventricular dysfunction occurs, and anthracyclines are discontinued, patients may have a good prognosis with standard medical therapy. However, if diagnosed later in the disease course, mortality rates of 20% have been reported.

ADDITIONAL READING

Keefe DL. Anthracycline-induced cardiomyopathy. *Semin Oncol* 2001;28 (suppl 12):2–7.

Mason JW, Bristow MR, Billingham ME, et al. Invasive and noninvasive methods of assessing andriamycin cardiotoxic effects in man: superiority of histopathologic assessment using endomyocardial biopsy. *Cancer Treat Rep* 1978;62:857–864.

Shaddy RE, Olsen SL, Bristow MR, et al. Efficacy and safety of metoprolol in the treatment of doxorubicin-induced cardiomyopathy in pediatric patients. *Am Heart J* 1995;129:197–199.

Singal PK, Iliskovic N. Doxorubicin-induced cardiomyopathy. *N Engl J Med* 1998;339:900–905.

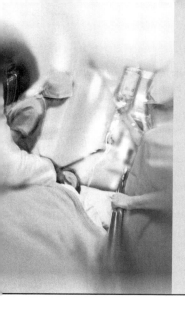

3

5-Fluorouracil-Induced Cardiotoxicity

DEFINITION

5-fluorouracil (5-FU) is an antimetabolite that inhibits DNA synthesis. It may cause potentially life-threatening cardiotoxicity that manifests as myocardial infarction or ischemia, ventricular arrythmia, or sudden death.

CLINICAL SETTING

Evidence of 5-FU cardiotoxity has been reported in up to 6% of patients during prolonged intravenous infusions utilized for treatment of various neoplasms, usually colorectal, esophageal, and head and neck malignancies.

PATHOGENESIS

5-FU is a fluoropyrimidine antimetabolite cytotoxic drug that requires a complex, multi-step enzymatic activation process for interruption of tumor growth. This drug is cell-cycle specific, acting primarily in the S-phase of the cell cycle. A detailed discussion of the metabolic activation of 5-FU is beyond the scope of this text. However, thymidylate synthase is the key target enzyme within tumor tissue that is inhibited by 5-FU and is responsible for ultimate cytotoxicity. Inhibition of thymidylate synthase leads to accumulation of intermediate products (e.g., dUMP) that result in inhibition of DNA synthesis. 5-FU undergoes extensive metabolism by various enzymatic systems, with dihydropyrimidine dehydrogenase (DPD) being the key catabolic enzyme. In fact, deficiency of DPD may lead to life-threatening myelosuppression and mucositis manifested as profuse diarrhea and sepsis.

Historically, 5-FU has been the backbone of treatment for gastrointestinal malignancies (e.g., esophagus, stomach, colon) and breast cancer. Most often, 5-FU is administered by bolus or, more recently, by continuous intravenous infusion for treatment of esophageal and colonic cancers. Capecitabine, a newer oral prodrug that requires three-step activation to 5-FU, is being utilized more frequently to treat breast and gastrointestinal cancers, with similar effects.

5-FU, and more recently capecitabine, has been associated with cardiotoxicity which most commonly complicates prolonged intravenous infusions. This is seen most often during the initial cycle of chemotherapy. Mild cases of 5-FU cardiotoxicity may manifest as asymptomatic, non-specific electrocardiographic changes. However, life-threatening toxicity is typically associated with myocardial ischemia, angina, and ventricular arrhythmias. Although the exact pathogenesis is unclear, most authors suggest that direct endothelial toxicity from 5-FU may be responsible. It is postulated that coronary artery smooth muscle spasm induced by the catabolite, fluoroacetate, may result in myocardial ischemia, infarction, and arrhythmia induction. Some patients with 5-FU cardiotoxicity have been noted to have elevated serum endothelin-1 levels, a potent vasoconstrictor. The significance of this, however, is unclear. Although pre-existing coronary artery disease or thoracic radiation therapy are predisposing factors for 5-FU vasospasm, cases have been reported in angiographically normal arteries. Some authors have documented coronary artery vasospasm during angiography, supporting the notion that toxicity is related to smooth muscle constriction.

ETIOLOGY

Cases of 5-FU toxicity have been reported with the following 5-FU regimens:

- 5-fluorouracil
  - Reported with bolus and infusional regimens
- Capecitabine

SYMPTOMS AND SIGNS

Most symptoms and signs of cardiotoxicity result from myocardial ischemia and include:

- Angina pectoris
- Palpitations
- Dyspnea
- Diaphoresis
- Dizziness
- Tachycardia
- Ventricular gallop

DIAGNOSTIC STUDIES

Diagnosis of 5-FU cardiotoxicity requires a high index of suspicion but ancillary studies are necessary for the diagnosis:

- Electrocardiogram
  - ST-segment elevation (indicative of vasoocclusion due to spasm) or depression, sinus tachycardia, ventricular arrhythmias, conduction disturbances
- Echocardiogram
  - Depressed ejection fraction, dyskinesis of left ventricle
- Cardiac enzymes
  - Elevation in troponin or creatine phosphokinase
- Coronary angiography
  - Coronary artery spasm: can occur in normal coronary arteries, but underlying plaque may be present

TREATMENT

If 5-FU cardiotoxicity is suspected, cessation of the drug is imperative. Generally, the drug should not be resumed with further chemotherapy cycles, although some authors have successfully rechallenged patients with prophylactic arterial dilators. Pharmacologic agents that have been reported to treat vasospasm include intravenous nitroglycerin and calcium channel blockers (e.g., diltiazem, verapamil) and intracoronary nitroglycerin. Many authors recommend aspirin in the absence of a contraindication.

PROGNOSIS

Prognosis is favorable if 5-FU is discontinued before myocardial necrosis occurs; most cases resolving with supportive care.

ADDITIONAL READING

Chu E, McGowan M, Elfiky A, et al. Chemotherapeutic and biologic drugs. In: *Physicians' Cancer Chemotherapy Drug Manual* 2007. Chu E, DeVita VT, eds. Boston: Jones and Bartlett Publishers, 2007, pp. 15–378.

Labianca R, Beretta G, Clerici M, et al. Cardiac toxicity of 5-Fluorouracil: a study on 1083 patients. *Tumori* 1982;68:505–510.

Keefe DL, Roistacher N, Pierri MK. Clinical cardiotoxicity of 5-Fluorouracil. *J Clin Pharmacol* 1993;33:1060–1070.

Schnetzler B, Popova N, Lamb CC, et al. Coronary spasm induced by capecitabine. *Ann Oncol* 2001;12:723–724.

Shoemaker LK, Arora U, Rocha Lima MS. 5-Fluorouracil-induced coronary vasospasm. *Cancer Control* 2004;11:46–49.

Tsavaris N, Kosmas, Vadiaka M, et al. Cardiotoxicity following different doses and schedules of 5-Fluorouracil administration for malignancy–a survey of 427 patients. *Med Sci Monit* 2002;8:51–57.

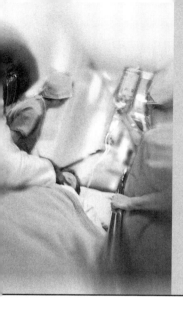

4

Complete Atrioventricular Block

DEFINITION

Atrioventricular (AV) block results from impaired transmission of the electrical impulse from the atria to the ventricular conduction system, which results in AV dissociation and impaired cardiovascular performance.

CLINICAL SETTING

Complete AV block (or complete heart block) is a rare occurrence in the cancer patient and usually occurs in the setting of widely metastatic disease that involves the heart, increased vagal tone, or certain medications.

PATHOGENESIS

Most cases of complete AV block in patients with cancer complicate widespread metastatic disease that secondarily involves the AV node. The AV node is an anatomic area of specialized excitatory and conductive cardiomyocytes located within the right atrium in the region of atrial septum. Spontaneous electrical impulses generated within the intrinsic cardiac pacemaker, the sinoatrial node, spread along specialized conduction pathways to reach the AV node. Once within the AV node, the impulse is delayed before reaching the ventricles; this delay is manifest at the PR interval on the normal surface electrocardiogram.

Although virtually any malignancy can metastasize to the heart, melanoma seems to have the highest propensity to spread to the myocardium. Lung and breast cancers can not only spread hematogenously, but also involve cardiac tissue by contiguous extension. Lymphoma and leukemia are frequently found to involve the heart at autopsy. Whatever the underlying neoplasm, the pathogenesis of malignancy-associated AV block results from neoplastic cell infiltration of the AV node, although inflammation and fibrosis may play a role as well. Radiation therapy has been reported to cause fibrosis in the region of the AV node. Doxorubicin and cyclophosphamide infusion have been reported to cause complete AV block and may result from AV nodal inflammation, local release of vasoactive substances, endothelial damage to AV-node microvasculature, or intense drug-induced nausea and vomiting resulting in heightened vagal tone.

ETIOLOGY

Etiologies of complete AV block in cancer patients include:

- Melanoma
    - Melanoma is the tumor with the highest incidence of cardiac metastasis
- Non-Hodgkin's lymphoma
- Cardiac angiosarcoma
- Doxorubicin
- Cyclophosphamide
    - Usually high-dose therapy used for hematopoietic stem cell transplantation
- Thoracic or mediastinal radiation (especially for Hodgkin's lymphoma)
- Stem cell transplantation
    - Dimethylsulfoxide cryopreservative-induced

SYMPTOMS AND SIGNS

Complete AV block can present with sudden cardiac death or the following clinical manifestations:

- Dyspnea
- Chest discomfort
- Nausea
- Vomiting
- Lightheadedness
- Syncope
- Bradycardia
- Hypotension
- Cool extremities

DIAGNOSTIC STUDIES

Bradycardia and hypotension should prompt consideration of complete AV block in any patient with metastatic cancer or who has a history of anthracylcine administration. Useful diagnostic studies include:

- Electrocardiogram
    - Typical findings include bradycardia and AV dissociation in which the atria and ventricles beat at their own rates, each driven by their intrinsic pacemakers

- Echocardiogram
  - Myocardial mass or infiltration involving the atrium or the area of the interventricular septum
  - Anterior wall hypokinesis and atrial-ventricular dyssynchrony may also be noted
- Cardiac magnetic resonance imaging
  - Useful to detect myocardial metastasis
- Computed tomography

TREATMENT

Patients with documented complete AV block should be admitted to a cardiac care unit, have adequate vascular access, and have transcutaneous pacing patches applied. Some patients may require temporary transvenous pacing or a permanent pacemaker if a cardiac metastasis is the etiology. Treatment of the underlying malignancy with chemotherapy should be considered, especially in a chemotherapy-sensitive disease such as lymphoma where control of disease may resolve the heart block.

PROGNOSIS

Untreated AV block can result in cardiogenic shock and death. Patients with an otherwise treatable malignancy may have a favorable prognosis after permanent pacemaker implantation.

ADDITIONAL READING

Ando M, Yokozawa T, Sawada J, et al. Cardiac conduction abnormalities in patients with breast cancer undergoing high-dose chemotherapy and stem cell transplantation. *Bone Marrow Transplant* 2000;25:185–189.

Cohen IS, Bharati S, Glass J, et al. Radiotherapy as a cause of complete atrioventricular block in Hodgkin's disease. *Arch Intern Med* 1981;141:676.

Kilickap S, Akgul E, Aksoy S, et al. Doxorubicin-induced second degree and complete atrioventricular block. *Europace* 2005;7:227–230.

Klatt EC, Heitz DR. Cardiac metastases. *Cancer* 1990;65:1456–1459.

Ozyunco U, Sahin M, Altin T, et al. Cardiac metastasis of malignant melanoma: a rare cause of complete atrioventricular block. *Europace* 2006;8:545–548.

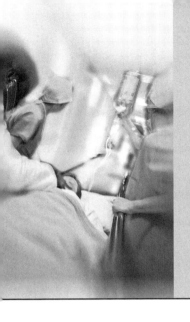

5

Torsades de Pointes

Definition

Torsades de pointes ("twisting about the points"), or polymorphic ventricular tachycardia, is a malignant ventricular arrhythmia characterized by QRS complexes of varying amplitude that twist around the isoelectric baseline of the electrocardiogram.

Clinical Setting

Torsades de pointes is closely associated with prolongation of the QT interval, which is the interval that encompasses ventricular depolarization and repolarization. Prolongation of the QT interval in the cancer patient may occur in the setting of electrolyte derangements, cardiomyopathies, use of class I anti-arrhythmics for underlying heart disease, or with the use of certain antimicrobial or chemotherapeutic agents.

Pathogenesis

Prolongation of the QT interval is a common electrocardiographic manifestation of any state that results in delayed repolarization, such as hypokalemia and drugs that act as class I anti-arrhythmic agents. If the next cycle of ventricular depolarization occurs before repolarization is complete (R on T phenomenon), ventricular tachycardia or Torsades de pointes may ensue. Additionally, any drug that prolongs action potential duration or induces early after depolarizations or ectopy may induce Torsades. Since this arrhythmia is a form of ventricular tachycardia, cardiac output abruptly declines leading to hypotension and cardiac arrest. Underlying cardiomyopathy may increase the risk of Torsades in the setting of electrolyte depletion (e.g., hypokalemia or hypomagnesemia) or drugs that prolong the QT interval.

ETIOLOGY

Etiologies of Torsades de pointes that are peculiar to the patient with cancer include:

- Electrolyte derangements
  - Hypokalemia and hypomagnesemia secondary to chemotherapy-induced vomiting and diarrhea
  - Diuretics used to treat edema from volume overload, taxanes, or all-trans retinoic acid syndrome
  - Renal wasting of magnesium and potassium due to acute myeloid leukemia, platinum analogues, or ifosfamide
- Cardiomyopathy
  - Anthracycline or traztuzumab-induced
- Chemotherapeutic agents
  - Arsenic trioxide used to treat promyelocytic leukemia
    - May result from arsenic-induced autonomic neuropathy resulting in sympathetic imbalance
- Supportive care agents
  - Haloperidol, ondansetron
- Antimicrobial agents
  - Azole antifungal agents, quinolones, erythromycin

SYMPTOMS AND SIGNS

Patients with Torsades may be asymptomatic if the arrhythmia spontaneously remits or if sudden death occurs. Otherwise, some of the clinical findings include:

- Palpitations
- Lightheadedness
- Syncope
- Dyspnea
- Chest discomfort
- Irregular and diminished pulse
- Hypotension

DIAGNOSTIC STUDIES

A high index of suspicion for Torsades should alert the clinician to place the patient on continuous telemetric monitoring. However, diagnostic studies include:

- Electrocardiogram
  - Prolongation of the QT interval, prominent U waves if hypokalemia or hypomagnesemia is present
  - Irregular QRS complexes of varying morphology

- Holter monitor
  - May be useful in patients with risk factors who complain of non-specific symptoms

TREATMENT

Prompt airway and hemodynamic control are imperative. Patients with cardiopulmonary arrest should be intubated, if applicable, and concurrent treatment for the Torsades de pointes should be instituted. Defibrillation is the treatment of choice if the patient is hemodynamically unstable. Intravenous magnesium sulfate may be utilized as well.

Isoproterenol infusion shortens the QT interval, and may be helpful for intermittent, refractory cases as may an overdrive pacemaker. Correction of hypokalemia and hypomagnesemia and discontinuation of non-essential QT-altering drugs are important treatment adjuncts.

PROGNOSIS

Prognosis for Torsades de pointes depends upon rapid diagnosis and treatment before hemodynamic collapse occurs. In the setting of a reversible factor such as electrolyte depletion or medication effect, prognosis is favorable with correction of the triggering event. Patients receiving arsenic trioxide should have their QT interval and electrolytes monitored regularly during treatment.

ADDITIONAL READING

Marinella MA, Burdette SD. Hypokalemia-induced QT interval prolongation. *Am J Emerg Med* 2000;35:405.

Tatesu H, Asou N, Nakamura M, et al. Torsades de pointes upon fluconazole administration in a patient with acute myeloblastic leukemia. *Am J Hematol* 2006;81:366–369.

Unnikrishnan D, Dutcher JP, Varshneya N, et al. Torsades de pointes in 3 patients with leukemia treated with arsenic trioxide. *Blood* 2001;97:1514–1516.

Viskin S. Long QT syndromes and Torsades de pointes. *Lancet* 1999;354:1625–1633.

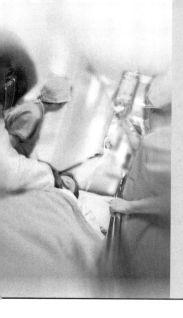

6

Superior Vena Cava Syndrome

DEFINITION

Superior vena cava (SVC) syndrome is a clinical constellation of symptoms and signs that result from elevated upper body venous pressures due to extrinsic compression or intraluminal obstruction of the SVC, most often due to malignancy.

CLINICAL SETTING

Most patients with the SVC syndrome have known cancer, but it may be the first manifestation of malignancy with thoracic involvement. Some patients develop SVC syndrome in the setting of central venous catheter use or hypercoagulability, both of which are prevalent in the cancer patient.

PATHOGENESIS

The SVC is a thin-walled vein that collects and drains venous blood from the head, upper extremities, and torso. Anatomically, the SVC is formed by the confluence of the brachiocephalic veins. In turn, the brachiocephalic veins are formed by the conjunction of the subclavian and jugular veins. The SVC commences at approximately the level of the sternal angle, which courses along the right side of the ascending aorta to empty into the right atrium. The distal two centimeters of the SVC are contained within the pericardial sac. Due to the compliant nature of the SVC in the vicinity of several rigid mediastinal structures, it is easily compressed by extrinsic mass lesions, most commonly metastatic or primary thoracic neoplasms. Enlarged lymph nodes can also occlude the low-pressure SVC. Occlusion of the SVC by intraluminal thrombosis also leads to impaired flow and venous return. Superior vena cava thrombosis can occur secondary to tumoral-induced vascular damage, vessel wall invasion, or from an indwelling vascular catheter. Generally, SVC obstruction above the azygous vein orifice is better tolerated than obstruction caudad to the orifice. The azygous vein is the primary collateral flow system for the SVC and is formed by contributions from ascending lumbar and subcostal veins. Collateral flow via the azygous system is allowed since there are numerous anastomses between the SVC, azygous vein, and lumbar veins. Furthermore, other collateral vessels for the SVC include the mammary, vertebral, lateral thoracic, esophageal, and paraspinous venous systems. If SVC obstruction occurs cephalad to the azygous vein, blood is diverted through chest wall veins into the thoracic and iliac veins, which ultimately reaches the heart via the inferior vena cava (IVC) and azygous venous system. Phenotypically, this scenario is manifest as dilation of veins over the chest wall and breasts. If the SVC is obstructed between the azygous vein and the heart, the only possible way of blood return is via the IVC.

Impaired venous return leads to collateralitization of the azygous system and increased central venous pressure, sometimes reaching as high as 20 to 40 mmHg (normal range 2 to 8 mmHg). Increased venous pressure results in edema formation of the upper body soft tissues, nasopharynx, larynx, ocular vasculature, and occasionally, the brain, which can prove fatal on rare occasions. Severe laryngeal edema can lead to airway compromise and acute obstructive respiratory failure. As such, the symptoms of SVC syndrome result primarily from increased venous pressures and tissue and organ edema.

ETIOLOGY

Approximately 65% of cases of SVC syndrome are due to malignant diseases, most commonly lung cancer. However, with the increased use of central venous catheters for the administration of cytoxic chemotherapy, thrombosis of the SVC is not uncommon. Some of the causes of SVC syndrome in the cancer patient include:

- Superior vena cava thrombosis
  - Secondary to central venous catheter
  - Hypercoagulability secondary to malignancy
  - Venous stasis and endothelial damage resulting from tumor compression or erosion of the SVC
- Lung cancer
  - Usually in smokers
    - Non-small cell cancers (e.g., adenocarcinoma, squamous, and large cell carcinomas) account for 50% of cases of malignant SVC syndrome
    - Small cell lung cancer
- Lymphoma
  - Non-Hodgkin's and Hodgkin's lymphoma
- Metastatic cancer
  - Breast cancer most common
  - Gastrointestinal cancer

- Germ cell tumor
  - Usually male patients with mediastinal mass
- Thymoma
  - May be associated with myasthenia gravis
- Mesothelioma
  - Typically in setting of prior asbestos exposure

Symptoms and Signs

Most patients have subacute symptoms of a few weeks duration. Rapid onset of SVC occlusion may increase the risk for cerebral edema. More than 95% of patients are symptomatic at presentation and manifest various characteristic physical findings, often in combination:

- Sensation of "fullness" within the head
- Dyspnea
- Facial swelling
- Cough
- Visual blurring
- Headache
- Dizziness
- Arm swelling/edema
- Hoarseness
- Dilated chest wall veins
- Distended neck veins
- Facial plethora
- Conjunctival injection
- Engorged retinal veins on fundoscopic examination
- Stridor
- Confusion
- Papilledema

Diagnostic Studies

Any patient, especially a smoker, with symptoms of SVC syndrome noted to have elevated jugular venous pressure and dilated chest wall veins should undergo imaging to confirm the diagnosis; tissue procurement is also vital if there is no prior diagnosis of malignancy. The most useful diagnostic studies include:

- Chest radiograph
  - Typically reveals a right upper thoracic or paratracheal mass
  - Pleural effusion common
- Contrast-enhanced computed tomography scan
  - Findings usually include thoracic mass, lymphadenopathy, pleural effusions, and a slit-like superior vena cava
  - Contrast filling of collateral vessels such as azygous system
  - Thrombosis may be present, especially if a catheter is present

- Positron emission tomography (PET) scan
  - May be useful in delineating benign from malignant disease, cancer staging, and response to treatment
- MRI
  - May be useful if iodinated contrast is contraindicated
- Venogram
  - Gold standard but cumbersome, uncomfortable, and carries risk of venous thrombosis
- Invasive diagnostic modalities for tissue diagnosis. The least invasive maneuver should be the first.
  - Thoracentesis and cytologic analysis if pleural effusion is present
  - Lymph node biopsy or aspiration
    - If lymphoma is suspected, excisional node biopsy is optimal
  - Bronchoscopy with endobronchial brushings or transbronchial biopsy
  - Percutaneous CT-guided biopsy
    - High-yield procedure and generally technically feasible in most patients
  - Mediastinoscopy
  - Video-assisted thoracoscopic surgery (VATS)

TREATMENT

Treatment of SVC syndrome is typically not truly emergent unless evidence of airway compromise or cerebral edema is present. Most patients can be managed in an expectant and thoughtful manner, while simultaneously pursuing tissue diagnosis. The crux of treatment is radiation therapy, especially for radiation-sensitive diseases such as lung cancer. Patients with highly chemotherapy-sensitive tumors, such as lymphoma, small cell carcinoma, or germ cell tumor, can be treated with chemotherapy alone if the patient is otherwise stable. Patients with impending airway obstruction from laryngeal edema or severe central nervous system dysfunction from cerebral edema may benefit from emergent placement of an SVC endovascular stent preceded by angioplasty. Patients with radioresistant tumors such as mesothelioma or metastatic renal cell carcinoma may also improve following stent deployment. General supportive measures should be instituted as well and include elevation to the head of the bed to facilitate dependant venous drainage; corticosteroids (e.g., dexamethasone) to decrease airway or cerebral edema; loop diuretics; and anticoagulation in the presence of SVC thrombus.

PROGNOSIS

Overall, prognosis of patients with SVC syndrome is poor, with a median survival of 6 months. However, patients with chemotherapy-sensitive neoplasms, such as small cell cancer, lymphoma, and germ cell tumor, may enjoy prolonged survival or even cure. Survival among patients with neoplastic SVC syndrome is not substantially different than those patients with the same cancer type and disease stage who do not develop SVC syndrome.

ADDITIONAL READING

Courtheoux P, Alkofer B, Al Refai M, et al. Stent placement in superior vena cava syndrome. *Ann Thorac Surg* 2003;75:158–161.

Laskin J, Cmelak AJ, Roberts J, et al. Superior vena cava syndrome. In: Abeloff MD, Armitage JO, Niederhuber JE, et al., eds. *Clinical Oncology*. 3rd ed. Philadelphia: Elsevier Churchill Livingstone, 2004, pp 1047–1061.

Marinella MA. Superior vena cava syndrome. In: *Recognizing Clinical Patterns: Clues to a Timely Diagnosis*. Philadelphia: Hanley and Belfus, 2002.

Rice TW, Rodriguez RM, Light RW. The superior vena cava syndrome: clinical characteristics and evolving etiology. *Medicine (Baltimore)* 2006;85:37–42.

Wilson LD, Detterback FC, Yahalom J. Superior vena cava syndrome with malignant causes. *N Engl J Med* 2007;356:1862–1869.

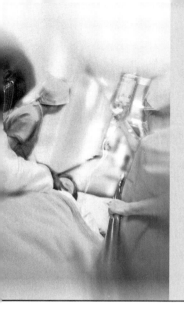

7

Marantic Endocarditis

Definition

Marantic, or non-bacterial thrombotic, endocarditis is a potentially devastating complication of advanced cancer that is characterized by bland, fibrin-laden vegetations involving the mitral and aortic valves that may result in catastrophic embolic phenomena.

Clinical Setting

The majority of cancer patients with marantic endocarditis have widely metastatic adenocarcinomas, typically mucin-producing, often in the setting of low-grade disseminated intravascular coagulation (DIC).

Pathogenesis

Patients with cancer, especially those with adenocarcinoma, often exhibit hypercoagulability resulting from tumor cell production of procoagulant species such as cysteine proteases and tissue factor which activate the clotting cascade ultimately resulting in thrombus formation. Circulating monocytes interact with malignant cells causing release of proinflammatory cytokines such as tumor necrosis factor, interleukin (IL)-1, and IL-6, which results in endothelial damage of blood vessels and the heart. Additionally, tissue factor plays a role in the coagulation cascade by forming a complex with factor VIIa which activates the common coagulation pathway resulting in the formation of a fibrin clot. Pathologic clotting in the setting of malignancy may manifest as deep venous thrombosis, pulmonary embolism, arterial occlusion, or DIC. An uncommon complication of advanced malignancy is the formation of sterile, fibrin-rich vegetations on the cardiac valvular surfaces, a phenomenon known as marantic endocarditis. Microtrauma to cardiovalvular endothelium in the setting of carcinoma can trigger the tissue factor-VIIa cascade resulting in the formation of bland fibrin-rich vegetations. Vegetations on the aortic or mitral valves may dislodge and enter the arterial circulation, culminating in end-organ damage in the brain, coronary circulation, mesenteric vasculature, or extremities. As such, marantic endocarditis may present as stroke, myocardial infarction, mesenteric infarction, or lower extremity gangrene, respectively. Furthermore, release of proinflammatory cytokines often results in systemic inflammation manifesting as fever, weight loss, night sweats, anorexia, and fatigue. Microvascular emboli may invoke capillary occlusion and a vasculitis-like picture within the acral areas and kidneys.

ETIOLOGY

The cancers most frequently associated with marantic endocarditis include:

- Pancreatic adenocarcinoma
- Gastric carcinoma
- Lung cancer
  - Especially adenocarcinoma and bronchioloalveolar carcinoma
- Ovarian carcinoma
- Breast carcinoma

SYMPTOMS AND SIGNS

Patients may be asymptomatic and present suddenly with neurologic, abdominal, or cardiac symptoms depending on the ultimate destination of the embolus. Some of the symptoms of marantic endocarditis include:

- Constitutional symptoms
  - Fever
  - Malaise
  - Anorexia
  - Weight loss
- Neurologic
  - Hemiparesis
  - Aphasia
  - Ataxia
  - Confusion
  - Dysarthria
  - Dysphagia
  - Diplopia
  - Coma
- Subungual and subconjuctival splinter hemorrhages
- Livedo reticularis

- Angina pectoris
- Flank pain and hematuria
  - Suggestive of acute renal infarction from renal artery embolus
- Abdominal pain
  - Acute mesenteric ischemia
- Acute arterial insufficiency of the lower extremities
  - Pain, pallor, diminished pulses, cool feet

DIAGNOSTIC STUDIES

Diagnosis of marantic endocarditis requires a high index of suspicion and should be suspected in any patient with underlying malignancy who develops sudden neurologic or stroke-like symptoms, angina, abdominal pain, or symptoms of extremity ischemia. Helpful diagnostic studies include:

- Complete blood count and coagulation studies
  - Anemia, prolonged prothrombin time (PT) and partial thromboplastin time (PTT), thrombocytopenia, hypofibrinogenemia, elevated D-dimer, and schistocytes if DIC is present
- Urinalysis
  - Often reveals hematuria and proteinuria
- Echocardiography
  - Transesophageal echocardiography is more sensitive to detect smaller valvular vegetations, which typically involve the mitral and/or aortic valves
- Magnetic resonance imaging and angiography of the brain
  - May reveal recent cerebral infarction or embolic vascular occlusion
  - Areas of infarction involve the bilateral cerebral hemispheres and reflect a central embolic source
- Visceral computed tomographic angiography (CTA) and conventional computed tomography (CT)
  - Emboli to the mesenteric arteries may appear as a filling defect or vessel cut-off
  - Low density areas in the liver, spleen, and kidneys from embolic arterial infarction

TREATMENT

Since marantic endocarditis frequently complicates the course of disseminated, usually incurable cancer, supportive care is paramount. In some patients, treatment of the underlying cancer with chemotherapy may be considered. Anticoagulation is suggested by many authors, especially if concurrent hypercoagulability-related venous or arterial thrombosis is present. Some studies suggest improved outcomes with low-molecular weight heparins in patients with malignancy, possibly due to anti-cancer effects of this drug class.

Prognosis

Prognosis of patients with acute stroke, mesenteric ischemia, or myocardial infarction from systemic emboli is very poor. From an oncologic standpoint, since most patients have widespread disease, lifespan is typically measured in weeks.

Additional Reading

Blanchard DG, Ross RS, Dittrich HC. Nonbacterial thrombotic endocarditis: assessment by transesophageal echocardiography. *Chest* 1992;102:954–956.

Chen L, Li Y, Gebre W, et al. Myocardial and cerebral infarction due to nonbacterial thrombotic endocarditis as an initial presentation of pancreatic adenocarcinoma. *Arch Pathol Lab Med* 2004;128:109–111.

Edoute Y, Haim N, Rinkevich D, et al. Cardiac valvular vegetations in cancer patients: a prospective echocardiographic study of 200 patients. *Am J Med* 1997;102: 252–258.

Singhal AB, Topcuoglu MA, Buonannao FS. Acute ischemic stroke patterns in infective and nonbacterial thrombotic endocarditis: a diffusion-weighted magnetic resonance imaging study. *Stroke* 2002;33:1267–1273.

Vassallo R, Remstein ED, Parisi JE, et al. Multiple cerebral infarctions from nonbacterial thrombotic endocarditis mimicking cerebral vasculitis. *Mayo Clin Proc* 1999;74:798–802.

Young RSK, Salneraitis EL. Marantic endocarditis in children and young adults: clinical and pathological findings. *Stroke* 1981;12:635–639.

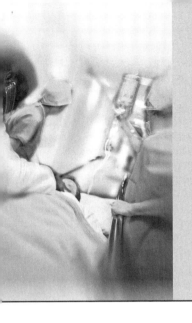

8

Venous Gas Embolism

Definition

Venous gas embolism (VGE) denotes the presence of gas (typically ambient air) within the systemic venous circulation that may lead to catastrophic hemodynamic collapse.

Clinical Setting

The majority of cases of VGE occurring in cancer patients are iatrogenic in nature and result from ambient air entering central venous catheters, although various surgical procedures may also result in VGE.

Pathogenesis

The circulating blood column contains a variety of dissolved gases, notably oxygen and carbon dioxide. The entry of gas—typically ambient air but also carbon dioxide, nitrous oxide, or nitrogen—into the venous circulation is enhanced by the incising of noncollapsing veins and the subatmospheric pressure present within this compartment. Noncollapsing veins that may serve as a portal-of-entry during medical and surgical procedures include the epiploic veins, dural venous sinuses, and veins in the throat, which may entrain air during neurosurgical and head and neck procedures, respectively. Air may also gain access via central venous catheters or through the myometrium during the puerperium. In the cancer patient, VGE is most likely to occur through placement or manipulation of a central venous catheter or port. During inspiration, intrathoracic pressure declines, enhancing entrainment of ambient air into an open catheter lumen. Pathologic venous entrainment of ambient air (VGE) results in the formation of multiple air bubble emboli, which resemble a string of pearls. These air bubbles have the tendency to coalesce, forming sizes large enough to occlude not only the microvasculature but also larger vessels such as the pulmonary outflow tract. Upon reaching the right heart and pulmonary circulation, the workload of the right ventricle increases abruptly, as does pulmonary arterial vascular resistance. As a result of acute right heart strain and pulmonary hypertension, pulmonary venous volume declines leading to decreased left ventricular preload and cardiac output. If untreated, malignant ventricular arrhythmias, cardiovascular collapse, and shock rapidly ensue. If large amounts of gas or air (>50 milliliters) enter the venous circulation, acute asystole may occur. Additionally, ventilation-perfusion mismatch results in intrapulmonary shunting, exacerbating pulmonary vasoconstriction, pulmonary hypertension, hypoxemia, and hypercapnia, all of which increases cardiac workload further. If a patent foramen ovale is present, cerebral ischemia and infarction may result from entry of air bubbles into the arterial circulation.

ETIOLOGY

Any procedure or condition that creates an interface between the ambient environment and the venous circulation may result in VGE. Etiologies of VGE in the cancer patient include:

- Central venous catheters
  - During catheter insertion, or if hub is open or damaged, air may enter the catheter in a spontaneously breathing patient due to the negative intrathoracic pressure generated with inspiration
  - Volume depleted and cachectic patients at higher risk
- Hemodialysis catheters
- Laparoscopic surgery
  - May occur with pneumoperitoneum
- Endoscopic procedures
  - Esophagogastroduodenoscopy
  - Colonoscopy
  - Endoscopic retrograde pancreatography (ERCP)
- Orthopaedic surgical procedures
  - Hip arthroplasty for pathologic fracture
  - Spine surgery
- Video assisted thoracoscopic surgery (VATS)
- Radical prostatectomy for prostate cancer
- Neurosurgical procedures performed in the sitting position
  - Air may enter the dural venous sinuses or epiploic veins during craniotomy

SYMPTOMS AND SIGNS

In an obtunded, sedated, or intubated patient, symptoms may go unnoticed, and the only clinical clue to VGE may be an acute drop in blood pressure or oxygen saturation. If the patient is connected to mechanical ventilation or is undergoing general anesthesia, a sudden decline in end-tidal carbon dioxide may be the only indicator of VGE. Other symptoms and signs include:

- Inspiratory gasp
- Dyspnea
- Lightheadedness
- Chest pain
- Tachypnea
- Apnea
- Tachycardia
- Confusion
- Seizures
- Cyanosis
- Cool extremities
- Harsh, "mill wheel" cardiac murmur
  - A splashing sound best ausculatated over the precordium or epigastrium that results from air in the cardiac chambers and great vessels

DIAGNOSTIC STUDIES

The diagnosis of VGE may be made clinically in any cancer patient with a central venous catheter who develops sudden hypotension, hypoxia, tachycardia, and the classic "mill wheel" murmur. However, if the diagnosis is unclear helpful ancillary studies include:

- Decreased end-tidal carbon dioxide
  - Can be measured only if patient is intubated
- Chest radiography
  - Insensitive, but if air embolus is large, may reveal hyperlucency in the right ventricle
- Air bubbles upon aspiration of central venous catheter
- Electrocardiogram
  - Acute right bundle branch block or right axis deviation if pulmonary hypertension is severe
- Echocardiogram
  - May reveal intracardiac air and right ventricular dilation and strain
  - Transesophageal route more sensitive

TREATMENT

If VGE is suspected in the correct clinical setting, immediate treatment measures include prevention of further air entry into the circulation via the Valsalva maneuver and stopping the source of air exposure. Immediately placing patient into the left lateral decubitus (Durant's maneuver) and Trendelenburg position allows air to migrate to right ventricular apex, away from outflow tract. Administration of oxygen (100% FiO2) facilitates resorption of air. Some authors advocate syringe aspiration of blood and air from the central venous catheter, if present. General supportive measures include volume expansion, inotropic support with dobutamine, and mechanical ventilation. Hyperbaric oxygen therapy, often cumbersome and difficult to obtain, may be useful in refractory cases or in the setting of paradoxical VGE with cerebral ischemia.

PROGNOSIS

If not recognized and treated, VGE may result in rapid cardiovascular collapse and death. Small amounts of air entering the venous circulation may be tolerated without sequelae in the patient with no pre-existing cardiac disease. If stroke occurs from the presence of a patent foramen ovale, permanent neurologic dysfunction may result.

ADDITIONAL READING

De Angelis J. A simple and rapid method for evacuation for embolized air. *Anesthesiology* 1975;43:110–111.

McGee DC, Gould MK. Preventing complications of central venous catheterization. *N Engl J Med* 2003;348:1121–1133.

Murphy BP, Harford FJ, Cramer FS. Cerebral air embolism resulting from invasive medical procedures. *Ann Surg* 1985;201:242–245.

Muth CM, Shank ES. Gas embolism. *N Engl J Med* 2000;342:476–481.

Palmon SC, Moore LE, Lundberg J, et al. Venous air embolism: a review. *J Clin Anesth* 1997;9:251–257.

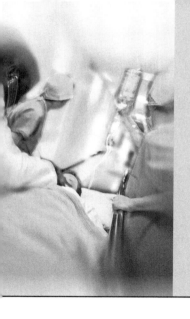

9

Tracheo-innominate Fistula

DEFINITION

Tracheoinnominate fistula (TIF) is an uncommon, but deadly, complication of tracheostomy that results from tracheostomy tube-induced pressure necrosis and erosion of the innominate artery which results in massive arterial bleeding and fatal exsanguination.

CLINICAL SETTING

The incidence of TEF is < 1% in patients with tracheostomy tubes placed for a variety of conditions and typically occurs in the presence of an overinflated cuff, a low-lying tube, or excessive tube movement. The majority of cases occur between 3 and 4 weeks following tracheostomy.

PATHOGENESIS

The innominate (brachiocephalic) artery is the largest branch of the aortic arch and is approximately 4–5 centimeters long before dividing into the right common carotid and right subclavian arteries. The artery arises from the convex portion of the aortic arch behind the sternal manubrium and ascends passing in anatomic proximity to the trachea, where it crosses at approximately the ninth tracheal ring. If a tracheostomy tube is placed below the third tracheal ring, if the balloon is overinflated, or if there is excessive tube movement, gradual pressure necrosis of the tracheal mucosa may ensue with eventual erosion through the tracheal wall and into the innominate artery, resulting in a TIF. Increased cuff pressures (>20 mmHg) can lead to impaired tracheal mucosal blood flow by exceeding capillary perfusion pressure. Prolonged endotracheal intubation and radiation therapy to the neck region may also play a pathophysiologic role. If erosion into the inominate artery occurs, exsanguinating hemorrhage may result. Smaller amounts of blood emanating through the tracheostomy tube may precede massive hemorrhage, a phenomenon known as a sentinel bleed.

ETIOLOGY

In the cancer patient, several scenarios in which TIF may occur include:

- Tracheostomy tube placement for advanced head and neck cancer or prolonged mechanical ventilatory support
- Radiation therapy to the neck area in patients with head and neck malignancy
  - Risk increased in patient with concurrent tracheostomy tube or large necrotic neoplasm
- Prolonged mechanical ventilation and endotracheal tube placement in cancer patients with respiratory failure

SYMPTOMS AND SIGNS

Patients with tracheostomy tubes may have difficulty in relaying symptoms due to impaired speech function. Additionally, patients receiving mechanical ventilation via an endotracheal tube cannot verbally communicate. Clinical manifestations such as the following should suggest TIF:

- Minor hemoptysis or blood-tinged tracheal secretions
  - More than 50% of patients who develop TIF report or are noted to exhibit this symptom or sign, a phenomenon known as a "sentinel" hemorrhage
- Bright red blood per tracheostomy—may be massive
  - TIF until proven otherwise
- Cough
- Dyspnea
- Tachycardia
- Hypotension
  - May result from hemorrhagic shock

DIAGNOSTIC STUDIES

Any patient who develops blood-tinged tracheal secretions or frank tracheal bleeding in the first several weeks following tracheostomy or who is receiving protracted mechanical ventilation should be suspected of having a TIF. The diagnosis is clinical. Immediate transfer to the operating suite for fiberoptic or rigid bronchoscopy is indicated if TIF is suspected.

TREATMENT

In the presence of massive tracheostomy bleeding, immediate tamponade of the innominate artery is required while awaiting definitive treatment. Overdistention of the tracheostomy cuff or insertion of a finger into the tracheal stoma to compress the innominate artery against the sternum are indicated to produce temporary vessel tamponade. Insertion of an endotracheal tube with cuff inflation distal to the stoma to protect the distal airway from blood aspiration should be considered. Definitive treatment of TIF, however, remains surgical exploration with debridement and repair of the fistula and innominate artery, respectively.

PROGNOSIS

Without operative repair, the mortality rate of a TIF is 100%. Therefore, diagnosis of TIF needs to be entertained in at-risk patients who are noted to have bloody tracheal discharge and appropriate surgical referral instituted.

ADDITIONAL READING

Brewster DC, Moncure AC, Darling RC, et al. Innominate artery lesions: problems encountered and lessons learned. *J Vasc Surg* 1985;2:99–112.

Epstein SK. Late complications of tracheostomy. *Respir Care* 2005;50:542–549.

Grant CA, Dempsey G, Harrison J, et al. Tracheo-innominate artery fistula after percutaneous tracheostomy: three case reports and a clinical review. *Br J Anaesth* 2006;96:127–131.

Kapural L, Sprung J, Glunic J, et al. Tracheo-innominate artery fistula after tracheostomy. *Anesth Analg* 1999;88:777–780.

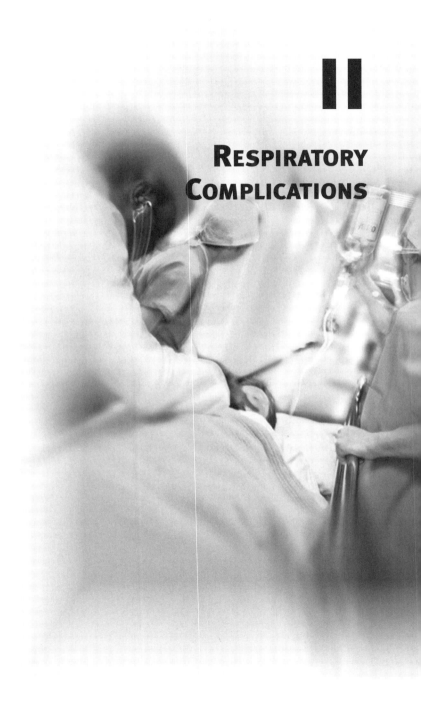

II

RESPIRATORY
COMPLICATIONS

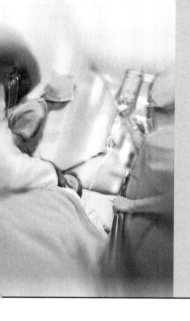

10

Acute Pulmonary Embolism

DEFINITION

Pulmonary embolism (PE) represents the life-threatening end of the venous-thromboembolism spectrum. A PE occurs when a venous thrombus, typically originating in the lower extremities, dislodges and migrates to the pulmonary artery circulation.

CLINICAL SETTING

Although pulmonary embolism can affect multiple segments of the general population, the presence of cancer, treatment with systemic chemotherapy, recent cancer surgery, and immobility all provide the clinical setting for a PE to occur.

PATHOGENESIS

The pathogenesis of venous thromboembolism is complex and only a brief overview of the pathogenic mechanisms in the cancer patient will be discussed. Virchow's triad underlies the formation of venous thrombosis and consists of a hypercoagulable state, venous stasis, and endothelial disruption. Patients with cancer frequently fulfill the triad, which makes this population especially prone to venous thromboembolism. Various tumor types, especially mucin-secreting adenocarcinomas of the lung or abdomino-pelvic viscera, secrete thrombogenic substances such as tissue factor or cysteine proteases that can activate the clotting cascade, resulting in thrombus formation and propagation. Venous stasis due to nodal or tumoral compression of venous outflow, poor mobility, recent surgery, or a bedbound state from cancer-associated debility, increase local blood viscosity, further enhancing the risk. The third part of Virchow's triad, endothelial disruption, is often fulfilled in the cancer patient due to venous endothelial damage from vascular catheters, chemotherapy, surgical procedures, or tumor-invasion of the vasculature.

Most cases of PE result from embolization of thrombi from the lower extremity and pelvic veins, although thrombi of the upper extremity veins associated with central venous catheters may also embolize. Although PE may be asymptomatic, large, central emboli occluding the bifurcation of the main pulmonary trunk ("saddle embolus") may result in sudden death due to acute right heart failure and hemodynamic collapse. Large pulmonary emboli not causing sudden death can lead to acute pulmonary hypertension, cor pulmonale, hypoxic pulmonary vasoconstriction, and impaired left ventricular filling. All of these increase the risk of death due to arrhythmia, respiratory failure, or cardiac failure.

ETIOLOGY

As alluded to, the cancer patient has many co-existing factors that increase the risk of venous thrombosis and pulmonary embolism:

- Immobility
  - Recent surgery
  - Generalized debility
  - Spinal cord compression
  - Pathologic fracture
- Venous trauma
  - Vascular catheters
  - Surgery
  - Peri-venous tumor or lymph node
- Malignancy
  - Adenocarcinoma
    - Pancreas
    - Ovary
    - Stomach
    - Colorectal
    - Lung
    - Breast
    - Prostate
  - Glioblastoma multiforme
  - Lymphoma
  - Acute promyelocytic leukemia
- Chemotherapy drugs
  - L-asparaginase
  - Thalidomide
  - Cisplatinum

Symptoms and Signs

Pulmonary embolism often presents with non-specific symptoms and signs. This can make the diagnosis a challenge, even to the most experienced of clinicians. Up to 10% of patients with acute PE die within the first hour and often present with syncope and clinical signs of shock. However, a variety of clinical manifestations may occur, making it important to consider PE in any cancer patient with otherwise unexplainable symptoms and signs, which include:

- Dyspnea
  - Occurs in approximately 75% of patients with symptomatic PE
- Pleuritic chest pain
  - If present with dyspnea and hemoptysis, PE should be considered the diagnosis until proven otherwise
- Hemoptysis
- Cough
- Palpitations
- Leg pain and swelling
- Sense of impending doom
- Confusion
- Hypotension
- Tachypnea
- Pulmonary rales
- Tachycardia
- Ventricular gallop
- Jugular venous distention
  - If cor pulmonale is present

Diagnostic Studies

Since many conditions in the cancer patient can mimic the presentation of acute PE (e.g., pneumonia, pleural effusion, pericardial tamponade), diagnostic accuracy is imperative, although not without challenges. Some of the most useful diagnostic studies include:

- Electrocardiogram
  - Sinus tachycardia, right bundle branch block, right ventricular strain pattern, S1Q3T3 pattern, atrial fibrillation
- Chest radiography
  - Often normal but may reveal pleural effusion, wedge-shaped infiltrate, or peripheral venous oligemia (Westermark sign)
- Ventilation-perfusion (VQ) scan
  - Helpful only if negative or high probability
  - Often non-specific in patients with underlying pulmonary metastasis, pneumonia, or pre-existing lung disease

- Spiral computed tomography
  - Emerging as the diagnostic study of choice due to rapid imaging time, wide-availability, and ability to detect other etiologies for cardiopulmonary symptoms
  - Sensitivity and specificity in the 80% to 90% rates for more central emboli but less sensitive for peripheral emboli
- Pulmonary angiography
  - Gold standard but invasive and may increase risk of venous thrombosis
  - Intravascular "cut off" or filling defect is diagnostic
- Echocardiogram
  - May reveal right ventricular dilatation and hypokinesis, increased pulmonary artery pressures, or dilation of the pulmonary arteries if hemodynamically significant PE is present
  - Presence of right ventricular dysfunction portends a twentyfold increase in mortality
- Compression venous ultrasound
  - If a thrombus is visualized in the correct clinical setting, PE may be diagnosed
- Cardiac troponin and B-natriuretic peptide
  - May be elevated due to increased myocardial strain and volume overload
- Arterial blood gas
  - Non-specific, but often reveals hypoxemia, hypercarbia, and a widened A-gradient
- Serum D-dimer
  - Not typically helpful in the patient with cancer due to low specificity, but if negative, PE is virtually excluded

TREATMENT

When the clinical suspicion for acute PE is high, especially in the setting of hemodynamic changes, treatment should not be delayed while awaiting diagnostic studies. Treatment of acute PE in the cancer patient is often difficult due to the frequent presence of cardiopulmonary dysfunction, multiple co-morbidities, thrombocytopenia, drug interactions, bleeding risk from coagulopathy, and brain metastasis, which may hemorrhage with systemic anticoagulation. Systemic anticoagulation with a heparin compound is the preferred initial treatment in the hemodynamically stable patient without a contraindication. Unfractionated heparin is historically the gold-standard anticoagulant drug for PE, but due to alterations in serum proteins with systemic malignancy, the anticoagulation effect is often unpredictable resulting in subtherapeutic anticoagulation effect or bleeding. Low molecular weight heparins (LMWH) such as enoxaparin or dalteparin are more efficacious than heparin in the cancer patient and have the advantages of a predictable dose response, no need to follow coagulation parameters, and ease of use. Some data suggest an anti-neoplastic effect of the LMWH agents. Fondaparinux is an anti-factor Xa inhibitor that has proven equally effective as heparin for the treatment of PE; this agent is contraindicated with significant renal failure. Warfarin, although widely utilized for chronic anticoagulation, possesses erratic anticoagulation response in malnourished cancer patients or patients with hepatic metastasis. There are also numerous potential drug interactions that may increase bleeding risk. Resistance to warfarin is common in metastatic cancer, with some patients developing recurrent thromboses despite therapeutic anticoagulation. Thrombolytic therapy is indicated in patients with hemodynamic instability or right ventricular dysfunction on echocardiography. Rapid clot lysis with streptokinase or recombinant tissue plasminogen activator induces a significant bleeding risk due to metastatic disease, age, and coagulapathy. Vena caval filter interruption is useful when anticoagulation is contraindicated or if PE occurs despite adequate anticoagulation. Catheter embolectomy is an interventional radiologic procedure in which a suction catheter is advanced into pulmonary artery for clot disruption and removal. It may be considered in the cancer patient with hemodynamic compromise, shock, or large clot burden, in whom thrombolytic therapy is contraindicated

PROGNOSIS

Patients presenting with syncope or shock have a high mortality rate and often die within the first hour of onset. In the absence of significant cardiopulmonary dysfunction, most patients respond favorably to acute anticoagulation and supportive care. However, studies demonstrate that cancer patients with venous thromboembolism have a reduced life expectancy compared to similar cancer patients without thromboembolism. Cancer patients with venous thrombosis or PE have a fourfold to eightfold higher risk of dying after an acute event than patients without malignancy. The overall 1-year survival rate in patients with cancer-related venous thromboembolism is 10% to 15%.

ADDITIONAL READING

Blann AD, Lip GYH. Venous thromboembolism. *BMJ* 2006;332:215–219.

Carlbom DJ, Davidson BL. Pulmonary embolism in the critically ill. *Chest* 2007; 132:313–324.

Hyers TM. Venous thromboembolism. *Am J Repir Crit Care Med* 1999;159:1–14.

Kearon C. Diagnosis of pulmonary embolism. *CMAJ* 2003;168:183–194.

Kucher N. Catheter embolectomy for acute pulmonary embolism. *Chest* 2007;132:657–663.

Lee AYY, Levine MN. Venous thromboembolism and cancer: risks and outcomes. *Circulation* 2003;107:I-17–I-21.

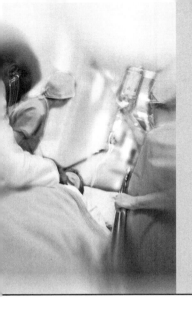

11

Pulmonary Tumor Embolism

DEFINITION

Tumor embolism (TE) is a life-threatening, and frequently overlooked, complication of advanced malignancy that results from a mass of tumor material embolizing to the pulmonary vasculature via the systemic venous circulation, resulting in a clinical syndrome similar to venous thromboembolism.

CLINICAL SETTING

Most cases of TE occur in the setting of advanced thoracic or visceral cancers, with some autopsy studies revealing frequencies up to 26% in advanced cancer patients. Indeed, the diagnosis is only rarely made ante-mortem.

PATHOGENESIS

Pulmonary TE is a life-threatening and often fatal complication of advanced cancer and shares pathogenetic features with thrombotic pulmonary embolism. Tumor cells within the abdominal cavity or thorax that reach the venous circulation may induce thrombosis, forming a growing mass of tumor cells and fibrin clot. Indeed, adenocarcinoma cells can directly activate the clotting cascade by an interaction with factor VIIa and tumor-derived tissue factor. Renal cell carcinoma and hepatocellular carcinoma are unique in that the primary tumor mass may directly invade the renal veins and hepatic veins, respectively, in a serpiginous fashion and result in TE. In any event, TE occurs when the tumor-laden complex reaches the inferior vena cava and travels to the pulmonary artery which may result in cardiac collapse if the mass is large enough, or subacute cor pulmonale if a significant portion

(>50%) of smaller pulmonary vasculature is occluded. Oxygen exchange is impaired, as is right ventricular function due to pulmonary hypertension, which occurs in thrombotic pulmonary embolism. The other route in which TE may reach the pulmonary vasculature is via lymphatic spread into the thoracic duct and then the superior vena cava.

ETIOLOGY

The majority of cases of TE occur in patients with advanced or metastatic carcinomas of the thorax or abdomen, some of which include:

- Contiguous spread of tumor mass into the vena cava
  - Renal cell carcinoma
  - Hepatocellular carcinoma
  - Adrenal carcinoma
- Venous or lymphatic spread by embolic tumor material
  - Breast cancer
  - Lung cancer
  - Gastric cancer
  - Colorectal cancer
  - Gynecologic cancer

SYMPTOMS AND SIGNS

Rarely, TE may go undetected clinically and present with sudden death in a manner similar to thrombotic PE. However, many patients have non-specific symptoms and signs:

- Dyspnea
- Cough
- Hemoptysis
- Chest pain
- Fatigue
- Tachycardia

DIAGNOSTIC STUDIES

Diagnosis of TE requires a very high index of suspicion since more common cardiopulmonary complications in the cancer patient present in similar fashion. Many diagnoses of TE are made at autopsy where tumor emboli and fibrin thrombi are found in the small, muscular pulmonary arteries and occasionally pulmonary lymphatics. In the case of macroemboli from renal cell or hepatocellular carcinoma, large plugs of tumor material may be found occluding main and segmental pulmonary arteries reminiscent of thrombotic PE. Nonetheless, diagnostic studies may include:

- Chest radiography
  - Often normal or non-specific findings

- Computed tomography
  - Pulmonary arterial filling defects (rare), pleural effusion
- Electrocardiogram
  - Sinus tachycardia, right bundle branch block, right ventricular strain
- Echocardiography
  - Dilation of the right ventricle or evidence of pulmonary hypertension if TE burden is significant
- Ventilation-perfusion lung scan
  - Multiple subsegmental perfusion defects, may be normal
- Pulmonary arteriogram
  - Most useful to exclude venous thromboembolism
  - May reveal large, occlusive emboli in the case of renal cell or hepatocellular carcinoma or delayed filling of subsegmental vessels
- Swan-Ganz pulmonary arterial blood aspiration for cytology
  - Requires a right-sided pulmonary artery catheter; 10-20 cc of blood aspirated for cytologic analysis
- Lung biopsy
  - Gold standard, but often not obtained ante-mortem
  - Reveals tumor cell emboli with surrounding fibrin material involving the small muscular pulmonary arteries and, occasionally, lymphatics

TREATMENT

Since TE is rarely diagnosed before death, no reliable trials of specific treatment exist. In cases where the diagnosis is established, chemotherapy directed at the underlying primary tumor may be utilized if the patient's performance status is adequate. Supportive care for hypoxia and hypoxic pulmonary hypertension should be treated with oxygen.

PROGNOSIS

Prognosis in the setting of TE is very poor due to the systemic nature of disease and often poor condition of patients with this disorder. As such, survival of most patients is typically measured in weeks.

ADDITIONAL READING

Bhuvaneswaren JS, Venkitachalam CG, Sandhyamani S. Pulmonary wedge aspiration cytology in the diagnosis of recurrent tumour emboli causing pulmonary arterial hypertension. *Int J Cardiol* 1993;39:209–212.

Kane RE, Hawkins HK, Miller JA. Microscopic pulmonary tumour emboli associated with dyspnea. *Cancer* 1975;36:1473–1482.

Masson RG, Krikorian J, Lukl P et al. Pulmonary microvascular cytology in the diagnosis of lymphangitic carcinomatosis. *N Engl J Med* 1989;321:71–76.

Wong CH, Suvarna SK, Ciulli F, et al. Small cell lung carcinoma presenting as acute cardiovascular collapse due to tumour cell embolisation. *Respiration* 2000; 67:323–326.

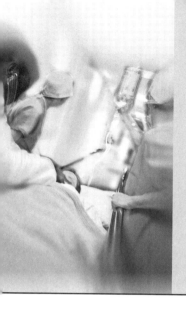

12

Lymphangitic Carcinomatosis

DEFINITION

Lymphangitic carcinomatosis (LC) represents intrapulmonary lymphatic spread of cancer cells that results in impaired gas exchange and pulmonary hypertension.

CLINICAL SETTING

Most cases of LC occur in the setting of metastatic carcinomas of various primary sites but may occasionally be the first manifestation of cancer.

PATHOGENESIS

The hallmark of LC is the spread of tumor cells within the pulmonary lymphatic circulation from microembolization (in a manner similar to tumor embolism), retrograde spread of tumor cells from involved lymph nodes, local lymphatic invasion from a primary lung cancer, or transdiaphragmatic tumor cell spread. Pathologically, LC results in firmness of lung tissue noted at autopsy. Histologic specimens characteristically reveal tumoral filling of septal and peribronchial lymphatic vessels. Mechanisms of hypoxia and pulmonary hypertension of LC include coexistent vascular tumor emboli, vascular compression by tumor-distended lymphatic vessels, and a reactive vasculopathy secondary to LC. Additionally, plugging of the lymphatic system leads to abnormal alveolar distention and parenchymal rigidity thereby increasing the work of breathing, which contributes to the refractory dyspnea so characteristic of LC. Restrictive lung physiology may also result from occult LC, and may pose a diagnostic dilemma.

Etiology

A variety of cancers have been reported with LC, some of the more common include:

- Breast cancer
- Gastric cancer
- Pancreatic cancer
- Prostate cancer
- Colorectal cancer
- Lung cancer
- Ovarian cancer

Symptoms and Signs

The presence of LC should be considered in any solid tumor patient who develops progressive, unrelenting dyspnea that is not explained by more common etiologies and does not improve with standard treatments. On rare occasion, acute respiratory failure may result, but the presentation is most often subacute in nature. Some of the more common symptoms and signs include:

- Dyspnea
- Cough
- Chest discomfort
- Fatigue
- Cyanosis
- Tachypnea
- Tachycardia
- Pulmonary rales

Diagnostic Studies

Diagnosis of LC may prove difficult and requires a high index of suspicion, diagnostic integration of symptoms, and selected diagnostic studies:

- Chest radiograph
  - A coarse, diffuse reticulonodular infiltrate, often involving the lower lung zones, is typical but may be normal in over one-half of cases
  - Kerley B lines are common and represent tumor-plugged lymphatic vessels
    - The presence of Kerley B lines in the absence of congestive heart failure is very suggestive of LC
- High-resolution computed tomography
  - More sensitive than standard computed tomography and does not require intravenous contrast
  - Typical findings of LC include nodular thickening of the bronchovascular bundles, thickening of interstitial lines, beaded interlobular septae, ground glass infiltrates, and air bronchograms

- Bronchoscopy with bronchoalveolar lavage or biopsy
  - Cytologic washings may reveal tumor cells; transbronchial biopsy may reveal neoplastic cell clusters in the lymphatic spaces, interlobular interstitium, alveoli, and peribronchovascular areas
- Swan-Ganz pulmonary artery catheter blood aspiration for cytology
  - As discussed in the section of tumor embolism, aspiration of 10-20 cc of venous blood from a pulmonary artery catheter may yield the diagnosis
- Pulmonary function testing
  - Restrictive impairment common finding with impaired DLCO
- Open lung biopsy or video-assisted thoracoscopic surgery (VATS)
  - Has much higher yield than transbronchial biopsy, but is more invasive and may be hazardous in patients with poor performance status

TREATMENT

Directing treatment at the primary tumor type may be palliative, especially in chemotherapy or hormone-sensitive diseases such as breast cancer. Supportive care, such as oxygen, is necessary in all patients.

PROGNOSIS

Generally, LC portends a very poor prognosis in patients with otherwise incurable neoplasms, and is often a preterminal event.

ADDITIONAL READING

Fujita J, Yamagishi Y, Kubo A, et al. Respiratory failure due to pulmonary lymphangitis carcinomatosis. *Chest* 1993;103:967–968.

Hauser TE, Steer A. Lymphangitis carcinomatosis. *Ann Intern Med* 1951;34:881.

Janower ML, Blennerhasset JB. Lymphangitic spread of metastatic cancer to the lungs. A radiologic-pathologic classification. *Radiology* 1971;101:267–273.

Masson RG, Krikorian J, Luki P, et al. Pulmonary microvascular cytology in the diagnosis of lymphangitic carcinomatosis. *N Engl J Med* 1989;321:71–76.

Munk PL, Muller NL, Miller R, et al. Pulmonary lymphatic carcinomatosis CT and pathologic findings. *Radiology* 1988;166:705–709.

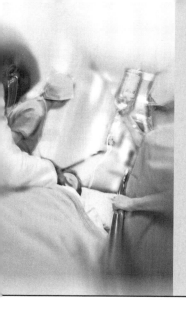

13

Acute Radiation Pneumonitis

DEFINITION

Acute radiation pneumonitis is an inflammatory reaction involving the lung parenchyma and interstitium that results from thoracic radiation therapy occurring during, or within weeks of receiving, radiotherapy.

CLINICAL SETTING

Most cases of acute radiation pneumonitis complicate thoracic radiotherapy for cancers of the lung, breast, esophagus, or lymphomas and occur within 1 to 3 months.

PATHOGENESIS

Acute radiation pneumonitis (as opposed to chronic radiation fibrotic injury) results from ionizing radiation-induced damage to various macromolecules, including DNA, peptides, lipids, and enzyme systems. Ionizing radiation may cause tissue damage directly by releasing energy sufficient to cause breakage of chemical bonds within these macromolecules or indirectly due to the interaction of radiation with tissue water. Additionally, local radiation enhances release of inflammatory cytokines, such as tumor necrosis factor (TNF), interleukins, and platelet derived growth factors which induce the inflammatory and, ultimately, the fibrogenic reaction characteristic of radiation lung injury. The acute inflammatory reaction is characterized by vascular congestion, intra-alveolar fibrinous exudation, and injury to type II pneumocytes. Local infiltration by neutrophils increases acute damage by liberation of cytotoxic chemical species. This acute injury may be followed in the coming weeks by hyperplasia of mucosal lining cells leading to increased secretions as well as sloughing of endothelial and epithelial cells. The net result of this acute inflammatory-exudative reaction is impaired pulmonary function and diminished gas exchange. The concurrent use of radiosensitizing chemotherapy such as bleomycin, gemcitabine, taxanes, and cyclophosphamide may further aggravate the tissue injury. Microvascular injury leading to capillary thrombosis may also contribute to the pathogenesis.

ETIOLOGY

Thoracic radiotherapy utilized for a variety of neoplasms may be associated with acute radiation pneumonitis:

- Lung cancer
- Breast cancer
- Esophageal cancer
- Non-Hodgkin's lymphoma
- Hodgkin's lymphoma

SYMPTOMS AND SIGNS

Acute radiation pneumonitis may present with any or all of the following symptoms and signs:

- Cough, usually non-productive
- Dyspnea
- Fever
- Pleuritic chest pain
- Malaise
- Weight loss
- Tachypnea
- Pulmonary rales
- Pleural rub

DIAGNOSTIC STUDIES

Acute radiation pneumonitis can be confused with more common processes such as tumor progression, bacterial pneumonia, or aspiration pneumonitis. Some of the following diagnostic tests may be helpful in establishing the diagnosis:

- Chest radiograph
  - Classically, reveals patchy alveolar infiltrates corresponding to radiation portals exhibiting a straight or non-anatomic line of demarcation from uninvolved lung
  - Pleural effusion or perivascular haziness on occasion
- Computed tomography
  - More sensitive than chest radiography; the straight line effect more prominent

- Blood count
  - Leukocytosis and anemia common
- Fluorodeoxyglucose (FDG) positron emission tomography (PET) scan
  - Acute radiation injury typically enhances, as does tumor and infection, making specificity of PET scanning limited
- Lung biopsy
  - Via transbronchial, open lung biopsy, or video-assisted thoracoscopic surgery (VATS)
  - Reveals infiltration of inflammatory cells, alveolar infiltration with inflammatory debris, and epithelial cell desquamation

TREATMENT

Exclusion of other common processes such as bacterial pneumonia, congestive heart failure, or pulmonary embolism is essential. If the clinical and radiographic picture is consistent with acute radiation pneumonitis, supportive care with oxygen is indicated if the patient is hypoxic. Corticosteroids such as prednisone may quell the inflammatory reaction with doses of 60 mg daily followed by a slow taper.

PROGNOSIS

Most cases of acute radiation pneumonitis resolve with minimal sequelae with steroids and supportive therapy, although some patients may experience a protracted recovery. A subset of patients may enter into a fibrotic phase, which may cause significant morbidity or mortality due to lack of effective treatment.

ADDITIONAL READING

Abratt RP, Morgan GW. Lung toxicity following chest radiation in patients with lung cancer. *Lung Cancer* 2002;35:103–109.

Churg A. Pulmonary disease in the immunocompromised host. In: Thurlbeck WM, ed. *Pathology of the Lung*. New York: Thieme Medical Publishers, 1988, pp 247–262.

Crawford SW. Noninfectious lung disease in the immunocompromised host. *Respiration* 1999;66:385–395.

Morgan GW, Pharm B, Breit SN. Radiation and the lung: a reevaluation of the mechanisms mediating pulmonary injury. *Int J Radiat Oncol Biol Phys* 1995;31:361.

Movas B, Raffin TA, Epstein AH, et al. Pulmonary radiation injury. *Chest* 1997;111:1061–1076.

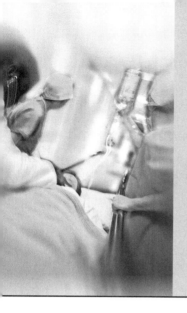

14

Diffuse Alveolar Hemorrhage

Definition

Diffuse alveolar hemorrhage (DAH) is the end result of a variety of clinical insults and is characterized by bleeding into the alveolar space resulting from damage to the pulmonary parenchyma or vasculature.

Clinical Setting

Although most cases of DAH in cancer patients occur in the setting of stem cell or bone marrow transplantation, this syndrome can complicate acute leukemia, chemotherapy administration, and various opportunistic infections.

Pathogenesis

Since the pathogenesis of DAH is complex and multifactorial, only a brief overview will be provided. Pulmonary capillaritis underlies most cases of DAH, resulting in vascular disruption and subsequent hemorrhage. Significant bleeding into the alveolar space can cause an acute decline in hematocrit with symptomatic anemia. A peculiar phenomenon of DAH is an increased DLCO that results from increased carbon dioxide diffusion through the intra-alveolar hemoglobin. In the setting of hematopoietic stem cell transplantation, DAH may result from intensive conditioning chemotherapy and total body irradiation as well as acute graft versus host disease. Damage to pulmonary endothelium may be the culprit in these cases. In the non-transplant setting, DAH frequently occurs in patients with acute leukemia, although it may be subclinical and confused with other causes of respiratory complications. Autopsy studies have noted some degree of DAH in 54% of acute leukemia patients, with severe pulmonary compromise occurring in 12% of these patients. Certain vasophilic organisms, most notably *Aspergillus* species, can erode the pulmonary vessels resulting in alveolar hemorrhage and massive hemoptysis. Necrotizing Gram-negative organisms such as *Pseudomonas aeruginosa* and *Stenotrophomonas maltophilia* have also been implicated especially in the setting of thrombocytopenia, which is nearly universal in the acute leukemia population. Platelet counts of fewer than 20,000 cells/mm^3 in conjunction with fever may increase the risk of DAH as may concurrent coagulopathy. Another proposed pathogenic mechanism of DAH is acute hemorrhagic pulmonary edema related to volume overload. Although DAH is a diagnosis of exclusion, it remains the most common cause of non-infectious pulmonary infiltrates in some studies.

ETIOLOGY

Diffuse alveolar hemorrhage can be associated with many infectious and non-infectious etiologies in the cancer population:

- Pulmonary infections
  - Fungal: *Aspergillus* species
  - Bacterial: *Pseudomonas aeruginosa*, *Stenotrophomonas maltophilia*, Klebsiella species, *Staphylococcus aureus*
  - Viral: Cytomegalovirus, Adenovirus
  - Parasitic: *Strongyloides stercoralis*
- Chemotherapy damage to endothelium
  - Cyclophosphamide, BCNU
- Acute myeloid leukemia
  - Pulmonary leukostasis
  - Monocytic leukemia
  - Acute promyelocytic leukemia
    - Disseminated intravascular coagulation (DIC)
    - Retioic acid syndrome
- Pulmonary edema
- Thrombocytopenia
- Coagulopathy/DIC
- Hematopoietic stem cell transplantation
- Massive aspiration pneumonitis
- Idiopathic

SYMPTOMS AND SIGNS

Patients with DAH may not manifest symptoms or may only have non-specific symptoms that, in the setting of severe illness, may be difficult to attribute to DAH. However, many patients exhibit the following:

- Cough
- Dyspnea

- Hemoptysis (occurs in less than 50% of patients)
- Fever
- Tachypnea
- Tachycardia
- Hypotension
- Pallor
- Pulmonary rales

Diagnostic Studies

Diagnosis of DAH requires a very high index of suspicion and exclusion of more common pulmonary complications. Useful diagnostic tests include:

- Chest radiography
  - Diffuse infiltrates common, but non-specific
- Computed tomography
  - Diffuse or lobar infiltrates common, often in an alveolar pattern
- Complete blood count
  - Severe anemia may be present if hemorrhage is severe
  - Thrombocytopenia common in setting of chemotherapy or hematologic malignancies
- Pulmonary function studies
  - Restrictive pattern with increased DLCO
- Bronchoscopy with bronchoalveolar lavage
  - Bronchoscopy may be helpful if the patient can tolerate the procedure and may reveal diffuse oozing of blood in the bronchial tree without focal source
  - Bronchoalveolar lavage often bloody or blood-tinged
    - Hemosiderin-laden macrophages on cytologic analysis suggestive of subacute hemorrhage
- Lung biopsy
  - Depending on stability of patient, transbronchial, thoracoscopic, or thoractomy routes are options for tissue diagnosis
    - Histology reveals hemorrhage into alveolar spaces. If concurrent infection is present, organisms may be noted

Treatment

Supportive care, airway protection, and hemodynamic support are indicated as general measures of treatment for DAH. Correction of coagulopathy and thrombocytopenia, as well as directing treatment at the underlying malignant process and/or infection, is of vital importance. Some authors recommend high-dose corticosteroids, although there are no randomized trials and treatment is not without risk. Anecdotal reports suggest possible benefit with recombinant factor VIIa for refractory cases of DAH.

PROGNOSIS

Since most patients who develop DAH have underlying hematopoietic neoplasms and often have significant respiratory dysfunction requiring mechanical ventilation, prognosis is quite poor, with many patients not surviving hospitalization.

ADDITIONAL READING

Bodey GP, Powell R Jr, Hersh EM, et al. Pulmonary complications of acute leukemia. *Cancer* 1966;19:781.

Blatt J, Gold SH, Wilely JM, et al. Off-label use of recombinant factor VIIa in patients following bone marrow transplantation. *Bone Marrow Transplant* 2001;28: 405–407.

Crawford SW. Noninfectious lung disease in the immunocompromised host. *Respiration* 1999;66:385.

Gupta S, Jain A, Fanning TV, et al. An unusual cause of alveolar hemorrhage post-hematopoietic stem cell transplantation: a case report. *BMC Cancer*. 2006;6:87.

Hildebrand FL, Rosenow EC, Habermann TM. Pulmonary complications of leukemia. *Chest* 1990;98:1233.

Smith LJ, Katzenstein AL. Pathogenesis of massive pulmonary hemorrhage in acute leukemia. *Arch Intern Med* 1982;142:2149.

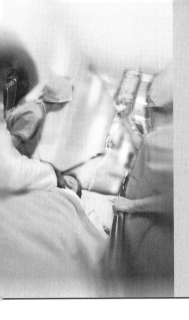

15

Invasive Pulmonary Aspergillosis

DEFINITION

Invasive pulmonary aspergillosis (IPA) is an acute fulminant, necrotizing pneumonic process. It is most often due to *Aspergillus fumigatus* that typically occurs in patients with prolonged severe neutropenia.

CLINICAL SETTING

Most cases of IPA occur in the setting of prolonged neutropenia and have recently undergone induction chemotherapy for acute leukemia or hematopoietic stem cell transplantation for hematologic neoplasia.

PATHOGENESIS

Aspergillus species are known for their angiotropic properties which result in necrotizing inflammation of not only the pulmonary parenchyma, but also the pulmonary vasculature. Aspergillosis is acquired through inhalation as this organism is frequently isolated from the hospital environment. Remodeling or demolition in the vicinity of patient wards may disperse the organism into ventilation ducts and the ambient air. Once in the alveolar space, the organism may damage parenchyma and result in necrotizing pneumonia. Invasion of blood vessels leads to vascular thrombosis and hemorrhagic infarction, which augments the growth of the organism within the necrotic tissue. Blood vessel destruction can lead to massive, and sometimes fatal, hemoptysis. Neutropenia is the major risk factor for the development of IPA, and explains the predominance of cases in patients with hematologic malignancies. Selective pressure for growth of *Aspergillus* species from broad spectrum antimicrobial use and the nearly ubiquitous presence of *A. fumigatus* in the environment set the stage for infection. As neutropenia resolves, the infarcted, devitalized areas of lung are infiltrated with neutrophils which subsequently release tissue-damaging enzymes that lead to cavitation. Erosive cavitation into a major vessel can induce massive hemoptysis. A unique feature of IPA is that recovery of the neutrophil compartment augments the tissue damage which can ultimately prove fatal. Bleeding from IPA is often exacerbated by disseminated intravascular coagulation (DIC) or thrombocytopenia induced by chemotherapy and leukemic bone marrow infiltration.

ETIOLOGY

Most cases of IPA result from disease-related and treatment-induced neutropenia in the setting of a hematopoietic malignancy:

- Acute myelogenous leukemia
- Acute lymphocytic leukemia
- Hematopoietic stem cell transplantation
- Myelodysplastic syndrome
- Lymphoma
- Myeloma
- Bone marrow failure syndromes resulting in protracted neutropenia
  - Aplastic anemia
  - Chemotherapy

SYMPTOMS AND SIGNS

Directly attributing symptoms and physical findings to IPA may be difficult since patients most prone to IPA are often very ill with multiple acute co-morbidities. However, the most common findings include:

- Hemoptysis
- Cough
- Pleuritic chest pain
- Fever
- Dyspnea
- Tachypnea
- Tachycardia
- Pulmonary rales
- Pleural friction rub
- Cyanosis

DIAGNOSTIC STUDIES

Various diagnostic modalities, non-invasive and invasive, are typically required to make the diagnosis of IPA:

- Chest radiography
  - Findings may include focal or multi-focal cavitary infiltrates or opacities
  - The classic "air crescent" sign, which represents a rim of air surrounding a nodular area, is very suggestive of IPA and results from air entering a cavity from erosion into the bronchial tree
- Computed tomography
  - Much more sensitive than chest radiography in the diagnosis of IPA
  - The classic "halo sign" represents ground glass attenuation surrounding a pulmonary nodule; the ground glass radiographically represents parenchymal hemorrhage and the nodule represents tissue necrosis
    - The likelihood of observing a "halo sign" is approximately 96% in the first 1–2 days of infection, but markedly diminishes by 2 weeks; as such the finding of this sign in the appropriate clinical setting is highly suggestive of IPA
  - If the nodule enlarges and cavitates, the "air crescent" sign may appear
- Sputum stain and culture
  - Fungal stains may reveal *Aspergillus* organisms but this method is not sensitive and typically not helpful
- Complete blood count
  - Neutropenia is very common but a normal or increasing neutrophil count is common once the clinical manifestations of IPA appear
  - Thrombocytopenia common
- Bronchoscopy
  - Bronchoscopic lavage and biopsy may reveal evidence of *Aspergillus* organisms on fungal smear, culture, or histologic analysis
- Lung biopsy
  - Many patients with suspected IPA are too ill or thrombocytopenic to undergo transbronchial or operative lung biopsy. However, biopsy should be considered to establish a diagnosis
    - Typical histologic findings include necrosis, thrombosis of small blood vessels, hemorrhagic infarction, as well as angio-invasion by fungi

TREATMENT

Untreated, IPA is nearly universally fatal. As such, early diagnosis and treatment are necessary. In at-risk patients with prolonged neutropenia, fever, and pulmonary infiltrates that do not respond to traditional antibiotics, empiric antifungal therapy with amphotercin B or voriconazole should be considered. Large areas of necrotic lung, especially if associated with hemoptysis, may require surgical resection to eradicate the infection and prevent fatal hemoptysis. Bronchial artery embolization may be considered to control hemoptysis in a patient unfit for surgery or to rapidly control bleeding. Correction of thrombocytopenia and coagulopathy with platelet concentrates and frozen plasma should be administered if appropriate.

Recombinant factor VIIa has been utilized to control bleeding associated with IPA, but no controlled studies are available for this indication.

PROGNOSIS

The most important factor in determining prognosis is control of the underlying hematologic malignancy and recovery of the neutrophil count. Patients with protracted neutropenia and ongoing evidence of active leukemia have an extremely high mortality rate despite anti-*Aspergillus* therapy. Massive, uncontrolled hemoptyis also portends a dismal prognosis.

ADDITIONAL READING

Aurora R, Milite F, Vander Els NJ. Respiratory emergencies. *Semin Oncol* 2000; 27:256–269.

Corr P. Management of severe hemopytis from pulmonary aspergilloma using endovascular embolization. *Cardiovasc Intervent Radiol* 2006;29:807–810.

Fernando HC, Stein M Benfield JR, et al. Role of bronchial artery embolization in the management of hemoptysis. *Arch Surg* 1998;133:862–866.

Hachen R, Sumoza D, Hanna H, et al. Clinical and radiologic predictors of invasive pulmonary aspergillosis in cancer patients. *Cancer* 2006;106:1581–1586.

Hildebrand FL, Rosenow EC, Habermann TM, et al. Pulmonary complications of leukemia. *Chest* 1990;98:1233–1239.

Lee YR, Choi YW, Lee KJ, et al. CT halo sign: the spectrum of pulmonary diseases. *Br J Radiol* 2005;78:862–865.

White B, Martin M, Kelleher S, et al. Successful use of recombinant factor VIIa (novoseven) in the management of pulmonary hemorrhage secondary to aspergillus infection in a patient with leukemia and acquired factor VII deficiency. *Br J Haematol* 1999;106:254–255.

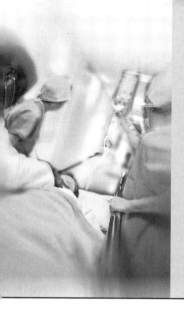

16

Transfusion-Associated Acute Lung Injury

DEFINITION

Transfusion-associated acute lung injury (TRALI) is a life-threatening clinical syndrome complicating transfusion therapy characterized by acute dyspnea, hypoxia, fever, and non-cardiogenic pulmonary edema.

CLINICAL SETTING

The incidence of TRALI is approximately 1 in 5,000 transfusions and occurs in acutely ill patients who are administered various types of blood products including packed red cell concentrates, fresh frozen plasma, platelets, or cryoprecipitate; patients with hematologic malignancies seem to be particularly at high risk.

PATHOGENESIS

The pathogenesis of TRALI is complex, but primarily immunologic in nature. The most widely published pathogenetic explanation attributes TRALI to donor-derived antibodies directed at recipient neutrophils that, when activated within the pulmonary vasculature, release cytokines leading to increased pulmonary vascular permeability and exudation of protein-rich fluid into the alveolar space. Additionally, many authors believe that patients who develop TRALI must have an underlying inflammatory or surgical illness that results in activation of the pulmonary endothelium causing intravascular sequestration of neutrophils. This is followed by a second "hit" in the form of a blood product transfusion laden with specific antibodies directed at the sequestered pulmonary neutrophils. Lipophilic compounds in the transfused blood product may also contribute to the capillary damage and leak characteristic of

TRALI. Multiparous female blood donors are especially likely to harbor various paternally-derived anti-leukocyte antibodies that subsequently target host neutrophil specific (e.g., NA2, NB1, NB2) epitopes or human leukocyte antigen (HLA) class I and II antigens. Binding of these antibodies to their host neutrophil targets leads to an immunologic cascade culminating in pulmonary vascular injury and increased permeability leading to non-cardiogenic pulmonary edema.

Autopsy studies of patients who have died as a result of TRALI have revealed massive pulmonary edema fluid within the alveolar space as well as neutrophil aggregation within the pulmonary microcirculation. This pulmonary vascular sequestration of neutrophils commonly leads to acute leukopenia, which can be a valuable diagnostic clue to TRALI. The edema fluid is characteristically protein-rich, in keeping with capillary leakage of plasma proteins.

ETIOLOGY

Any type of blood product administration can cause TRALI:

- Packed red blood cells
- Whole blood
- Fresh frozen plasma
- Platelets
- Cryoprecipitate
- Intravenous immune globulin (IVIG)

SYMPTOMS AND SIGNS

The majority of cases of TRALI manifest during transfusion or within 1 to 2 hours afterward; some patients may not have symptoms until 6 hours later. The most common clinical findings include:

- Acute-onset dyspnea
- Fever
- Cough
- Frothy, clear pulmonary secretions (especially notable if endotracheal tube in place)
- Tachypnea
- Accessory respiratory muscle use
- Cyanosis
- Hypotension
- Tachycardia
- Pulmonary rales
- Decreased breath sounds

DIAGNOSTIC STUDIES

The diagnosis of TRALI is primarily clinical and should be suspected in any patient who develops sudden dyspnea, respiratory distress, and hypoxia during or shortly after receiving a transfusion. However, TRALI can be difficult to differentiate from acute volume overload/pulmonary edema or aspiration pneumonitis. Helpful diagnostic studies include:

- Chest radiograph
  - Diffuse, bilateral fluffy/alveolar infiltrates
    - May have predilection for upper lobes
    - Cardiomegaly and pleural effusions often absent
- Arterial blood gas
  - Typically reveals hypoxia and respiratory alkalosis
- Complete blood count
  - Transient leukopenia is common and results from pulmonary sequestration of neutrophils
- B-natriuretic peptide (BNP)
  - Normal in TRALI due to non-cardiogenic nature of pulmonary edema
- Pulmonary arterial flotation or central venous catheter
  - Not typically indicated for diagnosis but, if present, findings compatible with hypovolemia or euvolemia (pulmonary wedge pressure $<$ 18 mmHg)
  - Low or normal central venous pressure
- Echocardiogram
  - Normal or hyperdynamic left ventricular function with absence of segmental wall motion abnormalities
- Measurement of edema fluid protein content
  - Feasible only if endotracheal tube present, in which copious amounts of frothy fluid can often be aspirated
  - Simultaneous edema fluid protein/plasma protein ratio $>$0.75

Treatment

The majority of patients who develop TRALI present with sudden, profound respiratory distress. Immediate airway stabilization is vital. As many as 72% of patients require endotracheal intubation and mechanical ventilation. If the patient is alert and can protect his airway, a non-invasive measure such as bilevel continuous positive airway pressure (BiPAP) can be attempted. All patients require some type of oxygen and often require intravenous fluid support if hypotension or evidence of volume depletion is evident. Diuretic therapy for TRALI-induced pulmonary edema can be hazardous, or even fatal, since exacerbation of volume depletion can lead to hypovolemic shock. Most cases of TRALI resolve spontaneously with supportive care within 48–72 hours. By then, the chest radiograph should show significant improvement, which is typically not the case in other forms of acute pulmonary injury. Corticosteroids have been used anecdotally, but the literature does not support their use for TRALI. The implicated blood product should be analyzed by the blood bank and the patient should not receive transfusions from that donor in the future.

PROGNOSIS

Although the majority of patients recover spontaneously without sequelae, TRALI carries a mortality rate of 5% to 8%. However, other authors have reported mortality rates of up to 25% which may relate to the underlying disease and lack of recognition of TRALI and treatment for another process.

ADDITIONAL READING

Hilbert G, Gruson D, Vargas F, et al. Noninvasive ventilation in immunosuppressed patients with pulmonary infiltrates, fever, and acute respiratory failure. *N Engl J Med* 2001;344:481–487.

Kopko PM, Marshall CS, MacKenzie MR, et al. Transfusion-related acute lung injury: report of a clinical look-back investigation. *JAMA* 2002;287:1968–1971.

Looney MR, Gropper MA, Matthay MA. Transfusion-related acute lung injury: a review. *Chest* 2004;126:249–258.

Silliman CC, Ambruso DR, Boshkov LK. Transfusion-related acute lung injury. *Blood* 2005;105:2266–2273.

Tsalis K, Ganidou M, Blouhos K, et al. Transfusion-related acute lung injury: a life-threatening transfusion reaction. *Med Sci Monit* 2005;11:CS19–22.

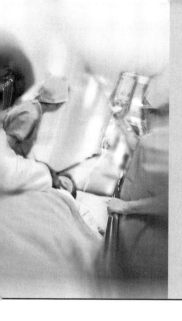

17

Pneumothorax

DEFINITION

Pneumothorax is the presence of air in the pleural space and is characterized as primary in the absence of underlying disease and secondary in the presence of underlying thoracic pathology. In the absence of trauma or iatrogenic injury, pneumothoraces are defined as spontaneous in nature. Iatrogenic pneumothorax results from diagnostic or therapeutic procedures.

CLINICAL SETTING

Pneumothorax in the cancer patient is usually secondary or iatrogenic in nature and occurs in the setting of pre-existing lung disease, opportunistic infections, thoracic neoplasia, or various invasive procedures and therapies.

PATHOGENESIS

Regardless of etiology, pneumothorax results when air enters the potential space that exists between the visceral and parietal pleura. If the air has no escape mechanism, a tension pneumothorax results. The intrapleural space exists at subatmospheric pressure as a net result of the normal physiologic tendency of the thoracic cage to expand and the lung to collapse from elastic recoil. When there is a break in the pleura from underlying lung disease or iatrogenic injury, air travels along a pressure gradient along the pleural space until equilibrium occurs with lung collapse. Ventilation-perfusion balance is disrupted, a degree of physiologic shunt occurs, and vital capacity decreases. All of these contribute to the symptoms and hypoxia. A rapidly life-threatening situation known as tension pneumothorax occurs when pleural pressure exceeds atmospheric pressure from unidirectional air entry from the lung to the pleural space without an exit point. Pressure within the thorax reaches dangerous levels, impeding venous return, cardiac output, and oxygen exchange, and ultimately leads to circulatory collapse if not treated.

The cancer patient may develop spontaneous secondary pneumothorax as a result of underlying smoking-induced chronic obstructive pulmonary disease (COPD), necrotizing infections, pneumocystis pneumonia (PCP), subpleural tumor necrosis, or iatrogenic injury. In the case of COPD, rupture of subpleural blebs and in the case of neoplasm or infection, erosion into a bronchiole or pleural space results in pneumothorax.

ETIOLOGY

Etiologies of pneumothorax in the cancer patient can result from tumor itself, from cancer or therapy-related complication, or from diagnostic or therapeutic procedures:

- Tumor-related
  - Pleural or parenchymal sarcoma metastasis
  - Bronchogenic carcinoma: rarely can be presenting manifestation
    - Squamous cell carcinoma
      - Accounts for over 50% of lung cancer-induced pneumonthoraces
      - Results from propensity of squamous cancer to cavitate
    - Adenocarcinoma
    - Small cell carcinoma
    - Bronchioalveolar carcinoma
- Underlying lung disease
  - COPD: common in lung cancer patients
- Radiation-induced
  - May result from pleural scarring
- Infection
  - Invasive aspergillosis
  - Necrotizing bacterial pneumonia
    - *Pseudomonas aeruginosa, staphylococcus aureus,* anaerobes
  - *Pneumocystis jirovecii* pneumonia (PCP)
    - May occur with hematologic malignancies, Hodgkin's disease, or treatment with steroids or nucleoside analogues
- Pulmonary embolism with infarction
- Iatrogenic or therapy-related
  - Central venous catheter placement
  - Thoracentesis
  - Transthoracic needle lung biopsy
  - Transbronchial lung biopsy
  - Nerve blocks

Symptoms and Signs

Spontaneous pneumothorax is usually acutely symptomatic but iatrogenic pneumothorax may be more insidious. Typical symptoms and signs of pneumothorax in general include:

- Pleuritic chest pain
- Dyspnea
- Cough
- Tachycardia
- Tachypnea
- Diminished breath sounds
- Hyper-resonance to percussion
- Hypotension
  - Indicative of tension pneumothorax
- Cyanosis
  - Indicative of tension pneumothorax
- Tracheal deviation
  - Indicative of tension pneumothorax

Diagnostic Data

- Chest radiography
  - Initial study of choice
  - Reveals radiolucent pleural line with lack of peripheral markings
  - Tension pneumothorax may reveal deviation of tracheal air column
- Computed tomography
  - More sensitive for detecting pleural air; may also reveal evidence of etiology such as necrotizing pneumonia or malignancy

Treatment

If tension pneumothorax is suspected (sudden dyspnea, tracheal deviation, hypotension), immediate needle-catheter decompression into the second anterior intercostal space is indicated without diagnostic studies, to prevent fatal circulatory collapse. If there is no evidence of tension with a small <15%) pneumothorax, observation and oxygen, which increases the resorption of air by the pleura, may suffice. In the setting of a large pneumothorax or if the patient has significant underlying pulmonary disease, decompression and drainage of the air is indicated. Simple catheter aspiration with a 50-milliliter syringe connected to a large bore catheter-over-needle device may be attempted if the pneumothorax is small and the patient is hemodynamically stable. Insertion of a one-way Heimlich valve, a small device that can be placed at bedside by a radiologist or pulmonologist, may be considered if the patient is hemodynamically stable. This method may be especially useful for iatrogenic pneumothorax following needle-puncture of pleura.

Many patients require tube thoracostomy connected to a water-seal. Smaller tubes (8 to 16 French tube) may be effective, although patients with significant lung disease or pleural fluid may require placement of a 20 to 28 French tube. Video-assisted thoracoscopic surgery (VATS) may be useful for pneumothorax resulting from rupture of a subpleural necrotic tumor/bleb or a concomitant pleural effusion (hydropneumothorax). Pleurodesis or resection of subpleural pathology and drainage of pleural effusion may afford relief and prevent recurrence and can be performed at the time of VATS or tube thoracostomy insertion.

PROGNOSIS

Patients with a small to moderate pneumothorax have a good prognosis with appropriate treatment. However, some patients will manifest persistant air leaks that may necessitate prolonged tube thoracostomy or surgical intervention. Patients with underlying COPD and advanced malignancy have a poorer prognosis due to their underlying lung dysfunction and disease state. The prognosis for a tension pneumothorax is grim if the thorax is not immediately decompressed as described above.

ADDITIONAL READING

Arnett JC, Hatch HB. Pneumothorax associated with bronchogenic carcinoma. *Chest* 1976;70:796.

McKellan MD, Miller SB, Parsons PE, et al. Pneumothorax with *pneumocystis carinii* pneumonia in AIDS: incidence and clinical characteristics. *Chest* 1991; 100:1224–1228.

Sahn SA, Heffner JE. Spontaneous pneumothorax. *N Engl J Med* 2000;342: 868–874.

Steinhauslin CA, Cuttat JF. Spontaneous pneumothorax: a complication of lung cancer? *Chest* 1985;88:709–713.

Young WF, Humphries RL. Pneumothorax. In: *Emergency Medicine: A Comprehensive Study Guide*. 5th ed. Tintanalli JE, Kelen GD, Stapczynski JS, eds. New York: McGraw-Hill, 2000, pp. 471–474.

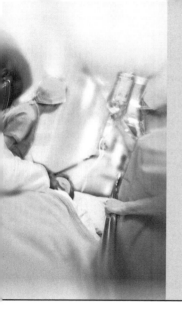

18

Spontaneous Hemothorax

DEFINITION

Spontaneous hemothorax (SH), a rare but life-threatening complication of primary or metastatic thoracic malignancy, results from spontaneous hemorrhage within the pleural space. SH is defined as a pleural fluid hematocrit exceeding 50% of the peripheral blood.

CLINICAL SETTING

Spontaneous hemothorax in the oncology population typically results from metastatic sarcomas or lung cancer. A variety of other neoplasms have been implicated, most often in patients with widely metastatic disease.

PATHOGENESIS

Tumoral involvement of the lung parenchyma, pleura, mediastinal structures, and thoracic skeleton is not an uncommon complication of metastatic malignancy or primary intrathoracic neoplasms. Although SH is a rare complication of cancer, it is vital to recognize it since death from hemorrhagic shock or respiratory failure can occur rapidly. The pathogenesis of SH results from rupture of a metastatic tumor deposit into the pleural space and often occurs in the setting of vascular neoplasms such as angiosarcoma. As tumors grow, the central area often undergoes necrosis due to poor oxygenation which may lead to spontaneous tumor rupture and subsequent hemorrhage. Underlying coagulopathy from disseminated intravascular coagulation (DIC), anticoagulant therapy, or the anti-vascular endothelial growth factor agent, bevacizumab, may potentiate tumoral hemorrhage.

Enlarging neoplasms may secondarily invade large pulmonary vessels or the microvasculature resulting in massive hemorrhage and shock. Tumor implants involving the parietal or visceral pleura may spontaneously bleed, since the neovascularization involving most cancers is "leaky" and disorganized, which may contribute to spontaneous hemorrhage. Transdiaphragmatic invasion of the pleural space from hepatic angiosarcoma or hepatocellular carcinoma are other mechanisms of SH. A unique etiology of SH in the patient with acute leukemia is invasive pulmonary aspergillosis due to the vasotropic nature of this organism that may result in blood vessel erosion and hemorrhage.

Etiology

Although the most common etiologies of SH in the hospital setting result from trauma or iatrogenic injury, causes reported among cancer patients include:

- Coagulopathy
  - May result from DIC or anticoagulant therapy
- Pulmonary infarction/necrosis complicating pulmonary embolism
- Invasive pulmonary aspergillosis
- Sarcoma, usually metastatic in nature
  - Angiosarcoma of skin, soft tissue, viscera
  - Chondroblastoma of rib
  - Synovial sarcoma
  - Ewing sarcoma
  - Neurofibrosarcoma
    - Often reported in patients with neurofibromatosis
- Lung carcinoma
  - Large cell, adenocarcinoma, bronchioloalveolar
- Mesothelioma
- Pulmonary blastoma
  - Rare primary lung tumor arising from pulmonary blastema similar to the origin of Wilms' tumor
- Teratoma of mediastinum
- Meningioma of mediastinum
- Choriocarcinoma
- Renal cell carcinoma
- Breast carcinoma
- Hepatocellular carcinoma
  - May result from lung metastasis, tumoral diaphragmatic erosion, or rib metastasis

Symptoms and Signs

The diagnosis of SH should be considered in any cancer patient, especially those with metastatic disease, who present with any of the following manifestations:

- Sudden dyspnea
- Sharp chest pain
- Hemoptysis
- Cough
- Syncope
- Fever
- Tachycardia
- Hypotension
- Diminished breath sounds
- Dullness to percussion over involved hemithorax

DIAGNOSTIC STUDIES

Diagnosis of SH requires a high index of suspicion since similar symptoms may be attributed to more common disorders such as malignant pleural effusion, pneumonia, or pulmonary embolism. The most helpful diagnostic studies include:

- Chest radiography
  - Most common finding is unilateral pleural effusion, which may obliterate the entire hemithorax
  - Mass lesion(s) may be noted
- Computed tomography
  - More sensitive for detecting hemorrhage in the pleural space, adenopathy, or evidence of primary or metastatic malignancy
  - Contrast extravastion
- Complete blood count
  - Severe anemia common
- Coagulation studies
  - Elevated prothrombin time (PT) or partial thromboplastin time (PTT) in setting of DIC or anticoagulant therapy
- Thoracentesis
  - Hemorrhagic pleural fluid or gross, non-clotting blood
  - Hematocrit of pleural fluid exceeds 50% that of a simultaneous peripheral hematocrit

TREATMENT

Patients with suspected SH and signs of hemorrhagic shock should have large-bore vascular cannulas inserted for administration of crytalloids and red cell transfusions for volume resuscitation. Underlying coagulopathy should be treated with vitamin K, fresh frozen plasma, or cryoprecipitate. Recombinant factor VIIa may be considered for refractory bleeding but data is lacking. Drainage of the pleural space should be considered to relieve respiratory embarrassment and may be performed with a large-bore thoracentesis catheter or tube thoracostomy, which is preferable in the setting of ongoing bleeding. Some authors recommend intrapleural sclerosing agents. Surgical intervention with thoracotomy or video-assisted tho-racoscopic surgery (VATS) may be needed to identify the bleeding site and achieve hemostasis. Transarterial embolization may be effective in controlling hemorrhage from a parenchymal, skeletal, or pleural tumor mass.

PROGNOSIS

Death due to hemorrhagic shock may complicate SH if bleeding is not controlled. Long-term prognosis depends on the etiology of SH, with metastatic tumors such as lung carcinoma or angiosarcoma having a dismal prognosis with survival often measured in weeks to months.

ADDITIONAL READING

Ausin P, Gomez-Caro A, Rojo RP, et al. Spontaneous hemothorax caused by lung can-cer. *Arch Bronconeumol* 2005;41:400–401.

Chou SH, Cheng YJ, Kao EL, et al. Spontaneous hemothorax: an unusual presen-tation of primary lung cancer. *Thorax* 1993;48:1185–1186.

Park SI, Choi E, Lee HB, et al. Spontaneous pneumomediastinum and hemopneu-mothoraces secondary to cystic lung metastasis. *Respiration* 2003;70:211–213.

Shiota S, Nakaya Y, Sakamoto K, et al. Spontaneous hemothorax secondary to im-mature teratoma of the mediastinum. *Intern Med* 1999;38:726–728.

Tan CK, Wu KC, Wu RH, et al. Spontaneous hemothorax caused by metastasis of a rib tumor. *CMAJ* 2008;178:679.

Varsano S, Edelstein E, Gendel B, et al. Bilateral and unilateral spontaneous mas-sive hemothorax as a presenting manifestation of rare tumors. *Respiration* 2003;70:214–218.

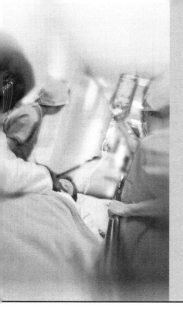

19

Reexpansion Pulmonary Edema

DEFINITION

Reexpansion pulmonary edema (RPE) is a form of noncardiogenic pulmonary edema that complicates rapid lung reexpansion following removal of a pleural effusion or decompression of a pneumothorax.

CLINICAL SETTING

Within the oncology population, the most cases of RPE follow large-volume thoracentesis for malignant pleural effusion, although any procedure producing rapid lung reexpansion can cause RPE.

PATHOGENESIS

Pleural effusions are common in patients with metastatic malignancy, most often occurring in the setting of breast and lung cancers, and may become quite large—exceeding two liters within a hemithorax. With prolonged large effusions, significant lung atelectasis occurs, which results in poor oxygen exchange and diminished blood flow into the collapsed portion of lung. Upon rapid removal of a large volume (typically >1500 milliliters) of pleural fluid, the collapsed lung reexpands into the caudad hemithorax. The pathogenesis of RPE is postulated to result from rapid lung reexpansion in conjunction with alterations in pulmonary vascular permeability. Proposed pathogenic mechanisms for this increase in vascular permeability include: chronic lung parenchymal hypoxia, prolonged lung collapse, intrathoracic negative pressure generated during pleural fluid drainage, increases in the pressure gradient between the alveoli and capillary unit, rapid increase in parenchymal blood flow following reexpansion, altered lymphatic flow, and loss of lung surfactant.

This increase in pulmonary capillary permeability results in rapid flow of fluid into the interstitium and alveoli impairing oxygen exchange. It is important to emphasize that RPE is a form of non-cardiogenic pulmonary edema and not related to volume overload or congestive heart failure. Therefore, typical treatments for cardiogenic pulmonary edema or volume overload, such as loop diuretics, have minimal effect. Most cases of RPE occur in the lung ipsilateral to the pleural drainage procedure. Rarely, cases of contralateral RPE have been reported which have been attributed to local release of vasoactive mediators (e.g., histamine and prostaglandins) or reflex neural mechanisms. Rapid lung reexpansion of a pneumothorax may cause RPE via similar mechanisms.

ETIOLOGY

Significant lung collapse, followed by a reexpansion procedure, such as thoracentesis or chest tube thoracostomy, underlie most cases of RPE in the cancer population:

- Drainage of pleural effusion: especially if >1500 cc of fluid removed by thoracentesis or tube thoracostomy
  - Malignant pleural effusion
  - Congestive heart failure/volume overload
  - Nephrotic syndrome
  - All-trans retinoic acid syndrome (ATRA) syndrome
- Relief of endobronchial obstruction: RPE may follow endobronchial stent placement or bronchoscopic removal of mucous plug
  - Bronchogenic carcinoma
  - Metastatic tumor to bronchus
  - Melanoma
  - Renal cell carcinoma
  - Breast carcinoma
  - Mucous plug
- Tube thoracostomy for pneumothorax complicating
  - Central venous line or port placement
  - Percutaneous needle lung biopsy
  - Transbronchial lung biopsy
  - Barotrauma complicating mechanical ventilation
  - Spontaneous pneumothorax from tumor or infection

SYMPTOMS AND SIGNS

Development of any of the following symptoms and signs during or following thoracentesis or chest tube thoracostomy should prompt consideration of RPE:

- Dyspnea
- Chest discomfort
- Cough
- Frothy sputum
- Tachypnea
- Tachycardia
- Hypotension
- Unilateral pulmonary rales
- Accessory respiratory muscle use

DIAGNOSTIC STUDIES

Although RPE can often be surmised in the setting of sudden dyspnea after a large-volume thoracentesis, useful diagnostic modalities include:

- Chest radiography
  - Typically reveals unilateral alveolar and interstitial pulmonary edema
- Computed tomography
  - More sensitive at detecting unilateral pulmonary edema and to exclude other causes of respiratory insufficiency
- Arterial blood gas
  - Typically reveals hypoxemia and respiratory alkalosis; however, respiratory acidosis may also occur
- B-type natriuretic peptide (BNP)
  - Useful to exclude cardiogenic pulmonary edema/congestive heart failure

TREATMENT

Diagnosis of RPE requires a high index of suspicion and, once the diagnosis is suspected, general airway care and oxygen administration are initial treatment measures. Unlike cardiogenic pulmonary edema and volume overload, RPE does not respond well to diuretic therapy since the pathophysiology involves altered capillary permeability and changes in intrathoracic pressure and not intravascular fluid overload. Therefore, supportive care with oxygen, non-invasive or mechanical ventilation, and hemodynamic support are the primary treatment modalities. Some authors advocate corticosteroids to decrease pulmonary capillary fluid leakage, but no large studies support this treatment.

PROGNOSIS

If untreated, RPE can lead to acute respiratory failure and, if diuretics are administered, hypovolemic shock may ensue. Mortality rates approach 20% in some series. Long-term prognosis of patients successfully treated for RPE primarily depends on the stage and response of the underlying neoplasm.

ADDITIONAL READING

Feller-Kopman D, Berkowitz D, Boiselle P, et al. Large-volume thoracentesis and the risk of reexpansion pulmonary edema. *Ann Thorac Surg* 2007;84:1656–1661.

Mahfood S, Hix WR, Aaron BL, et al. Reexpansion pulmonary edema. *Ann Thorac Surg* 1988;45:340–345.

Pavlin J, Cheney FW. Unilateral pulmonary edema in rabbits after reexpansion of collapsed lung. *J Appl Physiol* 1979;46:31–35.

Sautter RD, Dreger WH, MacIndoe JH, et al. Fatal pulmonary edema and pneumonitis after re-expansion. *Chest* 1971;60:399–401.

Sherman SC. Reexpansion pulmonary edema: a case report and review of the literature. *J Emerg Med* 2003;24:23–27.

III

GASTROINTESTINAL AND HEPATOBILIARY COMPLICATIONS

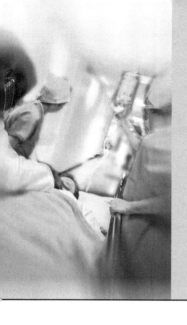

20

Tracheo-esophageal Fistula

DEFINITION

A tracheoesophageal fistula (TEF) exists when a fistulous communication is present between the thoracic esophagus and trachea.

CLINICAL SETTING

Acquired TEF is most often caused by malignant tumors of the esophagus or tracheo-bronchial tree and is typically a pre-terminal complication in the cancer patient. TEF may complicate 5% to 15% of cases of advanced esophageal carcinoma and 1% of cases of bronchogenic carcinoma.

PATHOGENESIS

Aggressive tumor growth originating in the esophagus, trachea, bronchus, or upper airway can erode through the esophagorespiratory mucosa and into neighboring structures, creating an open communication between the tracheobronchial tree and esophagus. Radiation therapy-induced tumor necrosis and previous local surgery may play a role as well. In any event, airway contamination occurs from entry of oral secretions, foodstuffs, ingested liquids, or gastroesophageal contents migrating through the fistulous connection into the lungs. Reflex bronchospasm may occur or, if particulate matter is large enough, airway obstruction may ensue culminating in acute respiratory failure. Aspiration pneumonitis and bacterial pneumonia are common complications which cause significant morbidity and mortality in patients with TEF. Hospitalized patients are particularly vulnerable to developing aspiration pneumonia due to resistant nosocomial organisms. Inflammatory and infectious pneumonitis leads to impaired gas exchange and severe hypoxia which, in conjunction with pulmonary sepsis, result in death.

ETIOLOGY

Malignancy-associated TEF is most often due to aerodigestive cancers or complications of their treatment:

- Esophageal carcinoma
  - Squamous cell carcinoma
  - Adenocarcinoma
- Bronchogenic carcinoma
  - Squamous cell carcinoma
  - Adenocarcinoma
  - Small cell carcinoma
- Radiation therapy of the esophagus or upper airway
  - External beam radiotherapy
  - Brachytherapy
- Post-operative necrosis or anastomotic breakdown
  - May result from local necrosis and tumor growth
- Prolonged endotracheal intubation
  - Pressure necrosis of tracheal wall with erosion into esophagus

SYMPTOMS AND SIGNS

Acute respiratory distress and respiratory failure may occur if a food bolus obstructs the trachea. Most patients with TEF present in a subacute manner with some or all of the following:

- Cough with drinking or eating
- Dyspnea
- Purulent sputum
- Chest pain
- Wheezing
- Dysphagia
- Weight loss
- Fever
- Stridor
- Tachypnea
- Pulmonary rhonchi and rales

DIAGNOSTIC STUDIES

Diagnosis of TEF requires a high index of suspicion but should be considered in any patient with advanced esophageal or lung cancer who presents with increasing respiratory distress, cough, fever, or recurrent pneumonia. Some helpful diagnostic studies include:

- Chest radiograph
  - May reveal evidence of lung consolidation or bilateral infiltrates

- Computed tomography
  - The fistulous connection may be visualized with water-soluble oral contrast media
  - Other findings may include a tracheoesophageal mass lesion or pulmonary infiltrates
- Barium or gastrograffin esophagram
  - Leakage of oral contrast media from the esophagus into the tracheobronchial tree is diagnostic of TEF
- Esophagogastroduodenoscopy (EGD)
  - May reveal ulceration involving tumoral tissue in the case of an esophageal cancer or a hole with airway secretions and air bubbles entering the esophagus in the case of a bronchogenic carcinoma
- Bronchoscopy
  - May reveal tumor tissue, ulceration, or an opening

TREATMENT

Almost without exception, development of TEF occurs in the setting of incurable malignancy and is a pre-terminal event. Therefore, palliation is the primary aim of therapy. Broad-spectrum antibiotics are indicated in the setting of pneumonia. Oxygen therapy and pain control are often necessary. Although surgical bypass procedures or closure of the fistula have been reported, patients with TEF are often very ill and of poor surgical risk. Placement of a metal esophageal or tracheobronchial stent has a technical success rate approaching 80% and is safe for sealing the fistulous connection in most patients. However, some patients fail to have relief of aspiration symptoms, closure of the fistula, or development of another TEF due to stent-induced pressure necrosis.

PROGNOSIS

Prognosis of patients with TEF due to esophageal or bronchogenic carcinoma is grim with most patients succumbing to their malignancy within weeks to months. Rapid death may ensue due to pneumonia and sepsis in some patients.

ADDITIONAL READING

Altorki NK, Migliore M, Skinner DB. Esophageal carcinoma with airway invasion: evolution and choices of therapy. *Chest* 1994;106:742–745.

Pairolero PC, Trastek VF, Payne WS. Esophagus and diaphragmatic hernias. In: *Principles of Surgery.* 5th ed. Schwartz SI, Shires GT, Spencer FC, eds. New York: McGraw-Hill, 1989, pp. 1103–1156.

Sharma A, Rehman MUR, Cowen ME. Management of a difficult malignant tracheoesophageal fistula. *Inter Cardiovasc Thor Surg* 2003;2:665–667.

Shin JH, Song HY, Ko GY, et al. Esophagorespiratory fistula: palliative treatment with covered expandable metallic stents in 61 patients. *Radiology* 2004; 232:252–259.

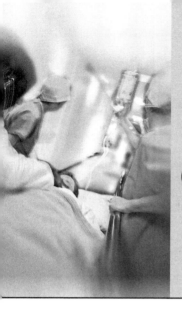

21

Gastrointestinal Bleeding

DEFINITION

Bleeding into the lumen of the gastrointestinal tract can be clinically defined as upper gastrointestinal bleeding (UGIB) when the bleeding source lies proximal to the ligament of Treitz and as lower gastrointestinal bleeding (LGIB) when the source lies distal to the ligament of Treitz, with most cases of LGIB originating in the colorectum.

CLINICAL SETTING

Gastrointestinal hemorrhage in the cancer patient can result from the same etiologies as encountered in the general population. However, the cancer patient often has multiple other risk factors predisposing them to hemorrhage related to luminal malignancy, specific cancer treatments, or therapies related to symptom control such as non-steroidal drugs. Thus, the clinical setting in which UGIB or LGIB occurs is often complicated in the cancer patient.

PATHOGENESIS

An exhaustive discussion of all of the pathogenetic factors implicated in cancer-related gastrointestinal hemorrhage is beyond the scope of this work. However, a few salient points related to UGIB and LGIB in the general cancer population will be discussed. In general, patients undergoing induction chemotherapy for hematologic malignancies such as acute leukemia are especially prone to develop upper or lower GIB due to stress-induced mucosal changes and chemotherapy-induced mucosal disruption and ulceration. Additionally, superimposed infection of the esophagus with *Candida* species or cytomegalovirus (CMV) may induce UGIB and colonic infection with CMV may be associated with LGIB in the leukemia and bone marrow transplant population. Emetogenic chemotherapy may induce a Mallory-Weiss tear. As will be discussed in another chapter, neutropenic enterocolitis or typhilitis can occasionally result in LGIB. Concurrent use of corticosteroids or non-steroidal anti-inflammatory drugs (NSAIDS) decrease prostaglandin-mediated gastric mucosal protection and may especially pose a dangerous risk in the already denuded gastric epithelium of the patient receiving cytotoxic chemotherapy. Septic shock and mechanical ventilation also decrease the local mucosal defenses of the upper gastrointestinal tract and add to the risk of UGIB. Chemotherapy-related thrombocytopenia or concurrent coagulopathy due to leukemia or disseminated intravascular coagulation (DIC) further enhance the risk and seriousness of gastrointestinal hemorrhage. Patients with premorbid use of NSAIDS or ethanol may be predisposed to UGIB when treatments for cancer are commenced. Another unique pathophysiologic cause of UGIB is rapid tumor necrosis of a gastric or bowel lymphoma which can result in life-threatening hemorrhage when chemotherapy is instituted. Massive bleeding from a primary gastric, small bowel, or colorectal carcinoma may occasionally occur if significant tumoral necrosis occurs and erodes a vessel. Administration of the anti-vascular agent, bevacizumab, may also invoke tumoral or bowel wall necrosis and result in hemorrhage. Rarely, a metastatic tumor to the gastrointestinal tract, usually lung, kidney, or melanoma, can result in acute UGIB or LGIB. Patients with myeloproliferative disorders or splenic vein thrombosis from pancreatic carcinoma may develop variceal bleeding due to splenomegaly and portal hypertension.

ETIOLOGY

The etiologies of gastrointestinal hemorrhage in the cancer patient are diverse and depend not only on premorbid disease, but also the underlying neoplasm and specific therapies directed at the malignancy. Some of the etiologies of UGIB and LGIB in the cancer patient include:

- Upper GIB
  - Tumor necrosis
    - Esophagus, gastric, small bowel, or colorectal carcinoma
    - Primary gastric lymphoma
    - Metastatic tumors
      - Bronchogenic carcinoma, renal cell carcinoma, melanoma, breast carcinoma
  - Erosive esophagitis
    - Acid-induced, pill esophagitis (e.g., bisphosphonates, potassium chloride)
  - Infectious esophagitis
    - *Candida* species, CMV

- ○ Radiation esophagitis
- ○ Erosive or stress gastritis
  - ■ Associated with critical illness, sepsis, hypotension, mechanical ventilation
- ○ Peptic ulcer disease
- ○ Corticosteroids and NSAIDS
- ○ Chemotherapy
  - ■ Many drugs can induce enteric mucositis and include cytarabine, fluoropyrimidines, taxanes
- ○ Esophageal or gastric varices
  - ■ Underlying cirrhosis, portal vein thrombosis, splenic vein thrombosis (gastric varices), splenomegaly due to myeloproliferative disorders
- • Lower GIB
  - ○ Tumor necrosis
    - ■ Small bowel or colorectal carcinoma
    - ■ Primary small bowel or colorectal lymphoma
    - ■ Metastatic tumors
      - — Bronchogenic carcinoma, renal cell carcinoma, melanoma, breast carcinoma
  - ○ Chemotherapy enteritis
    - ■ Many chemotherapeutic drugs can induce enteric mucositis and include cytarabine, fluoropyrimidines, and taxanes
  - ○ Infectious enteritis
    - ■ CMV, *Clostridium difficile,* Gram-negative enteric bacilli
  - ○ Radiation enteritis
  - ○ Ischemic colitis
  - ○ Neutropenic enterocolitis/typhilitis
    - ■ Most commonly occurs in the setting of induction chemotherapy for acute leukemia
  - ○ Diverticular disease
  - ○ Malignant arterial-enteric fistula

Symptoms and Signs

Most often, UGIB presents with hematemesis and melena while LGIB presents with hematochezia. However, a brisk UGIB may present with hematochezia due to the rapid transit of blood through the intestinal lumen. A variety of symptoms and signs however, may occur:

- • UGIB
  - ○ Hematemesis
    - ■ Can be bright red or "coffee ground" in color
  - ○ Melena

- ○ Hematochezia
  - ▪ Rapid upper gastrointestinal bleeding can present with hematochezia due to the cathartic effect of blood on intestinal transit
  - ▪ Often associated with hemodynamic instability
- ○ Abdominal pain
- ○ Vomiting
- ○ Orthostatic dizziness
- ○ Weakness
- ○ Pallor
- ○ Tachycardia
- ○ Hypotension
- LGIB
  - ○ Melena
    - ▪ May occur if bleeding originates in the small bowel or proximal colon
  - ○ Hematochezia
  - ○ Abdominal pain
  - ○ Diarrhea
  - ○ Weakness
  - ○ Pallor
  - ○ Tachycardia
  - ○ Hypotension

DIAGNOSTIC STUDIES

In general, diagnosis of gastrointestinal hemorrhage is clinical, but various diagnostic tests are typically indicated to determine the anatomic site and etiology of bleeding:

- Nasogastric tube placement
  - ○ Bleeding site within the esophagus or stomach typically results in bloody or "coffee ground" aspirate of stomach contents
    - ▪ However, incompetence of the pyrlous may allow small intestinal blood to reflux into the stomach
- Esophagogastroduodenoscopy (EGD)
  - ○ Procedure of choice to investigate UGIB sources within the esophagus, stomach, and duodenum
  - ○ Massive bleeding may obscure mucosal detail
  - ○ EGD can be therapeutic during same session
- Colonoscopy
  - ○ Procedure of choice to investigate the colon and distal ileum
  - ○ Can be therapeutic during same session
- Computed tomography
  - ○ Not indicated routinely to investigate gastrointestinal hemorrhage in many cases, although may be helpful in the cancer patient, for example:

- May reveal primary tumor mass within the gastrointestinal lumen, perforation, bowel wall inflammation, fistula formation, or esophageal or gastric varices
- Nuclear bleeding scan
  - May localize a slow bleeding source within the large bowel
- Mesenteric angiography
  - May identify arterial source of mucosal bleeding or a hypervascular metastasis (e.g., renal cell carcinoma) but if the bleeding rate is <0.5 ml/min, the source may not be visualized

TREATMENT

Fundamental treatment principles for any significant gastrointestinal hemorrhage include insertion of two large bore peripheral venous cannulas or central venous access and prompt resuscitation with crystalloids or packed red blood cells. Correction of thrombocytopenia or coagulopathy is vital. In cases of UGIB, intravenous proton pump inhibitors are effective at decreasing gastric acid secretion and inhibiting further acid-related mucosal damage. If an UGIB does not cease spontaneously, therapeutic EGD may be indicated. For instance, esophageal varices can be banded or injected with a sclerosing agent and active arterial bleeding, a visible vessel, or an adherent clot over bleeding site may benefit from endoscopic laser, electrocoagulation, or heater probe application. Therapeutic colonoscopic procedures similar to those performed via EGD may be an option with LGIB. In cases of esophageal variceal hemorrhage, intravenous administration of vasopressin reduces portal venous flow through splanchnic arteriolar vasoconstriction; however, coronary vasospasm may limit the usefulness of vasopressin in the setting of cardiovascular disease. If hemorrhage remains uncontrolled with any of the above measures, angiography with arterial coil or foam embolization is usually effective at controlling bleeding, but can occasionally lead to transmural necrosis of the involved segment of gastrointestinal tract. Indications for surgical control of gastrointestinal bleeding include failure of medical therapy and transfusion of six or more units of blood. However, the overall prognosis of the patient's underlying neoplasm and risk for surgery may preclude an operation. Anecdotal reports of successful cessation of refractory hemorrhage have been reported with infusion of recombinant factor VIIa.

PROGNOSIS

Moderate bleeding from stress-induced gastritis or self-limited bleeding from any source carries a favorable prognosis depending on the patient's underlying disease response to treatment. Massive UGIB or LGIB in a patient with advanced or metastatic cancer and a poor performance status carries a dismal prognosis and is often a terminal event.

ADDITIONAL READING

Blair SL, Schwarz RE. Critical care of patients with cancer: surgical considerations. *Crit Care Clin* 2001;17:721–741.

Kemeny MM, Brennan M. The surgical complications of chemotherapy in the cancer patient. *Curr Probl Surg* 1987;24:613–675.

Klein MS, Ennis F, Sherlock P, et al. Stress erosions: a major cause of gastrointestinal hemorrhage in patients with malignant disease. *Am J Dig Dis* 1973;18:167–173.

Marinella MA. Metastatic lung cancer presenting as lower gastrointestinal hemorrhage. *Heart Lung* 2007;36:454–455.

Marinella MA. Fatal tumor lysis syndrome and gastric hemorrhage with metastatic small cell lung cancer. *Med Pediatr Oncol* 1999;32:464–465.

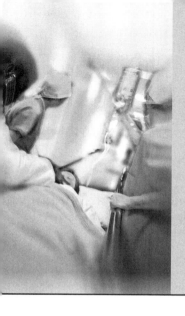

22

Ileus and Intestinal Pseudo-Obstruction

DEFINITION

Ileus refers to a non-obstructive, functional hypomotility disorder involving the gastrointestinal tract (with a predilection for the small bowel) that frequently complicates a variety of medical and surgical illnesses. Colonic ileus or intestinal pseudoobstruction, also known as Ogilvie's syndrome, refers to a dilated, adynamic, non-obstructed colon, which can lead to perforation.

CLINICAL SETTING

The vast majority of cancer patients with small intestinal ileus and colonic pseudoobstruction are acutely ill, hypomobile, or post-operative, and often have coexisting electrolyte derangements, are receiving gut-slowing medications, or are undergoing cytotoxic chemotherapy.

PATHOGENESIS

Acutely or critically ill patients commonly develop gastroparesis and small intestinal ileus due to a variety of factors such as sepsis, hypotension, respiratory failure, drugs, and electrolyte derangements. Hypotension may result in impaired blood flow to the gut resulting in hypomotility. Narcotic drugs impair smooth muscle contraction, frequently leading to slow bowel transit and ileus. Hypomagnesemia, hypokalemia, and hypercalcemia are common electrolyte derangements in cancer patients and all lead to impaired bowel motility and ultimately, ileus. Hyperglycemia, volume depletion, and acute infection, all of which are very common in the acutely ill, also decrease gastrointestinal motility. The chemotherapeutic agent, vincristine, is a well-known cause of autonomic neuropathy and ileus, which can rarely lead to perforation of a distended segment of bowel. Enteric mucositis related to chemotherapy may also induce hypomotility and ileus, especially during induction chemotherapy for acute leukemia. In total, ileus is often multifactorial and eventually results in vomiting and obstipation, which lead to further electrolyte and fluid losses as well as poor mobility due to abdominal discomfort and creates a viscous pathogenic cycle.

Acute colonic pseudoobstruction, or Ogilvie's syndrome, is a form of ileus localized to the large intestine, which can result in massive cecal and colonic dilatation. Ogilvie first described this syndrome in 1948 in two patients who developed nonobstuctive colonic dilatation and were found to have metastatic deposits involving the sympathetic plexus. Colonic dilation can be massive, and cecal diameters of >12 cm may perforate thereby causing abdominal sepsis and, often, death. The exact pathogenesis of Ogilvie's syndrome is unknown since not all patients have cancer or metastatic involvement of the gut sympathetic plexus. Amyloid infiltration of the myenteric plexus may lead to hypomotility. However, the risk factors are essentially the same as described for small intestinal ileus. Patients with underlying neurologic disease such as Parkinson's disease may be at especially high-risk for colonic pseudoobstruction in the setting of acute illness or cancer. A life-threatening complication of acute colonic pseudoobstruction is toxic megacolon, a clinical syndrome consisting of colonic dilatation in conjunction with systemic inflammatory toxicity manifested as fever, hypotension, and tachycardia. Patients with toxic megacolon are at high risk for septic shock and bowel perforation due to mucosal ischemia and transmural necrosis resulting from hypoperfusion of the bowel wall and mucosa.

ETIOLOGY

Etiologic factors implicated in small bowel ileus and colonic pseudoobstruction are similar and include:

- Recent surgery
  - Laparotomy, ovarian cancer debulking, pathologic hip fracture surgery
- Immobility/bedbound state
- Respiratory failure
- Hypotension
- Sepsis/infection
- Volume depletion
- Congestive heart failure
- Neurologic disease
- Electrolyte derangements
  - Hypokalemia, hypomagnesemia, hypophosphatemia, hypercalcemia
- Narcotic analgesics
- Anti-cholinergic drugs
  - Phenothiazines, antihistamines
- Chemotherapy-related
  - Autonomic neuropathy: vincristine, thalidomide
  - Mucosal inflammation/enteritis: cytarabine, taxanes

Symptoms and Signs

Patients with small bowel ileus typically present with vomiting and patients with colonic pseudoobstruction with abdominal pain and distention. However, there may be significant overlap with regard to symptoms and signs:

- Vomiting
- Nausea
- Anorexia
- Abdominal pain
- Constipation/obstipation
- Diarrhea
- Fever
- Tachycardia
- Hypotension
- Abdominal distention
- Tympany
- Abdominal tenderness
  - Peritoneal signs such as rebound tenderness, guarding, rigidity, or percussion tenderness are suggestive of transmural bowel wall ischemia or perforation
- Hypoactive or tinkling, high-pitched bowel sounds

Diagnostic Studies

The diagnosis of small or large bowel ileus can often be made on clinical grounds, but additional diagnostic studies are important to exclude mechanical bowel obstruction, free intraperitoneal air, or massive cecal distention that may require urgent decompression. The most useful diagnostic studies include:

- Flat plate and upright abdominal radiograph
  - Most useful initial diagnostic test
    - Features of ileus include dilation of the small and/or large bowel and cecal dilation; absence of colorectal air or a cut-off sign is more compatible with a mechanical obstruction
    - On upright views, patients with air-fluid levels within the small bowel are more likely to harbor a mechanical small bowel obstruction
    - Free subdiaphragmatic air indicates perforation
- Computed tomography
  - May be useful in diagnostically unclear cases in differentiating ileus versus mechanical obstruction with administration of water-soluble contrast which typically reveals a transition zone with mechanical obstruction
  - Also useful for detection of perforation, inflammatory masses, tumors, or air within the bowel wall (*pneumatosis intestinalis*)
- Gastrograffin enema
  - Water soluble compound injected under low pressure into the rectum to exclude mechanical large bowel obstruction

- Serum electrolytes
    - Imperative to obtain since correcting electrolyte abnormalities is vital in cases of ileus or pseudoobstruction

TREATMENT

General treatment principles include treatment of hypotension, hypoxia, volume depletion, infection, and electrolyte derangements with standard medical interventions. Avoidance of narcotic and anticholinergic drugs is important due to their adverse effect on bowel motility. Nasogastric suction is typically indicated for bowel decompression, but careful attention must be paid to avoid depletion of electrolyte-rich fluids, which can further exacerbate the ileus syndrome. Patients, if possible, should be mobilized out of bed. Prokinetic agents such as metoclopramide can be considered. Patients receiving vincristine require daily administration of cathartics to prevent obstipation.

In cases of colonic pseudoobstruction, frequent turning of the patient and insertion of a rectal tube may aid decompression. Neostigmine has been shown to be quite effective for colonic pseudoobstruction, but may be associated with severe adverse effects in the critically ill patient. Serial abdominal radiographs are helpful, and if the cecal diameter exceeds 12 cm, careful endoscopic decompression should be considered to decrease the risk of perforation. Placement of a percutaneous cecostomy decompression tube may be beneficial in critically ill patients unable to withstand colonoscopy and can remain in place for several days. The development of toxic megacolon may require urgent laparotomy with bowel resection, although the mortality rate remains high in patients with advanced cancer.

PROGNOSIS

The prognosis of small bowel ileus or colonic pseudoobstruction is variable and to a large extent depends on the patient's underlying cancer prognosis, as well as other co-morbid conditions. The development of toxic megacolon or bowel perforation typically leads to septic shock and carries a very high mortality rate in the cancer patient.

ADDITIONAL READING

Hayes-Lattin BM, Curtin PT, Fleming WH, et al. Toxic megacolon: a life-threatening complication of high-dose therapy and autologous stem cell transplantation among patients with AL amyloidosis. *Bone Marrow Transplant* 2002; 30:279–285.

Marinella MA. Acute colonic pseudoobstruction complicated by cecal perforation in a patient with Parkinson's disease. *South Med J* 1997;90:1023–1026.

Ponec RJ, Saunders MD, Kimmey MB. Neostigmine for the treatment of acute colonic pseudoobstruction. *N Engl J Med* 1999;341:137–141.

Schnoll-Sussman F, Kurtz RC. Gastrointestinal emergencies in the critically ill cancer patient. *Semin Oncol* 2000;27:270–283.

Sheth SG, LaMont JT. Toxic megacolon. *Lancet* 1998;351:509–513.

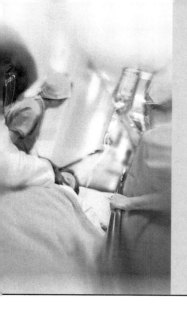

23

Small and Large Bowel Obstruction

DEFINITION

Small bowel obstruction (SBO) or large bowel obstruction (LBO) are present when gastrointestinal contents are inhibited from traversing the intestine due to occlusion of the bowel lumen because of an intraluminal mass lesion or an extraluminal process impinging on the bowel wall.

CLINICAL SETTING

Most cases of SBO in the cancer patient occur in the setting of intra-abdominal adhesions from prior abdominal surgery, intraluminal obstructing cancers, or extraluminal encasement of the bowel with metastatic tumor, as occurs in the setting of advanced ovarian cancer. In the case of LBO, the most frequent setting is a previously undiagnosed primary colon cancer.

PATHOGENESIS

The pathogenesis of SBO initially depends on whether the inciting process is an intraluminal mass lesion, such as a primary or metastatic neoplasm, or a process extrinsic to the bowel, most commonly peritoneal adhesions, internal hernias, or metastatic deposits involving the bowel wall. Patients with SBO typically present acutely due to the large amounts of intraluminal fluids and secretions that result in increased pressure and distention. A closedloop SBO, or strangulation, is present when the involved bowel segment is trapped or twisted, resulting in compromised arterial inflow and resultant bowel ischemia, necrosis, and ultimately, perforation and spillage into the peritoneal cavity. With a simple SBO, which can be partial or complete, intraluminal fluid sequestration results in volume and electrolyte depletion. Additionally, bowel distention leads to increased intraluminal pressure which can impede mucosal blood flow resulting in ischemia, necrosis, and bacterial translocation resulting in Gram-negative sepsis. Malignancy-associated SBO can result from intraluminal tumor (primary or metastatic), radiation-induced stricture formation, or coagulopathy-induced hemorrhage into the bowel wall. Most cases of LBO result from a large primary colon cancer and are more gradual in onset due to the larger luminal diameter of the colon and decreased fluid secretions.

Etiology

Cancer patients can develop SBO from the same benign processes as the general population, but are predisposed to many other cancer-related processes related to the primary tumor and treatments. Also, while LBO is most often due to a previously undiagnosed large primary colon cancer, other potential etiologies must be considered:

- SBO
  - Adhesion formation from prior abdominal surgery
  - Internal hernias (e.g., obturator, inguinal, incisional)
  - Intraluminal tumor
    - Primary tumor of small intestine
      - Carcinoma, lymphoma, carcinoid, leiomyosarcoma, gastrointestinal stromal tumor (GIST)
      - Can lead to primary occlusion of lumen or serve as a lead point for an intussusception
    - Metastatic tumor
      - Lung, kidney, breast, melanoma
  - Intramural hematoma
    - Warfarin-induced coagulopathy
    - Disseminated intravascular coagulation of any cause
    - Acquired factor VIII inhibitor
  - Radiation-induced stricture
  - Inflammatory enteritis with severe mucosal edema
  - Extrinsic compression of the bowel wall
    - Lymphoma, sarcoma, carcinoma
    - Enlarged lymph nodes
  - Encasement of the serosa with tumor (peritoneal carcinomatosis)
    - Very common with ovarian cancer
    - Gastric cancer/*linitis plastica*, colon cancer, pancreatic cancer
- LBO
  - Primary colonic carcinoma
  - Diverticulitis
  - Radiation-induced stricture
  - Inflammatory bowel disease
    - Associated with higher risk of colon cancer

Symptoms and Signs

The clinical presentation of SBO and occasionally LBO can resemble more prevalent and less urgent processes such as ileus, constipation, and chemotherapy-related vomiting and diarrhea. However, the most common symptoms and signs include:

- Vomiting
  - Typically bilious, but may become feculent in the case of a distal SBO or LBO
  - In the case of a proximal SBO, vomiting is early and severe; with a distal SBO, vomiting develops more gradually
- Nausea
- Anorexia
- Abdominal distention
  - More severe and gradual in onset with distal SBO due to the large amount of small bowel with intraluminal fluid and gas collection
  - Prominent feature of LBO
- Abdominal pain
  - May behave in a colicky, wave-like fashion
- Absent flatus
  - Suggestive of complete SBO or LBO
- Obstipation
  - Suggestive of complete SBO or LBO
- Abdominal tenderness
  - The presence of rebound tenderness, guarding, rigidity, or percussion tenderness suggest transmural ischemia with peritoneal inflammation and impending perforation
- High-pitched bowel sounds
- Tympany

Diagnostic Studies

While the diagnosis of SBO can be surmised on clinical grounds, the diagnosis requires definitive radiographic assessment to exclude ileus or pseudo-obstruction. However, it should be noted if the patient has evidence of frank peritoneal signs and/or is *in extremis,* immediate surgical consultation should be arranged for exploratory laparotomy, unless the patient is otherwise terminal from their cancer. Suggested diagnostic studies include:

- Abdominal flatplate and upright radiographs
  - Initial evaluation of choice
  - The most common findings of SBO include a dilated, fluid, and air-filled small intestine with air-fluid levels on the upright view with a paucity or absence of luminal gas distal to the obstruction
    - If tumor encasement is present on the bowel serosa, dilation may not occur and obscure the diagnosis of SBO

- ○ The most common findings of LBO include dilatation of the colon and absence of gas in the rectum
- ○ Indicators of bowel wall ischemia or necrosis include mucosal edema ("thumbprinting"), air in the bowel wall (*pneumatosis intestinalis*), portal venous gas, or free air under the hemidiaphragms
- Small bowel follow through (SBFT)
  - ○ May be useful in non-urgent cases; water-soluble contrast preferable to prevent barium inspissation
  - ○ Failure of contrast to opacify cecum at 24 hours is consistent with high-grade or complete SBO
- Gastrograffin enema
  - ○ May be useful in equivocal cases of LBO
  - ○ Water-soluble contrast gently injected rectally under low pressure may reveal intraluminal mass lesion
  - ○ If evidence of concurrent SBO found in addition to colonic obstruction, this is very suggestive of diffuse malignant carcinomatosis
- Computed tomography
  - ○ More sensitive to detection of SBO and LBO with intraluminal, water-soluble contrast
  - ○ May reveal intraluminal mass or extraluminal lesion compressing the small or large bowel as well as malignant carcinomatosis
  - ○ More sensitive than plain film radiography at detecting mucosal edema, *pneumatosis intestinalis*, portal venous gas, or signs of perforation

TREATMENT

The surgical dictum "do not let the sun set on a bowel obstruction" holds true for many cancer patients with evidence of a complete or closed loop SBO, especially if their primary disease process is under control or has a favorable prognosis. However, in patients with widely metastatic, incurable cancer or with diffuse carcinomatosis, palliative non-operative interventions as suctioning, anti-emetic agents, narcotic analgesia, and octreotide injections may be the best course of action. Octreotide, a somatostatin analogue, is highly effective at affording palliative relief of SBO via prolonged intestinal transit times and decreased gastrointestinal secretions. Intravenous corticosteroids have a palliative role in malignant SBO and LBO and produce benefit by decreasing bowel wall and tumoral edema, diminishing intraluminal salt and fluid secretion, and an anti-nausea effect. However, in patients who are operative candidates without evidence of acute abdomen or closed loop SBO, initial conservative management with *nil per os* status, intravenous fluids, and nasogastric suctioning can be attempted since many incomplete SBOs will spontaneously resolve. It is vital to remember that not all causes of SBO are cancer or cancer-related complications. Therefore, empiric denial of a cancer patient operative release of an SBO due to benign etiologies (e.g., adhesions, hernias) is inappropriate.

Other options for treatment of bowel obstruction in the non-terminal patient include intraluminal stent placement, external beam radiation therapy (especially for LBO-related rectal cancers), decompressive percutaneous endoscopic gastrostomy (PEG) tube, or surgical bypass. Placement of a PEG tube is generally well-tolerated and effective at controlling vomiting, nausea, and distention by providing a "venting" effect for luminal fluid and gas. Supportive care including anti-emetic therapy, electrolyte correction, and adequate hydration is appropriate in most patients. For the uncommon patient with obstruction due to a rapidly-growing, highly-treatable neoplasm such as lymphoma or germ cell cancer, institution of chemotherapy may result in dramatic tumor mass shrinkage and improvement in obstructive symptoms. Patients with ovarian cancer may be considered for chemotherapy depending on their clinical status if optimal surgical debulking is possible.

PROGNOSIS

Cancer patients with a good performance status who develop benign SBO have a favorable prognosis with conservative or, if needed, operative release. The most important factor, however, in determining prognosis in the cancer patient with bowel obstruction is the extent and prognosis of the primary neoplasm and response to treatment. Elderly, frail, malnourished, or otherwise incurable patients who present with bowel obstruction have a grim prognosis which probably warrants comfort measures.

ADDITIONAL READING

Helyer L, Easson AM. Surgical approaches to malignant bowel obstruction. *Support Oncol* 2008;6:105–113.

Khoo D, Hall E, Motson R, et al. Palliation of malignant intestinal obstruction using octreotide. *Europ J Cancer* 1994;30A:2–30.

Krouse RS, McCahill LE, Easson AM. When the sun can set on an unoperated bowel obstruction: management of malignant bowel obstruction. *J Am Coll Surg* 2002;195:117–128.

Ripamonti C, Conno FD, Bentafridda V, et al. Management of bowel obstruction in advanced and terminal cancer patients. *Ann Oncol* 1993;4:15–21.

Tang E, Davis J, Silberman H. Bowel obstruction in cancer patients. *Arch Surg* 1995;130:832–837.

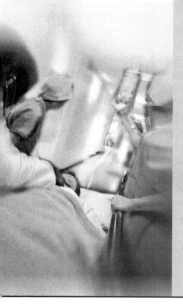

24
Gastrointestinal Perforation

DEFINITION

Perforation of the stomach or bowel occurs when a mucosal injury penetrates through all layers of the hollow viscus resulting in communication between the gastrointestinal lumen and peritoneal cavity.

CLINICAL SETTING

In the cancer patient, perforation of the gastrointestinal tract can result from benign causes or can be related to cancer-specific etiologies such as advanced tumor, chemotherapy, necrotizing infections, or iatrogenic injury.

PATHOGENESIS

Any process that leads to through-and-through perforation of the gastrointestinal tract creates an opening between the luminal contents and the peritoneal cavity, which can have catastrophic consequences such as peritonitis and sepsis. Location of the perforation can also influence the clinical effect of intraluminal leakage. For instance, the normal stomach harbors minute amounts of bacterial due to the acidic pH and, as such, spillage of gastric contents can invoke an extremely painful sterile inflammatory peritonitis. Likewise, perforation of the duodenum or proximal small bowel may invoke an alkaline, bilious peritonitis at the outset since this area of the gastrointestinal tract is typically sterile with a high pH. Gastric perforation may result from corticosteroid-, NSAID-, or *Helicobacter pylori*-related peptic ulcer disease. Malignant gastric ulcer may perforate in up to 4% of patients and be the presenting manifestation. An enlarging gastric carcinoma or lymphoma may spontaneously erode through the thin-walled stomach or, in the case of gastric lymphoma, rapid chemotherapy-induced tumor lysis may result in perforation. Unusual pathogenic mechanisms of gastric perforation include pressure necrosis from prolonged nasogastric intubation or a percutaneous gastrostomy tube as well as iatrogenic endoscopic damage to the gastric wall.

The most common location of small bowel perforation is the duodenum with classic duodenal ulcer remaining a common etiology in patients with malignancy. Due to tumoral involvement of the bowel wall, the cancer patient can develop small bowel perforation from primary tumors, such as adenocarcinoma, leiomyosarcoma, or lymphoma. Certain metastatic tumors, notably melanoma and renal cell carcinoma, have a predilection for involving the small intestine and may result in perforation via mural replacement by tumor and subsequent necrosis. Rarely, small bowel perforation has been reported when patients with an *in situ* small bowel neoplasm have received chemotherapy resulting in tumor and mural breakdown. Additionally, autopsy studies have revealed bowel perforation secondary to cytarbine-induction chemotherapy administered for acute leukemia. Colonic perforation in an adult should always lead to exclusion of a perforated colon or cecal carcinoma. Additional mechanisms of colonic perforation in the cancer patient include chemotherapy induced enteritis, neutropenic enterocolitis, toxic megacolon, or colonic pseudo-obstruction. In fact, any obstructive or non-obstructive process that results in colonic dilation can induce transmural ischemia via small vessel compromise resulting in necrosis and perforation. Patients with metastatic colon cancer who are treated with the anti-vascular endothelial growth factor (VEGF) antibody bevacizumab may develop colonic perforation if the cancer is left *in situ* as a result of local small vessel ischemia. Bevacizumab has also been associated with colonic perforation in patients treated for advanced lung cancer, likely as a result of the altered vascular physiology invoked with this drug. A dreaded complication of colonic perforation is spillage of fecal material into the peritoneal cavity which invokes a suppurative peritonitis which frequently leads to septic shock, especially in the setting of immunosuppression, chemotherapy, or corticosteroid use.

ETIOLOGY

The etiology of gastrointestinal perforation in the cancer patient varies somewhat anatomically. Some of the more commonly reported etiologies include:

- Gastric perforation
  - Peptic ulcer disease
    - *H. pylori*, NSAIDS, corticosteroids
  - Gastric carcinoma
  - Gastric lymphoma
    - May occur during chemotherapy
  - Metastatic tumor
    - Lung, renal cell, breast, melanoma

- Prolonged nasogastric intubation
  - PEG tube
  - Esophagogastroduodenoscopy/biopsy
- Small bowel perforation
  - Peptic ulcer disease
    - *H. pylori*, NSAIDS, corticosteroids
  - Primary tumor
    - Carcinoma, leiomyosarcoma, gastrointestinal stromal tumor (GIST), lymphoma
  - Chemotherapeutic agents
    - Taxanes, cytarabine, interleukin-2
  - Metastatic tumor
    - Lung, renal cell, breast, melanoma
- Colon perforation
  - Colorectal carcinoma
  - Diverticulitis
  - Colonic pseudo-obstruction
  - Toxicmegacolon
    - Chemotherapy related, *C. difficile*, underlying inflammatory bowel disease
  - Typhlitis
    - Inflammation of the ileocecal area in the setting of chemotherapy-induced neutropenia
  - Colonoscopy/biopsy
  - Barium enema
  - Metastatic tumor
    - Lung, breast, renal cell, melanoma
  - Stercoral ulceration
    - Occurs in setting of severe constipation as hard stool induces pressure necrosis of mucosa
  - Bevacizumab (anti-VEGF antibody)

Symptoms and Signs

Generally speaking, perforation of the stomach or duodenum presents in a sudden, crescendo-like fashion and should be considered in any cancer patient presenting with acute, intense abdominal pain. Colonic perforation may present with acute symptoms as well, but often the perforation will be contained by omental protection, thereby preventing the rapid development of generalized peritonitis. However, symptoms and signs of perforation may be masked by corticosteroid therapy or chemotherapy. With these caveats, the most common symptoms and signs of perforation in the cancer patient include:

- Abdominal pain
- Nausea

- Vomiting
- Abdominal distention
- Absent flatus
- Fever
- Pallor
- Tachycardia
- Hypotension
- Abdominal tenderness
- Peritoneal signs
  - Rebound tenderness, involuntary guarding, rigidity, percussion tenderness, absent bowel sounds, pain with heel tapping or cough

DIAGNOSTIC STUDIES

Any patient with sudden, excruciating pain at the onset should be presumed to have a perforated viscus until proven otherwise. If the patient is not otherwise terminal from his cancer, immediate abdominal exploration without diagnostic testing should be strongly considered. However, in otherwise stable patients who are not *in extremis,* a thoughtful diagnostic evaluation may include:

- Upright abdominal radiograph or chest radiograph
  - Classical finding in free infradiaphragmatic air, especially noticeable under the right hemidiaphragm
- Right lateral decubitus radiograph
  - Useful in bedbound patient who cannot sit up
  - Reveals free air between the liver edge and lateral abdominal wall
- Gastrograffin abdominal radiograph
  - In equivocal cases enteric administration of water-soluble contrast may reveal site of occult perforation
- Computed tomography
  - More sensitive for detection perforated viscus than plain radiography
  - May reveal evidence of other intra-abdominal complications of perforation such as abscess, portal venous air, impending obstruction, or *pneumatosis intestinalis*

TREATMENT

Although an in-depth discussion of the surgical management of gastrointestinal perforation is beyond the scope of this text, a few treatment principles will be discussed. First, adequate intravenous access, fluid resuscitation, and airway management are mandatory in cases of the acute abdomen. The patient should be *nil per os* and if evidence of sepsis exists, broad spectrum antibiotics that cover colonic pathogens should be provided. If the patient is otherwise a surgical candidate, perforation of the stomach or small bowel typically requires prompt surgical intervention to locate and repair the site of perforation. If the patient is too ill for surgery, some cases of upper gastrointestinal perforation can be managed with bowel rest, nasogastric suction, proton pump inhibitors, and antibiotics. Colonic perforation with suspected free spillage of intestinal contents in to the peritoneum typically requires urgent laparotomy and in some cases, colonic resection and colostomy. In cases of localized perforation that seem contained to a small area on imaging studies, conservative management may be offered. As an overriding rule, if the patient's cancer is under control, denying potentially life-saving surgery is not appropriate solely on the basis of even metastatic disease.

PROGNOSIS

Perforation due to a benign etiology such as peptic ulcer disease that is promptly treated surgically has a good prognosis. It is not uncommon for a patient to present with colonic perforation due to a locally advanced colon carcinoma. These patients may potentially be cured with surgical resection alone or, if node-positive, with adjuvant chemotherapy. Unfortunately, patients with extra-intestinal metastatic malignancy to the bowel have a very poor long-term prognosis, even with adequate surgical repair. In the patient with advanced terminal cancer who develops a perforation, aggressive comfort care should be instituted.

ADDITIONAL READING

Alwhouhayb M, Mathur P, Al Bayaty M. Metastatic melanoma presenting as a perforated small bowel. *Turk J Gastroenterol* 2006;17:223–225.

Gertsch P, Yip SKH, Chow LWC, et al. Free perforation of gastric carcinoma. *Arch Surg* 1995;130:177–178.

Gray J, Murren J, Sharma A, et al. Perforated viscus in a patient with non-small cell lung cancer receiving bevacizumab. *J Thorac Oncol* 2007;2:571–573.

Leidich RB, Rudolf LE. Small bowel perforation secondary to metastatic lung carcinoma. 1981;193:67–69.

Schnoll-Sussman F, Kurtz RC. Gastrointestinal emergencies in the critically ill cancer patient. *Semin Oncol* 2000;27:270–283.

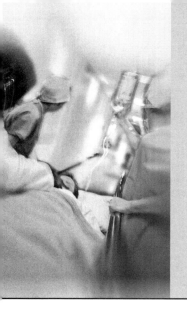

25

Typhlitis

DEFINITION

Typhlitis, or neutropenic enterocolitis, is a clinical syndrome consisting of right lower quadrant pain and fever resulting from mural inflammation of the ileocecal area that typically complicates chemotherapy-induced neutropenia in the setting of hematologic malignancy.

CLINICAL SETTING

The majority of cases of typhlitis occur in neutropenic patients being treated with cytotoxic therapy for acute leukemia, although the syndrome can also occur in patients receiving chemotherapy for solid tumors and various benign neutropenias.

PATHOGENESIS

The majority of cases of typhlitis complicate induction chemotherapy for acute myelogenous (AML) or acute lymphoid leukemia (ALL) due to the prolonged neutropenia that is universal to this setting. Most cases involve the cecum, but the terminal ileum and ascending colon are frequently involved. The pathophysiologic mechanism of typhlitis involves initial mucosal disruption, denudation, and ulceration due to chemotherapy; cytarabine is especially toxic to proliferating enteric mucosa. The ulceration then sets the stage for secondary bacterial invasion of the bowel wall with enteric Gram-negative, α-hemolytic streptococci, and anaerobic bacteria such as *Clostridium septicum*. Immunosuppression and granulocytopenia greatly impair the local host response to tissue damage and bacterial invasion, resulting in a necrotizing transmural process that can lead to perforation, acute abdomen, and septic shock. Areas of submucosal hemorrhage may occur due to vascular damage and thrombocytopenia. Although the majority of cases of typhlitis complicate hematologic malignancies, there have been an increasing number of reports in association with taxane administration for solid tumors, possibly due to local epithelial breakdown.

ETIOLOGY

Early cases of typhlitis were described in children receiving induction chemotherapy for ALL. However, several other malignant diseases treated with chemotherapy have been associated with typhlitis:

- Acute leukemia
  - AML, ALL
- Myelodysplastic syndrome
- Solid tumors treated with taxanes (paclitaxel, docetaxel), vinca alkaloids (vincristine, vinblastine), or anthracyclines (doxorubicin)
- Hematopoietic stem cell transplantation
  - Allogeneic, autologous
- Aplastic anemia
- Drug-induced agranulocytosis

SYMPTOMS AND SIGNS

Typhlitis should be considered in any neutropenic patient with fever and right lower quadrant pain. Common clinical findings regardless of etiology include:

- Abdominal pain
  - Most often involving the right lower quadrant, but may be generalized depending on extent of involvement
  - May be diminished if patient receiving corticosteroids
- Fever
- Diarrhea
  - May be watery or blood-tinged
- Nausea
- Vomiting
- Tachycardia
- Hypotension
- Abdominal distention
  - Can signify ileus or toxic megacolon
- Abdominal tenderness
- Peritoneal signs
  - Suggestive of transmural ischemia and impending or completed perforation
  - Rebound tenderness, involuntary guarding, rigidity, hypoactive bowel sounds, percussion tenderness, pain with heel tapping or coughing

- Palpable right lower quadrant mass
  - May represent distended boggy cecum, phlegmon, or abscess formation

DIAGNOSTIC STUDIES

Diagnosis of typhlitis requires a high index of suspicion and prompt diagnostic testing to differentiate from other causes of acute abdominal pain.

- Flat plate and upright abdominal radiograph
  - May reveal ileus pattern, a right lower quadrant soft tissue density, or *pneumatosis* of the cecum
  - Massive colonic dilation and mucosal edema ("thumbprinting") are suggestive of toxic megacolon.
  - Perforation suggested by infradiaphragmatic air
- Computed tomography
  - More sensitive than radiography
  - Findings include cecal dilatation, bowel wall thickening involving the ileocecal area, inflammatory fat stranding, *pneumatosis intestinalis*, and occasionally abscess formation, ascites, or free air
- Ultrasonography
  - Rapid to perform and may reveal thickened colonic wall, narrowed lumen, and ascites
- Colonoscopy
  - Generally contraindicated due to risk of perforation
  - Findings include hemorrhagic, ulcerated, friable mucosa

TREATMENT

Patients with typhlitis are often critically ill with evidence of sepsis, especially in the setting of induction chemotherapy for acute leukemia. Avoidance of surgery with conservative management is indicated for the majority of patients because of sepsis and concurrent thrombocytopenia and neutropenia, which increase operative risk. Nonetheless, if frank peritoneal signs or radiographic evidence of perforation or toxic megacolon is present, operative intervention is warranted. General non-operative therapy for typhlitis includes bowel rest and broad-spectrum antibiotics against enteric Gram-negative and anaerobic organisms. Transfusion of red cells and platelets as well as correction of coagulopathy are indicated. Drugs that slow bowel transit such as narcotics, anticholinergics, or antidiarrheals should be avoided. Some authors recommend granulocyte stimulating factor to enhance neutrophil recovery.

PROGNOSIS

Patients with mild to moderate typhlitis which responds to conservative care have a favorable prognosis, especially if the neutrophil count recovers in rapid fashion.

Patients with septic shock, vasopressor use, toxic megacolon, or bowel perforation have a poor prognosis and high mortality.

ADDITIONAL READING

Blijlevens NMA, Donnelly JP, DePauw BE. Mucosal barrier injury: biology, pathology, clinical counterparts and consequences of intensive treatment for haematological malignancy: an overview. *Bone Marrow Transplant* 2000;25:1269–1278.

Furonaka M, Miyazaki M, Nakajima M, et al. Neutropenic enterocolitis in lung cancer: a report of two cases and a review of the literature. *Internal Medicine* 2005;44:467–470.

Katz JA, Wagner ML, Gresik MV, et al. Typhlitis: an 18-year experience and postmortem review. *Cancer* 1990;65:1041–1047.

Sinicrope FA. Gastrointestinal complications. In: *Cancer Medicine 6. Volume 2.* Kufe DW, Pollock RE, Weichselbaum RR, et al., eds. Hamilton, Ontario: BC Decker, 2003, pp. 2573–2587.

Song HK, Kreisel D, Canter R, et al. Changing presentation and management of neutropenic enterocolitis. *Arch Surg* 1998;133:979–982.

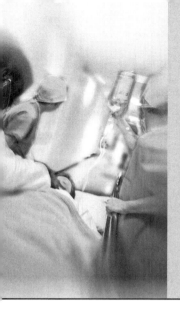

26

Pseudo-membranous Colitis

DEFINITION

Pseudomembranous colitis (PMC) is an inflammatory-infectious-exudative process involving the colon that results from overgrowth of the toxin-producing anaerobic bacterium, *Clostridium difficile*. Rarely, enteric infection with toxin-producing *Staphylococcus aureus* can cause PMC and appear phenotypically identical to *C. difficile*-associated PMC; this discussion focuses on PMC resulting from *C. difficile*.

CLINICAL SETTING

The vast majority of cases of PMC in the cancer patient are nosocomially-acquired and complicate administration of broad-spectrum antibiotics, although chemotherapy may also play a role in the pathogenesis.

PATHOGENESIS

Hospitalized patients are at risk for oral ingestion of *C. difficile* spores from contaminated fomites colonizing various hospital surfaces, including the hands of healthcare workers. The spores of this organism are hardy and can survive on inanimate objects within the hospital environment. Normally, the endogenous bacterial flora in the colon prevents sporulation and growth of *C. difficile*, but in patients with an altered colonic floral milieu, the organism may proliferate. Chemotherapeutic drugs, in the absence of concurrent antibiotics, have also been implicated in the development of PMC and are thought to somehow augment the local anaerobic microenvironment permitting *C. difficle* to proliferate. The mucosal injury resulting from *C. difficile* is related to cytotoxins that induce mucosal inflammation, ulceration, and necrosis. The hallmark of *C. difficile* colitis is the formation of mucosal pseudomembranes, which are yellowish exudative plaques comprised of cellular debris, fibrin, and products of local cytopathic effects. The diarrhea is toxin-mediated and may occasionally be bloody due to significant mucosal injury. The pathologic effects of *C. difficile* are mediated by three toxins: toxin A (an enterotoxin that induces fluid secretion and diarrhea); toxin B (a cytotoxin that causes cell epithelial cell injury and necrosis); and a motility altering factor. Diagnosis of PMC and *C. difficile*-associated diarrhea primarily relies on detection of these toxins in the stool, keeping in mind 3% of the general population is colonized with the organism. The diarrhea can lead to significant volume and electrolyte depletion leading to hypovolemic shock. Additionally, PMC can be associated with a life-threatening systemic inflammatory syndrome resembling septic shock that results from toxin-induced inflammatory mediators such as interleukin-8, substance P, and tumor necrosis factor-α. In fact, a small subset of patients (3% to 8%) may develop "fulminant" *C. difficile* colitis characterized by systemic toxicity, colonic dilatation, and hemodynamic instability that likely results from a patient's inability to mount an adequate immune response. Immunosuppressed patients with cancer or those receiving chemotherapy seem to be at increased risk for fulminant colitis, which is often fatal. Pathologic and autopsy colonic specimens of patients with fulminant PMC reveal hemorrhagic necrosis, marked inflammatory cell infiltration, and the presence of pseudomembranes. Proliferation of cytotoxins may reach the systemic circulation and produce extreme leukocytosis (leukemoid reaction), with levels exceeding 100,000 cells/mm^3 on occasion. A unique feature of PMC is the development of profound hypoalbuminemia as a result of protein-losing enteropathy induced by the toxin-induced cytopathic and secretory damage to enterocytes.

ETIOLOGY

The majority of cases of PMC in the cancer patient results from broad-spectrum antibiotic administration and occurs in hospitalized hosts. Commonly reported etiologies and contributors to the development of PMC include:

- Antibiotics
  - Clindamycin, cephalosporins, beta-lactams, quinolones
- Chemotherapy
  - Taxanes, methotrexate, doxorubicin, cyclophosphamide, bortezomib
- Prolonged hospitalization
- Advanced age
- Nasogastric tube/tube feedings

SYMPTOMS AND SIGNS

Although most cases of mild to moderate PMC are characterized by diarrhea, a variety of clinical findings may occur given the spectrum of severity:

- Diarrhea
  - Typically watery, but may be bloody
- Abdominal pain
- Nausea
- Constipation
  - May occur in as many as 10% of patients and delay diagnosis
- Fever
- Tachycardia
- Hypotension
  - Harbinger of fulminant colitis and shock
- Abdominal tenderness
  - Typically diffuse; the presence of peritoneal signs implies transmural necrosis and fulminant colitis
- Abdominal distention
  - May result from ileus induced by hypomobility, hypotension, volume depletion, electrolyte derangements, and narcotic usage
  - May result from colonic dysmotility in cases of fulminant disease

Diagnostic Studies

The diagnosis of PMC should be considered in any cancer patient with new-onset diarrhea, abdominal discomfort, or fever, whether or not antibiotics have been administered. Helpful diagnostic studies include:

- Stool toxin assays for A and B cytotoxin
  - Rapid, widely used, good sensitivity and specificity
  - May be negative in 12% of patients with fulminant colitis
- Stool culture
  - Slow turn-around, some patients colonized
- Tissue culture assay
  - Gold standard, but cumbersome and results not available rapidly
- Fecal leukocyte assay
  - Often positive, but non-specific
- "Sniff test"
  - Odor of stool in *C. difficile* patients reported to be unique and predictive
- Blood studies
  - Leukocytosis or leukemoid reaction characteristic of severe disease
  - Profound hypoalbuminemia indictative of a protein-losing enteropathy is a valuable clue in an ill patient with diarrhea
- Endoscopy
  - The classic finding on sigmoidoscopy or colonoscopy is adherent yellow pseudomembranes covering the colonic mucosa
  - Risk of perforation exists in patients with fulminant colitis

- Abdominal radiography
  - May reveal ileus pattern, colonic distention, or mucosal edema ("thumb-printing") in severe disease
- Computed tomography
  - Sensitive for diagnosing fulminant colitis
  - Common findings include colonic wall thickening or nodularity, peri-colonic tissue stranding, colonic dilatation, and ascites

TREATMENT

The preferred treatment for mild cases of PMC is oral metronidazole, which has efficacy rates of more than 90%. Relapses can be retreated with metronidazole or oral vancomycin. Patients unable to tolerate oral medications, or with an ileus, can be treated with intravenous metronidazole, which is secreted into the gut lumen. Intravenous vancomycin is ineffective. Antidiarrheal agents should be avoided since their use can induce colonic hypomotility and precipitate megacolon. Adequate hydration and electrolyte management are also essential. Patients with severe colitis who do not respond to first-line therapies may benefit from infusion of intravenous immune globulin. The development of fulminant colitis or toxic megacolon is an indication for colectomy, but carries a high mortality rate (57%) if surgery is performed once hypotension develops.

PROGNOSIS

The prognosis for most cancer patients with mild to moderate PMC is favorable with oral metronidazole treatment, although as many as 20% of patients experience relapse. The development of fulminant colitis or toxic megacolon carries a nearly 100% mortality rate without surgery, especially in the presence of hypotension or a leukocyte count of above 50,000 cells/mm^3.

ADDITIONAL READING

Adams SD, Mercer DW. Fulminant *Clostridium difficile* colitis. *Curr Opin Crit Care* 2007;13:450–455.

Burdette SD, Berstein JM. Does the nose know? The odiferous diagnosis of *Clostridium difficile*-associated diarrhea. *Clin Infect Dis.* 2007;44:1142.

Dallal RM, Harbrecht BG, Houjoukas AJ, et al. Fulminant *Clostridium difficile*: an underappreciated and increasing cause of death and complications. *Ann Surg* 2002;235:363–372.

Hassoun A, Ibrahim F. Use of intravenous immunoglobulin for the treatment of severe *Clostridium difficile* colitis. *Am J Geriatr Pharmacother* 2007;5:48–51.

Marinella MA, Burdette SD, Markert RJ, et al. Leukomoid reactions complicating *Clostridium difficile* colitis. *South Med J* 2004;97:959–963.

Moon SJ, Min CK, Lee DG, et al. Pseudomembranous colitis following bortezomib therapy in a myeloma patient. *Acta Haematol* 2007;117:211–214.

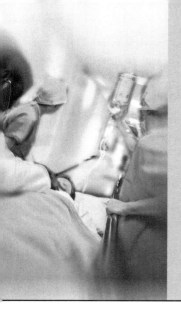

27

Fulminant Hepatic Failure

DEFINITION

Fulminant hepatic failure (FHF) is defined as liver failure in conjunction with encephalopathy developing within 8 weeks of symptom onset in the absence of antecedent liver disease.

CLINICAL SETTING

The development of FHF in the cancer patient is uncommon, but most commonly occurs in the setting of diffuse tumor infiltration of the hepatic parenchyma, an adverse drug reaction, or acute viral hepatitis.

PATHOGENESIS

The pathogenesis of FHF is complex, but a succinct overview as it pertains to the cancer patient will be presented. As noted, the hallmark of FHF is the rapid development of hepatic dysfunction manifested as markedly diminished synthetic and detoxification capabilities which account for the prominent clinical manifestations such as coagulopathy and encephalopathy, respectively. Underlying the pathophysiology of virtually all cases of FHF is massive hepatocyte necrosis, which markedly decreases the synthetic, metabolic, and detoxification machinery of the liver. Worldwide, the most common etiology of FHF is infection with hepatitis B. However, in Western nations other common causes of FHF include acetaminophen toxicity, idiosyncratic drug reactions, mushroom ingestion, metabolic diseases, and cardiac failure. Of course, the cancer patient is also at risk for some of these same diseases, but also from several other pathogenic processes specific to cancer or cancer-related therapies. For instance, cancer patients frequently ingest combinations of acetaminophen-narcotic agents, and may be at increased risk for inadvertent liver injury if the recommended dose is exceeded, if there is concomitant use of ethanol, or if there is underlying liver dysfunction related to malignancy. Acetaminophen is known to deplete hepatic antioxidant defense mechanisms which results in hepatocyte necrosis from electrophile-rich toxic intermediate species; regular alcohol use is known to decrease the dose threshold for this to occur. Many other cases of FHF are idiosyncratic in nature, but beyond the scope of this text.

Infiltration of the liver parenchyma with malignancy is a well-described etiology of FHF. The liver is the most common site of hematogenous metastasis in cancer patients, occurring in 36% of patients who die from cancer. Patients with extensive hepatocellular carcinoma involving the hepatic sinusoids may develop FHF. Additionally, a variety of metastatic neoplasms have been implicated in precipitating FHF, which have often been the initial manifestation of cancer. The proposed pathophysiology of malignancy-associated FHF has been elucidated from necropsy studies showing massive parenchymal destruction by direct tumor invasion or infarction and necrosis from local vascular occlusion by tumor. Obstruction of hepatic venules by tumor cells leads to hepatocyte necrosis and sinusoidal infiltration results in sudden ischemic injury and necrosis. In any event, when a critical mass of hepatocytes are lost, liver failure ensues due to deranged synthetic, metabolic, and detoxifying functions. Hematologic malignancies are the most commonly reported cause of FHF due to tumor infiltration, but many solid tumors have been implicated as well. Interleukin-2 release by tumor cells (especially from hematopoietic neoplasms) has been demonstrated to induce hepatocyte injury via the stimulation of Kupffer cells to release more cytokines (e.g., tumor necrosis factor) which activate circulating leukocytes and platelets causing them to adhere to and occlude the microvasculature resulting in ischemic necrosis. Another example of cytokine-induced liver injury is paraneoplastic FHF associated with nonmetastatic renal cell carcinoma. Overall, the decline in liver function resulting from FHF is usually due to liver failure rather than malignancy, a caveat that often precludes an attempt at cytotoxic therapy.

ETIOLOGY

The etiologies of FHF in the cancer patient are protean, however, some of the potential etiologies in the cancer patient include:

- Drug effects
  - Chemotherapeutic/anti-cancer agents
    - Cyclophosphamide
    - Methotrexate
    - Gemcitabine
    - Cytarabine

- L-asparaginase
- Imatinib
- Erlotinib
- Thalidomide
- Anti-androgens: flutamide, bicalutamide, cyproterone
- Acetaminophen
  - Lower threshold with advanced age, liver disease, ethanol use
- Valproic acid
- Trimethoprim-sulfamethoxazole
- Herbs/alternative medicines
  - Ma huang, Jin Bu Huan, germander
- Viral infections
  - Reactivation of hepatitis B with chemotherapy or rituximab
  - Adenovirus (following chemotherapy)
  - Varicella virus
- Hypotension and shock
  - "Shock liver" secondary to cardiogenic, septic, hypovolemic, or hemorrhagic shock
- Tumor-related
  - Hepatocellular carcinoma
  - Lymphoma
    - Reported with non-Hodgkin's and Hodgkin's lymphoma
  - Leukemia
  - Metastatic solid tumors
    - Bronchogenic carcinoma (small cell and non-small cell)
    - Melanoma
    - Breast
    - Gastric
    - Pancreatic
    - Colon
    - Urothelial
    - Carcinoma of unknown primary

Symptoms and Signs

By definition, symptoms and signs of FHF occur rapidly, often over days to a few weeks, with encephalopathic symptoms and signs predominating. However, many clinical findings are frequent:

- Malaise
- Anorexia
- Nausea/vomiting
- Abdominal discomfort
- Weight loss

- Dark urine
- Dysgeusia
- Anorexia
- Fever
- Confusion
- Jaundice
- Delirium/stupor
- Icterus
- Abdominal distention/ascites
- Abdominal tenderness
- Hepatomegaly
- Edema
- Asterixis
- Clonus
- Coma

DIAGNOSTIC STUDIES

Although the diagnosis of FHF can be clinically surmised based on rapid-onset jaundice and encephalopathy, various diagnostic studies are required for diagnosis and prognosis:

- Liver function studies
  - Elevated transaminase levels, hyperbilirubinemia
- Serum chemistries
  - Hypoalbuminemia
  - Elevated lactate dehydrogenase
    - Extreme elevation portends poor prognosis
  - Elevated creatinine
    - May indicate hepatorenal syndrome
  - Hypoglycemia
    - Indicates failure of hepatic gluconeogenesis
  - Hyperammonemia
  - Elevated serum lactate
    - Due to inability of liver to metabolize lactate
- Coagulation studies
  - Prolongation of partial thromboplastin (PTT) and prothrombin time (PT)
  - Hypofibrinogenemia
  - Decreased factor V level
- Leukocytosis
- Thrombocytopenia
- Viral serologic studies
  - Hepatitis A, B, C; cytomegalovirus; Epstein-Barr virus; herpesviruses; adenoviruses

- Abdominal ultrasound
  - May reveal hepatomegaly, focal hepatic metastasis, ascites
- Computed tomography
  - Common findings include hepatomegaly and focal metastatic lesions
  - Hepatomegaly without focal lesions reported with diffuse sinusoidal tumor infiltration
- Liver biopsy
  - Percutaneous route can be dangerous in the setting of coagulopathy
    - If deemed necessary, transjugular route may be safer
  - Findings include hepatocyte necrosis, tumoral invasion of sinusoids or vessels, and distinct tumor deposits

TREATMENT

Treatment of FHF in the setting of disseminated malignancy is frought with difficulty due to the need to control the underlying cancer, while avoiding further hepatic injury, and providing multi-system supportive care. General supportive measures for FHF include oxygenation, airway protection, fluid, glucose, amino acid and electrolyte replacement, as well as correction of coagulopathy with frozen plasma or cryoprecipitate. Lactulose may help with encephalopathic symptoms from changing the pH in the gut lumen, thereby enhancing ammonia removal. Infection and renal failure are very common in patients with FHF and need to be treated aggressively. There is no adequate treatment for hepatorenal syndrome outside of liver transplant, which is typically contraindicated in the setting of advanced cancer. Administering chemotherapy for chemotherapy-responsive neoplasms such as lymphoma and small cell carcinoma has led to reversal of liver injury in some patients, and should be considered if these tumor types are causing FHF due to diffuse liver involvement.

PROGNOSIS

Generally, cancer patients with FHF have a dismal prognosis, especially if the liver dysfunction results from solid tumor involvement. In one of the largest series on FHF due to hepatic tumor infiltration, 17 of 18 patients died. However, there have been reports of successful chemotherapy in patients with FHF resulting from various lymphomas and extensive stage small cell lung cancer. Patients with acidosis, low serum factor V, and marked coagulopathy have a grim prognosis with nil chance of survival.

ADDITIONAL READING

Cross TJS, Bagot C, Portmann B, et al. Imatinib mesylate as a cause of acute liver failure. *Am J Hematol* 2006;81:189–192.

Hamadani M, Benson DM, Copelan EA. Thalidomide-induced fulminant hepatic failure. *Mayo Clin Proc* 2007;82:638–639.

Ikeda K, Shiga Y, Takahashi A, et al. Fatal hepatitis B virus reactivation in a chronic myeloid leukemia patient during imatinib mesylate treatment. *Leuk Lymphoma* 2006;47:155–157.

Kaur B, Gottardo NG, Keil AD, et al. A rare case of adenoviral fulminant hepatic necrosis after chemotherapy. *Pediatr Hematol Oncol* 2002;19:361–371.

Kaira K, Takise A, Wantanabe R, et al. Fulminant hepatic failure resulting from small cell lung cancer and dramatic response to chemotherapy. *World J Gastroenterol* 2006;12:2466–2468.

Rowbotham D, Wendon J, Williams R. Acute liver failure secondary to hepatic infiltration: a single centre experience of 18 cases. *Gut* 1998;42:576–580.

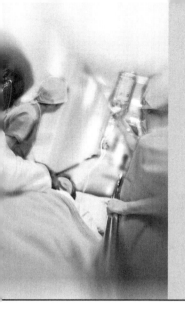

28

Ascending Cholangitis

DEFINITION

Ascending cholangitis (AC) is a clinical syndrome complicating benign or malignant obstruction of the biliary system that results in biliary stasis and subsequent bacterial infection, typically manifesting as septic shock.

CLINICAL SETTING

The most common etiology of AC is gallstones but many patients with malignancy are predisposed due to malignant biliary obstruction, peribiliary adenopathy, or the presence of a pre-existing biliary drain placed for palliative decompression.

PATHOGENESIS

Occlusion of the biliary ductal system (most often at the level of the common bile duct) underlies the development of AC. Intraluminal obstruction resulting from a hepatobiliary neoplasm, extrinsic biliary compression from a lymph node or mass, or occlusion of a pre-existing biliary stent or drain account for the majority of cases of AC in the cancer population. When bile flow into the duodenum is impaired, biliary stasis occurs, markedly increasing the risk of bacterial superinfection with gut flora (bactibilia). Additionally, biliary obstruction leads to increased intraductal pressure which results in reflux of infected bile into the liver and translocation of bacteria into the bloodstream, culminating in sepsis. Bacterial infection of bile is enhanced in the setting of immunosuppression, malignancy, and benign and malignant biliary strictures. In the presence of a biliary drainage tube, bacteria can deconjugate bilirubin and hydrolyze phospholipids resulting in sludge formation and drain occlusion. Biliary occlusion may also result in local immune dysregulation in the small intestine, favoring pathogenic bacterial proliferation. Resultant translocation of small bowel and biliary bacteria commence a systemic inflammatory response with cytokine-induced sepsis. If the biliary system is not decompressed, the viscous cycle of increased intraductal pressure with bacterial proliferation and translocation culminate in septic shock and ultimately, death.

ETIOLOGY

Although the cancer patient may develop biliary obstruction from underlying cholelithiasis, specific etiologies to this population include:

- Cholelithiasis
  - Most common etiology of AC in general population
- Biliary neoplasm
  - Cholangiocarcinoma
  - Gallbladder carcinoma
  - Ampullary carcinoma
- Pancreatic carcinoma
  - Especially at head of pancreas
- Hepatocellular carcinoma
- Biliary stricture
  - Benign or malignant
- Extrinsic compression
  - Lymphadenopathy/lymphoma
  - Metastatic carcinoma to surrounding organs
- Occlusion of pre-existing biliary stent or drain

SYMPTOMS AND SIGNS

Most patients with AC are acutely ill and manifest non-specific findings of sepsis syndrome. Charcot's triad is the classic presentation in patients with AC and consists of rigors, jaundice, right upper quadrant pain, or tenderness and is present in 50% to 100% of patients. Hypotension and delirium in conjunction with Charcot's triad constitute Reynold's pentad and is present in 10% to 20% of patients, but highly indicative of septic shock. However, patients with AC may present with various combinations of:

- Fever
  - Present in more than 90% of patients with AC
- Rigors
- Abdominal pain
  - Right upper quadrant or diffuse
- Nausea/vomiting
- Anorexia
- Dark urine

- Confusion
- Jaundice
- Tachycardia
- Hypotension
- Icterus
- Right upper quadrant tenderness
  - A minority of patients may exhibit peritoneal signs

DIAGNOSTIC STUDIES

The diagnosis of AC can typically be made in an at-risk cancer patient who presents with Charcot's triad or Reynold's pentad. However, since treatment relies on anatomic imaging studies, further evaluation is indicated. The most useful diagnostic studies in the diagnosis of AC include:

- Blood studies
  - Leukocytosis very common although leukopenia may complicate septic shock
  - Hyperbilirubinemia, elevated alkaline phosphatase, and transaminases
- Abdominal radiography
  - Only abnormal in 15% of patients but may reveal ileus or gallstones
- Right upper quadrant ultrasound
  - Initial test of choice due to portability and widespread availability
  - May reveal choledocholithiasis, biliary dilatation, mass lesions, or liver abscess
- Computed tomography
  - More sensitive than ultrasound for detecting etiology and level of biliary obstruction
  - Spiral scan improves sensitivity and specificity
  - Computed tomographic cholangiography is evolving
- Magnetic resonance cholangiopancreatography (MRCP)
  - Non-invasive method with sensitivity and specificity in the 85% range for detecting obstruction and tumors
- Endoscopic retrograde cholangiopancreatography (ERCP)
  - Very sensitive (90% to 100%) technique to identify etiology and site of biliary obstruction
  - Biliary drainage and endoscopic stent placement can be performed at time of diagnostic procedure
  - Allows brushing and cytology for diagnosis of malignancy
  - May result in cholangitis
- Percutaneous transhepatic cholangiography (PTC)
  - Performed under CT scan guidance but requires dilated intrahepatic bile ducts
  - Therapeutic drain can be placed during diagnostic procedure

- Endoscopic ultrasound (EUS)
  - Rapidly-growing diagnostic and therapeutic procedure that can identify biliary tract and pancreatic masses and adenopathy
  - Diagnostic needle aspiration/biopsy can be performed

TREATMENT

Cancer patients with AC have a high mortality rate if treatment is not instituted rapidly. Immediate fluid resuscitation and if needed, vasopressors, should be instituted. Broad-spectrum antibiotics effective against enteric Gram-negative bacilli, anaerobes, and enterococci (e.g., piperacillin-tazobactam) should be administered promptly after blood cultures have been obtained. Simultaneous imaging of the hepatobiliary system should be pursued to pinpoint the etiology of AC and assess for biliary ductal dilatation that may be amenable to endoscopic or percutaneous decompression. The cornerstone of treatment of AC is prompt decompression of the high-pressure within the biliary tree and improving biliary flow. Patients with hypotension require urgent decompression to avoid refractory septic shock and death. Options for rapid biliary drainage include a nasobiliary drain or endoscopic placement (via ERCP) of biliary stent. Studies show that both modalities are initially equally effective for acute treatment of AC. Percutaneous drainage via radiographic guidance is an option if intrahepatic dilatation is present, but hepatic parenchymal bleeding may pose a problem. Some authors have successfully utilized EUS-guided transduodenal puncture for placement of a biliary drain. Operative biliary bypass or drainage is reserved for the few patients in whom endoscopic, percutaneous, or nasobiliary drainage is unsuccessful or technically unfeasible. The surgical morbidity and mortality is substantial.

PROGNOSIS

The prognosis of AC in the cancer patient largely depends upon the cause of biliary obstruction (benign versus malignant) and the status of the underlying malignancy, along with the patient's performance status. Overall, patients with malignant biliary obstruction tend to have more severe AC and a worse outcome than patients with benign biliary obstruction who develop AC. Patients presenting with hypotension or Reynolds' pentad have an extremely high mortality rate even in the absence of malignant disease, and patients who do not respond to antibiotics and do not subsequently undergo drainage have a mortality approaching 100%.

ADDITIONAL READING

Hanau LH, Steigbigel NH. Acute (ascending) cholangitis. *Infect Dis Clin N Am* 2000;14:1–25.

Kumar R, Sharma BC, Singh J, et al. Endoscopic biliary drainage for severe acute cholangitis in biliary obstruction as a result of malignant and benign diseases. *J Gastroenterol Hepatol* 2004;19:994–997.

Puspok A, Lomoschitz F, Dejaco C, et al. Endoscopic ultrasound guided therapy of benign and malignant biliary obstruction: a case series. *Am J Gastroenterol* 2005;100:1743–1747.

Sharma BC, Kumar R, Agarwal N, et al. Endoscopic biliary drainage by nasobiliary drain or by stent placement in patients with acute cholangitis. *Endoscopy* 2005;37:439–443.

Weissglas IS, Brown RA. Acute suppurative cholangitis secondary to malignant obstruction. *Can J Surg* 1981;24:468–470.

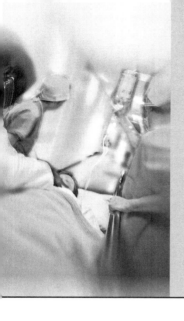

29

Acute
Pancreatitis

DEFINITION

Acute pancreatitis (AP), regardless of the etiology, is characterized by the inappropriate release and activation of pancreatic enzymes into the pancreatic parenchyma which result in pancreatic inflammation and, in severe cases, necrosis.

CLINICAL SETTING

The predominant etiologies of AP in the oncology population are identical to the general population, with the majority resulting from gallstones or ethanol consumption. However, the cancer patient may develop AP specifically related to malignancy, drugs, or iatrogenic injury.

PATHOGENESIS

Inappropriate release and activation of pancreatic enzymes leads to inflammation of the pancreatic interstitial tissues (interstitial pancreatitis) and later the parenchyma. Many benign and malignant disease processes and drugs can commence the cycle of enzyme activation, but the pathophysiologic end result is the same, despite the inciting factor. The spectrum of severity of AP ranges from mild, self-limited cases to fulminant disease associated with shock and pancreatic necrosis. Activation of trypsinogen to trypsin, the pivotal enzyme in the subsequent activation of pancreatic zymogens, commences the cascade of pancreatic damage. Lack of the rapid elimination of trypsin within pancreatic tissue also contributes to the pathogenesis. Activation of digestive enzymes such as lipases, induces pancreatic cellular injury and induces a systemic inflammatory response syndrome (SIRS) that is similar to the sepsis syndrome. This SIRS is mediated by various cytokines such as interleukins and tumor necrosis factor that can lead to widespread organ damage resulting in acute respiratory distress syndrome (ARDS), cardiac dysfunction, renal failure, and hematopoietic abnormalities. In fact, the most common cause of early death in patients with severe AP is multiple organ dysfunction syndrome (MODS) in a manner akin to sepsis. Marked hypoalbuminemia and vascular leak results in significant intravascular volume depletion from third-spacing of fluids. Intra-abdominal saponification of fats and calcium can lead to severe hypocalcemia with its attendant physiologic effects such as tetany and cardiovascular dysfunction.

Severe pancreatitis is often associated with pancreatic necrosis which results from necrotizing injury to the pancreatic parenchyma and disruption of the microcirculation. Inflammation and thrombosis of the pancreatic microcirculation accounts for the lack of contrast enhancement upon dynamic computed tomographic scanning. Pancreatic necrosis is often fatal, especially when superinfection of the devitalized tissue with enteric organisms occurs.

ETIOLOGY

The cancer patient may develop AP not only from the common etiologies, but also from precipitants unique to this population:

- Gallstones
- Alcohol
- Drugs
    - Anti-cancer drugs/chemotherapy
        - L-asparaginase
            - Most common cause of chemotherapy-related AP, occurring in up to 16% of patients
            - Mortality rates of 12% reported
        - Corticosteroids
        - Cytarabine
        - Cisplatinum
        - Methotrexate
        - Cyclophosphamide
        - Doxorubicin
        - Ifosfamide
        - Interleukin-2
        - Sorafenib
        - Estrogens
    - Miscellaneous
        - Thiazide diuretics, furosemide, azathioprine, tetracyclines, valproic acid, sulfa drugs
- Iatrogenic injury
    - ERCP
    - Pancreatic trauma during surgery
    - Transarterial chemoembolization (TACE) of the liver

- Metabolic factors
  - Hypercalcemia
  - Hypertriglyceridemia
- Neoplasm
  - Pancreatic carcinoma
  - Pancreatic lymphoma
  - Metastatic tumors
    - Small cell lung cancer (most common cause of metastasis-related AP)
    - Renal cell carcinoma
    - Breast cancer
    - Melanoma

Symptoms and Signs

Acute pancreatitis usually presents in rather sudden fashion and despite the multiple etiologies, symptoms and signs are similar.

- Abdominal pain
  - Usually epigastric and may be knife-like, radiating to the back
  - Patient often restless and does not lay still—unlike the case with acute peritonitis
- Nausea
- Vomiting
- Anorexia
- Visual changes
  - Rarely, severe pancreatitis can cause necrotizing retinopathy
- Fever
- Tachycardia
- Abdominal tenderness
  - Occasionally, peritoneal signs may be present
- Abdominal distention
  - May represent ileus or pancreatic ascites
- Subcutaneous nodules
  - In severe cases of AP, subcutaneous fat necrosis may occur
- Abnormal retinal vessels in case of retinopathy

Diagnostic Studies

Despite the many potential etiologies of abdominal pain in the cancer patient, AP should be considered in any patient with sudden abdominal pain and the following diagnostic studies considered:

- Serum amylase and lipase
  - Both are typically elevated, although lipase more specific for AP
  - Serum lipase remains elevated longer than amylase
- Complete blood count and coagulation studies
  - Leukocytosis common and has prognostic value
  - Elevated hematocrit signifies hemoconcentration and has prognostic value

- ○ Thrombocytopenia may occur if disseminated intravascular coagulation (DIC) present in severe cases
- ○ Elevated prothrombin time (PT), partial thromboplastin time (PTT), and hypofibrinogenemia signify DIC
- Serum chemistries
  - ○ Hypo- or hyperglycemia may be present; hyperglycemia has prognostic value
  - ○ Lactate dehydrogenase (LDH) elevation parallels pancreatic injury and has prognostic value
  - ○ Alanine aminotransferase (ALT) has prognostic value
  - ○ Hypocalcemia common due to saponification and hypoalbuminemia and has prognostic value
  - ○ Blood urine nitrogen often elevated and has prognostic value
- Abdominal radiograph
  - ○ No specific findings in most cases of AP but often reveals ileus pattern
  - ○ Pancreatic calcification signifies chronic pancreatic disease
- Abdominal ultrasound
  - ○ May reveal pancreatic edema, inflammation, or biliary dilatation in cases of obstructive disease, but overlying ileus limits usefulness
- Computed tomography
  - ○ Imaging test of choice to delineate interstitial or parenchymal pancreatitis or complications as obstruction, abscess, or pseudocysts
  - ○ Dynamic contrast-enhanced CT is the imaging test of choice to diagnose necrotizing pancreatitis and yields prognostic information
    - Normal pancreatic tissue enhances with contrast, but in cases of necrosis, contrast enhancement is absent due to microthrombosis
    - Some studies have revealed mortality rates of 23% in patients with CT evidence of necrosis
- Magnetic resonance cholangiopancreatography (MRCP)
  - ○ Difficult to perform in ill patients but a sensitive and non-invasive way to assess for biliary strictures, obstruction, and neoplasm
- Endoscopic retrograde cholangiopancreatography (ERCP)
  - ○ Invasive, but often procedure of choice if AP caused by gallstone impaction, stricture, or tumor due to ability to perform biliary drainage and stent placement
  - ○ May cause pancreatitis
- Endoscopic ultrasound (EUS)
  - ○ Rapidly-evolving technique that is very sensitive for detecting biliary causes of pancreatitis, including neoplasia

TREATMENT

Mild cases of AP may require only a few days of bowel rest, intravenous fluid therapy, and minimal narcotic analgesia. Removal of any precipitating drug is vital but makes it difficult to treat the underlying neoplasm, if present, and the chemotherapeutic agent is responsible. However, combination chemotherapy has been successful in the rare patient with pancreatic lymphoma-associated AP. Cancer-associated hypercalcemia can cause AP and requires aggressive hydration and often, bisphosphonates. Severe or necrotizing pancreatitis accompanied by SIRS or MODS requires treatment in an intensive care unit, often with mechanical ventilation, vasopressors, and nutritional support. Intravenous narcotic analgesia is required for severe pain. Adequate hydration is necessary but may prove difficult due to significant third-spacing from vascular leak. Coagulopathy and DIC is treated with frozen plasma if bleeding is evident. Patients with pancreatic necrosis may require needle aspiration to detect infection and require surgical debridement of devitalized tissue. Many authors recommend empiric antibiotics, notably imipenem, if pancreatic necrosis is noted on CT scan. In the case of gallstones, stricture, or a malignant etiology of AP, decompression and restoration of bile flow with ERCP is typically indicated.

PROGNOSIS

Most patients with mild AP recover without sequelae. However, severe cases of AP or the development of pancreatic necrosis is associated with high mortality rates, as high as 23% in some studies. Patients who undergo abdominal surgery within the first few days of AP onset have mortality rates of up to 65%. The status of the patient's underlying malignancy is a crucial factor in considering prognosis, especially in cases of metastatic or incurable cancers or in cases of hypercalemic-AP, which is often a pre-terminal event. Numerous scoring systems such as the APACHE index and Ranson's criteria have been developed to assist in determining prognosis, but will not be discussed here. Some general clinical indicators for increased morbidity and mortality include thirst, oliguria, hypoxemia, delirium, an elevated hematocrit, and failure to improve during the first 48 hours of illness.

ADDITIONAL READING

Baron TH, Morgan DE. Acute necrotizing pancreatitis. *N Engl J Med* 1999;340: 1412–1417.

Hung MC, Hung GY, Lin PC, et al. Acute pancreatitis associated with ifosfamide. *J Chin Med Assoc* 2007;70:176–179.

Kanno K, Hikichi T, Saito K, et al. A case of esophageal small cell carcinoma associated with hypercalcemia causing severe pancreatitis. *Fukushima J Med Sci* 2007;53:51–60.

Li M, Srinivas S. Acute pancreatitis associated with sorafenib. *South Med J* 2007; 100:909–911.

Saif MW, Khubchandani S, Walczak M. Secondary pancreatic involvement by a diffuse large B-cell lymphoma presenting as acute pancreatitis. *World J Gastroenterol* 2007;13:4909–4911.

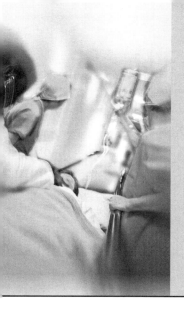

30

Hepatic Tumor Rupture

DEFINITION

Hepatic rupture occurs when tumor necrosis results in life-threatening bleeding into the hepatic parenchyma or peritoneal cavity (hemoperitoneum).

CLINICAL SETTING

Most cases of hepatic tumor rupture occur in patients with hepatocellular carcinoma or, less commonly, in the setting of large hepatic metastasis.

PATHOGENESIS

Large, necrotic hepatocellular carcinomas can occasionally erode into the hepatic arterial circulation resulting in massive parenchymal and often peritoneal bleeding. Most cases of spontaneous hepatic rupture occur in the setting of a large hepatocellular carcinoma, and occur most often in endemic countries such as Japan where rupture may occur in approximately 10% of cases. Since most cases of hepatocellular carcinoma complicate cirrhosis, rupture likely relates to central necrosis resulting from rapid tumor growth which is compounded by intratumoral venous congestion from portal hypertension as well as coagulopathy and thrombocytopenia. Hepatocellular carcinoma also has a propensity to invade the liver capsule, further increasing the risk for hemorrhage. Sudden increase in intratumoral pressure with coughing, deep palpation, or mild abdominal trauma may induce rupture. Spontaneous rupture of metastatic tumors to the liver may occur. The pathogenesis of metastatic tumor rupture is also related to tumor necrosis although increased intravascular pressure from tumor emboli and direct pressure against the liver capsule may contribute. Anticoagulant therapy may result in intratumoral bleeding and hemoperitoneum during bevacizumab administration in the presence of necrotic tumor.

ETIOLOGY

Any rapidly-growing tumor may result in hemorrhage, but the most commonly reported etiologies include:

- Hepatocellular carcinoma
- Metastatic tumors
  - Lung carcinoma
    - Reported with squamous, small cell, and adenocarcinoma
  - Gastric carcinoma
  - Esophageal carcinoma
  - Renal cell carcinoma
  - Colon carcinoma
  - Urothelial carcinoma
  - Melanoma
  - Sarcoma

SYMPTOMS AND SIGNS

Hepatic tumor rupture should be considered in any patient with known liver malignancy who develops sudden abdominal pain. The most common symptoms and signs include:

- Abdominal pain
  - Usually sudden and severe
- Nausea/vomiting
- Dizziness
- Syncope
- Tachycardia
- Hypotension
- Pallor
- Right upper quadrant mass
- Right upper quadrant or generalized abdominal tenderness
  - Hemoperitoneum typically causes peritoneal signs: guarding, rebound tenderness, or rigidity
- Hepatic rub or bruit
- Periumbilical (Cullen's sign) or flank ecchymosis (Grey-Turner's sign)
- Diminished pulses

DIAGNOSTIC STUDIES

Since rupture of a hepatic primary or metastatic tumor is uncommon, most clinicians do not consider the diagnosis. Therefore, if the etiology of abdominal pain in the cancer patient in unclear, the following diagnostic studies may be useful:

- Complete blood count
  - Anemia common

- Abdominal ultrasound
  - May reveal hepatic metastasis with surrounding fluid collection or evidence of ascites secondary to hemoperitoneum
- Computed tomography
  - Sensitive for detection of hemorrhage within a necrotic primary or metastatic tumor as well as ascites/hemoperitoneum
  - The finding of a liver lesion protruding from the liver surface and a discontinuous liver contour are suspicious for tumor rupture

TREATMENT

Spontaneous rupture of a liver neoplasm is frequently fatal due to rapid intraabdominal hemorrhage and hypovolemic shock. If the diagnosis is suspected, immediate large-bore venous catheters should be inserted for aggressive fluid and blood infusion while arranging rapid imaging studies. If clinically indicated, correction of coagulopathy and thrombocytopenia are important, as is reversal of warfarin or heparin effects with frozen plasma and protamine, respectively. Since the prognosis of most patients with liver metastasis or hepatocellular carcinoma is poor, immediate laparotomy may not be feasible and palliative terminal care should be considered. However, if the patient is felt to be a surgical candidate, laparotomy with identification and repair of the bleeding site or partial hepatectomy may be an option, although mortality rates are high. Another option is angiography with arterial embolization with coils or foam—a procedure known as transarterial embolization (TAE) which is effective at controlling hemorrhage in approximately 70% of patients.

PROGNOSIS

Hepatic tumoral hemorrhage is often a pre-terminal event, with most patients succumbing within 6 weeks, although prolonged survival has been reported in rare patients successfully treated with TAE.

ADDITIONAL READING

Chen CY, Lin XZ, Shin JS, et al. Spontaneous rupture of hepatocellular carcinoma: a review of 141 Taiwanese cases and comparison with nonrupture cases. *J Clin Gastroenterol* 1995;21:238–242.

Murakami R, Taniai N, Kumazaki T, et al. Rupture of a hepatic metastasis form renal cell carcinoma. *Clin Imaging* 2000;24:72–74.

Sakai M, Oguri T, Hattori N, et al. Spontaneous hepatic rupture due to metastatic tumor of lung adenocarcinoma. *Internal Medicine* 2005;44:50–54.

Urdaneta LF, Nielsen JV. Massive hemoperitoneum secondary to spontaneous rupture of hepatic metastases: report of two cases and report of the literature. *J Surg Oncol* 1986;31:104–107.

Yoshida H, Mamada Y, Taniai N, et al. Ruptured metastatic liver tumor from an α-fetoprotein-producing gastric cancer. *J Nippon Med Sch* 2005;72:236–241.

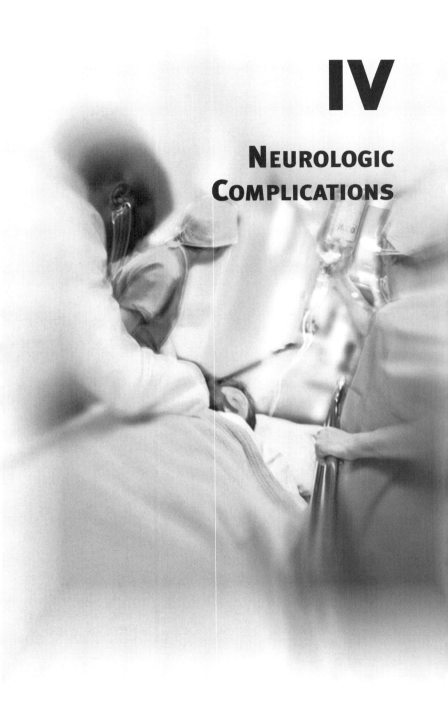

IV

NEUROLOGIC COMPLICATIONS

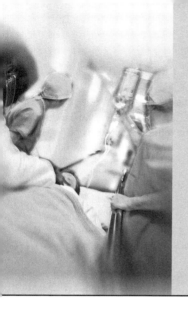

31
Spinal Cord Compression

DEFINITION

Malignant spinal cord compression (SCC) develops in as many as 14% of cancer patients and is characterized by tumoral compression of the spinal cord which results in neurologic dysfunction and paraplegia.

CLINICAL SETTING

The majority of patients with SCC have a known malignancy, most commonly cancer of the breast, lung, or prostate, although in 20% of patients, SCC can be the initial manifestation of cancer.

PATHOGENESIS

Malignant SCC typically occurs by one of three mechanisms: 1) growth of existing anterior vertebral body metastasis into the epidural space. This is by far the most common scenario; 2) collapse of the vertebral body with bone/tumor fragment displacement into the spinal canal and epidural space; and 3) growth of a paraspinal tumor mass through the neural foramina into the epidural space. The metastatic deposit gains access to the vertebral column via the arterial circulation or Batson's venous plexus, especially in the case of prostate or rectal cancers. The intervertebral disk is resistant to tumor involvement which helps to radiographically differentiate malignant SCC from that due to infection, which violates disc substance. Uncommon precipitants of SCC include subdural or intramedullary metastasis. In any event, the end result of any of these mechanisms is compression of the spinal cord proper with resultant neural damage. The primary mechanism of spinal cord damage is vascular in nature via tumoral compression of the epidural venous plexus, which results in increased vessel permeability and vasogenic cord edema. The increasing cord edema eventually exceeds capillary perfusion pressure leading to decreased blood flow to the neural tissue eventually causing white matter ischemia and infarction. The vasogenic spinal cord edema is the pathophysiologic target of corticosteroid therapy, the primary medical intervention for SCC. Arteriole compression and ischemia can also occur due to direct tumor compression against the spinal cord; rarely extradural compression of the artery of Adamkiewicz can cause sudden and devastating cord infarction.

The thoracic spinal cord is involved in approximately 70% of cases of metastatic SCC with the lumbar cord and cervical cord being involved in approximately 20% and 10%, respectively. However, 10% to 38% of patients with epidural SCC have multiple non-contiguous spinal cord lesions, which must be taken into account when imaging procedures are ordered. In general, cancers of the breast and lung tend to involve the thoracic spinal cord and tumors of the prostate, pelvis, and colon tend to involve the the lumbosacral cord segments. Lymphoma can involve any segment and primarily depends on the site of disease that often grows through the neural foramina. Rarely, spinal cord compression can be caused by an epidural hematoma or abscess.

ETIOLOGY

The majority of cases of SCC occur in patients with a known malignancy, but occasional patients may present with SCC as their initial manifestation of cancer. The most common causes of SCC likely to be encountered include:

- Metastatic carcinoma (*Note: Breast, lung, and prostate cancer each cause approximately 20% of cases of metastatic SCC*)
  - Breast
  - Lung
  - Prostate
  - Renal cell
  - Colorectal
  - Head and neck
  - Germ cell
  - Carcinoma of unknown primary site
- Lymphoma
- Sarcoma
- Melanoma
- Multiple myeloma
  - May cause SCC from vertebral fracture, plasmacytoma, or amyloidoma

SYMPTOMS AND SIGNS

The majority of patients with SCC are symptomatic and exhibit neurologic signs when examined in careful fashion:

- Back pain
  - Present in approximately 95% of patients and usually first symptom
  - May be acute or subacute and involve any area, but most commonly involves the midline thoracic or upper lumbar area
  - Helpful clues of malignant SCC pain:
    - Worse at night and with recumbancy (related to distention of the epidural venous plexus)
    - Exacerbated by movement, Valsalva maneuver, straight leg raise, or neck flexion
- Radicular pain
  - May radiate down the arm (cervical SCC), around the trunk in a band-like manner (thoracic SCC), or down the leg (lumbosacral SCC)
- Referred pain
  - Metastasis to the L1 vertebral cord area can refer pain to the sacroiliac joint which can be misdiagnosed as arthritis
- Weakness
  - Next most common symptom next to pain
  - Typically begins in the lower extremities and leads to difficulty ambulating and, eventually, paraplegia
- Sensory symptoms
  - Usually concurrent with development of muscle weakness and consists of paraesthesia/numbness or loss of sensation
  - Lhermitte's sign: parasthesia or shock-like sensation involving the spine and extremities in response to neck flexion; may occur with cervical SCC
- Urinary or fecal incontinence/retention
  - Occurs late in course and suggestive of lumbosacral or *cauda equina* involvement
- Impotence
- Ataxia
  - In isolation, suggests damage to the spinocerebellar tract
- Motor weakness/paraparesis
  - Typically begins in the lower extremities and is more significant in proximal muscle groups (especially iliopsoas) early in course of SCC
  - Can progress rapidly to complete paraplegia if not treated urgently
    - Ambulatory status at time of treatment institution is powerful prognosticator for retaining ability to ambulate
- Abnormal reflexes
  - Hyperreflexia, clonus
- Diminished anal sphincter tone
  - Suggestive of cauda equina involvement
- Horner's syndrome
  - Metastastic deposit in the cervical spine area involving the sympathetic plexus may produce miosis, anhidrosis, or ptosis

DIAGNOSTIC STUDIES

Any patient with known malignancy who presents with new-onset back pain should be considered to have SCC until proven otherwise, especially if neurologic dysfunction is present. Usually, minimal diagnostic imaging is required if the proper initial test is chosen:

- Magnetic resonance imaging (MRI)
  - Imaging study of choice to identify thecal sac and spinal cord compression, tumor involvement of vertebral body and para-vertebral area, and abnormal areas of enhancement of leptomeninges
  - Sensitivity and specificity rates of 93% and 97%, respectively
  - Entire neuroaxis should be imaged routinely since multifocal, synchronous lesions are common
- Computed tomography and myelography
  - Useful only if contraindication to MRI (e.g., pacemaker)
  - Can be useful, although less sensitive than MRI, at identifying cord compression and tumoral involvement
  - Myelography coupled with computed tomography increases yield at identifying site(s) of epidural compression
- Conventional myelography
  - Rarely utilized and carries risks with thrombocytopenia and coagulopathy
- Plain radiographs
  - Not helpful in identifying SCC, but in the presence of compatible clinical findings, the presence of blastic or lytic vertebral body and/or pedicle destruction is supportive of the diagnosis

TREATMENT

Treatment for SCC must be commenced without delay to prevent permanent neurologic injury, most notably, paraplegia. Indeed, ambulatory patients who are treated aggressively in a timely fashion are likely to retain their ability to ambulate; the converse is true as well. Immediate medical therapy for suspected SCC is intravenous corticosteroids, which should be administered before imaging studies are obtained. The only randomized study on this issue revealed that intravenous dexamethasone 10 mg once followed by 4 mg every 6 hours was effective at preventing neurologic deterioration. Therefore, intravenous dexamethasone is standard for patients with SCC and should continue with slow tapering. Radiation therapy has been the crux of therapy for metastatic SCC for years. The standard treatment does is 30 Gy delivered in 10 daily 3 Gy fractions. In patients unlikely to regain ambulation or who are otherwise terminal, steroids and radiation alone are indicated for palliation. However, patients who have at least a several month life expectancy should be considered for surgical decompression and stabilization. Patients with radiation-resistant neoplasms such as renal cell carcinoma, melanoma, and sarcoma should also have urgent surgical consulation and decompression if their medical status permits. Posterior laminectomy is almost never effective at stabilizing the spine since the majority of tumor mass involves the anterior body. An anterior or posterolateral incision with tumor debulking, corpectomy, and rod or cage stabilization is the preferred surgical approach to improve spine stability and integrity. An important phase III trial comparing aggressive decompression surgery followed by post-operative radiation versus standard 30 Gy radiation demonstrated significant improvement in ambulation rates and prolonged ambulation status in the surgical group. Many more patients who were unable to walk before treatment regained the ability to walk in the surgery group compared to the radiation-only group. Most patients with metastatic SCC should be evaluated by a spine surgeon, even if the patient is non-ambulatory at presentation. Patients with hypervascular metastases from renal cell or thyroid carcinoma usually require preoperative arterial embolization to prevent intra-operative hemorrhage. Chemotherapy is usually not utilized for metastatic SCC unless the underlying tumor is very chemosensitive as may be the case with some lymphomas, germ cell, small cell, or breast carcinomas.

PROGNOSIS

Overall, the prognosis of patients developing metastatic SCC is very poor with a mean survival of 3 to 6 months after diagnosis. However, patients with chemosensitive and radiosensitive tumors, small metastatic burden, and who are able to ambulate at presentation, may survive longer. Patients with lung cancer who develop SCC have a dismal prognosis. Patients who undergo anterior surgical decompression seem to have longer survival times than those patients who only receive radiotherapy; this is likely related to decreased frequency of paraplegia complications (e.g., sepsis, aspiration, venous thromboembolism).

ADDITIONAL READING

Byrne TN, Borges LF, Loeffler JS. Metastatic epidural spinal cord compression: update on management. *Semin Oncol* 2006;33:307–311.

Kwok K, DeYoung C, Garofalo M, et al. Radiation oncology emergencies. *Hematol Oncol Clin N Am* 2006;20:505–522.

Kwok Y, Tibbs PA, Patchell RA. Clinical approach to metastatic epidural spinal cord compression. *Hematol Oncol Clin N Am* 2006;20:1297–1305.

Patchell RA, Tibbs PA, Regine WF, et al. Direct decompressive surgical resection in the treatment of spinal cord compression caused by metastatic cancer: a randomized trial. *Lancet* 2005;366:643–648.

Schiff D. Spinal cord compression. *Neurol Clin N Am* 2003;21:67–86.

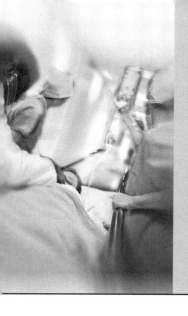

32

Intracerebral Hemorrhage

DEFINITION

Intracerebral hemorrhage (ICH) in the cancer patient is defined by bleeding within a parenchymal brain metastasis or, less commonly, bleeding into normal brain parenchyma as a result of various cancer-related complications.

CLINICAL SETTING

Most cases of ICH in the oncology population occur in the presence of known, widespread metastatic carcinoma, especially in the setting of thrombocytopenia or coagulopathy; ICH can occur in the setting of necrotic primary brain tumors as well.

PATHOGENESIS

The pathogenesis of ICH in the cancer patient is related to the presence of metastatic or primary brain lesions; the presence of abnormal vasculature; the administration of various drugs; or an underlying hematologic derangement in the presence of normal brain anatomy. The most common etiology of ICH in the patient with a solid tumor is hemorrhage within a metastatic focus. Any metastasis can develop ICH as can a primary brain tumor, especially glioblastoma multiforme, a tumor known for significant hypervascularity and necrosis. However, melanoma, choriocarcinoma, and renal cell carcinoma have the greatest propensity for bleeding, although lung cancer overall is the most common cause of ICH due to the prevalence of this disease in the population at large. The mechanism of metastatic tumor hemorrhage is rapid growth and necrosis, invasion of surrounding blood vessels by tumor, and rupture of newly formed vessels created by neoangiogenesis. Most cases of ICH occur in the tumor or surrounding parenchyma but may also involve the subdural, subarachnoid, or ventricular spaces depending on the anatomic location of the tumor. Curiously, simultaneous hemorrhage into multiple synchronous lesions may occasionally occur for unknown reasons.

Another anatomic reason for ICH is the rupture of an artery. This may occur due to vascular erosion by a neighboring tumor mass, rupture of a neoplastic aneurysm formed by tumor emboli that invade and weaken the arterial wall, or rupture of a mycotic aneurysm complicating bacteremia or fungemia. Bronchogenic carcinoma and choriocarcinoma are the most common etiologies of neoplastic aneurysms.

Various anti-cancer drugs and hematologic derangements can induce hemorrhage in otherwise normal brain tissue. L-asparginase is the most well-known cytotoxic agent associated with ICH and results from drug-induced depletion of fibrinogen and coagulation factors. Severe thrombocytopenia resulting from chemotherapy-induced thrombotic thrombocytopenic purpura (TTP) may complicate treatment with gemcitabine, cisplatin, bleomycin, or mitomycin-C and result in ICH. Finally, various hematopoietic derangements can result in ICH in the absence of brain pathology. Myeloproliferative disorders, acute leukemia, DIC-related coagulopathy, and chemotherapy or malignancy-induced thrombocytopenia may result in ICH. Acute promyelocytic leukemia is frequently associated with severe DIC and ICH is the most common cause of death during induction chemotherapy for this disease. Extreme leukocytosis ($>100,000$ cells/mm^3) associated with acute myeloid leukemia can result in sludging within the cerebral microvasculature and ICH.

ETIOLOGY

Malignancy-related ICH may result from various mechanisms with numerous etiologies:

- Primary of metastatic brain tumor
  - Primary brain tumors
    - Glioblastoma multiforme, oligodendroglioma
  - Metastatic brain tumors
    - Lung, breast, gastric, thyroid, hepatocellular, and renal cell carcinomas
    - Choriocarcinoma, germ cell tumors
    - Melanoma
    - Lymphoma
- Abnormal cerebral vasculature
  - Erosion of tumor into blood vessel
  - Neoplastic aneurysm
  - Mycotic aneurysm
  - Radiation-induced aneurysm
- Recent cerebral infarction (especially middle cerebral artery occlusion)

- Anti-cancer drugs
  - L-asparginase: depletion of fibrinogen and clotting factors
  - Mitomycin-C, cisplatin, bleomycin, gemcitabine: TTP-like syndrome
- Hematologic derangements
  - DIC related to sepsis, malignancy, or acute promyelocytic leukemia
  - Hyperleukocytosis/leukostasis secondary to AML
  - Myeloproliferative disorders
  - Anticoagulant therapy
  - Thrombocytopenia related to chemotherapy, DIC, TTP, or malignancy

Symptoms and Signs

Generally, symptoms and signs of ICH in the patient with an intratumoral hemorrhage are sudden but more gradual in cases of coagulopathies. However, clinical findings are often similar regardless of the etiology and include:

- Headache
  - Typically sudden and severe from the outset in cases of tumor hemorrhage or aneurysm rupture
- Vomiting
- Seizures
- Syncope
- Confusion
- Aphasia
- Bradycardia and hypertension (Cushing's reflex secondary to increased intracranial pressure)
- Apnea
- Focal weakness
- Pupillary abnormalities
- Babinski sign
- Hyperreflexia
- Decorticate or decerebrate posturing
- Coma

Diagnostic Studies

If ICH is suspected on clinical grounds in the patient with any type of malignancy, brain imaging is indicated:

- Computed tomography
  - Non-contrast CT scan is very sensitive and specific for acute parenchymal or subarachnoid hemorrhage and is initial imaging test of choice in suspected acute ICH
    - Posterior fossa may be missed due to bone artifact
  - Mass effect, edema, herniation, and ventricular hemorrhage may be noted

- Magnetic resonance imaging
  - Not as useful for acute imaging due to prolonged image times and need for patient to lie still
  - However, if no prior history of brain tumor is evident, gadolinium enhancement is useful to assess for metastatic or primary tumor
  - Also useful to assess for multiple brain metastasis or leptomeningeal involvement
  - Magnetic resonance angiography can be performed simultaneously if neoplastic or mycotic aneurysm is suspected

TREATMENT

Treatment of ICH is based on whether the presentation is acute, as in solid tumor hemorrhage, or more gradual, as typically occurs with hematologic diseases and coagulopathies. Patients who present with acute hemorrhage into a metastatic focus are often critically ill with neurologic and cardiorespiratory compromise and require intensive care unit admission. Intubation for airway protection may be necessary to prevent aspiration. Severe hypertension is common in cases of tumoral ICH and may require parenteral infusion of labetalol or nitroprusside. Correction of thrombocytopenia and coagulopathy is indicated with platelet and fresh frozen plasma infusion, respectively. Protamine is indicated if ICH complicates heparin therapy. If evidence of elevated intracranial pressure is evident, corticosteroids, hyperventilation (which temporarily induces cerebral vasoconstriction), and mannitol should be considered along with urgent neurosurgical consultation. In cases of a rapidly expanding hematoma, craniotomy with evacuation should be considered; ventricular drainage may be needed if obstructive hydrocephalus is present. In the uncommon scenario of hyperleukocytosis, acute leukopheresis and administration of hydroxyurea are effective at acute leukoreduction and decreasing leukostasis effects. In the setting of TTP, plasmapheresis should be considered. Patients with ICH secondary to acute promyelocytic leukemia with DIC should be treated aggressively with fresh frozen plasma, cryoprecipitate, and platelets as necessary along with institution of retinoic acid and chemotherapy. If a neoplastic or mycotic aneurysm is present, consideration of arteriography with embolization can be considered depending on the specific cirucumstances.

PROGNOSIS

The prognosis for patients who develop an ICH in the setting of widespread metastatic carcinoma or melanoma is very poor, and is often a terminal event. Patients who survive initially have survival measured in times of weeks or months. Patients with choriocarcinoma, germ cell tumors, promyelocytic leukemia, or lymphoma may experience dramatic response to chemotherapy and have prolonged survival.

ADDITIONAL READING

Graus F, Rogers LR, Posner JB. Cerebrovascular complications in patients with cancer. *Medicine (Baltimore)* 1985;64:16–35.

Mandybur TI. Intracranial hemorrhage caused by metastatic tumors. *Neurology* 1977;27:650–655.

Quinn JA, DeAngelis LM. Neurologic emergencies in the cancer patient. *Semin Oncol* 2000;27:311–321.

Rogers LR. Cerebrovascular complications in cancer patients. *Neurol Clin N Am* 2003;21:167–192.

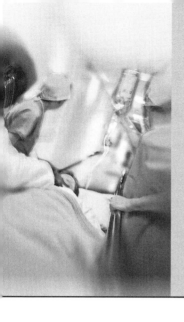

33

Status Epilepticus

DEFINITION

Status epilepticus (SE) is defined as continuous seizure activity lasting more than 30 minutes or two or more sequential seizures without full recovery of consciousness between the seizure episodes. Only tonic-clonic SE will be the focus of this section.

CLINICAL SETTING

There are numerous etiologies of seizures in the cancer population although in the majority of cases, SE occurs in patients with primary or metastatic brain tumors often in the setting of metabolic derangements or the use of narcotics or cytotoxic chemotherapy. Most patients have a known malignant disease, although SE can occasionally be the initial manifestation of cancer, especially in patients with primary brain tumors.

PATHOGENESIS

Untreated, SE is associated with significant morbidity and mortality due to not only neurologic injury, but also to various systemic effects that can result in dysfunction of many organ systems. Seizure development in cases of a brain mass lesion depends on tumor location, rate of growth, the number of lesions, and age. Tumor location is pivotal in influencing the risk of seizure generation and incidence is the highest with tumors located in the frontal, parietal, and temporal lobes and lowest in the occipital lobe. In addition, tumor involvement of the cortical gray matter increases risk. Slow-growing gliomas are more likely to present with seizures than a rapidly-growing glioblastoma. Overall, metastatic neoplasms are implicated in seizures more often than primary brain tumors due to their common occurrence. Metastatic tumors are more likely to present with seizures if there are multiple lesions or there is acute hemorrhage within the tumor. Nonstructural causes of seizures also can occur in the cancer patient and include metabolic derangements (e.g., hypoglycemia, hyponatremia), radiation therapy, chemotherapy, antibiotics, or opioids. Whatever the mechanism of seizure initiation, there is a risk for ongoing seizure activity and subsequent SE, although the risk may be higher in patients with a mass lesion rather than a reversible factor such as hypoglycemia.

Regardless of the cause of SE, the pathogenesis of cerebral and systemic injury is similar. Prolonged seizure activity creates an anaerobic and hypoxic environment within the brain and can lead to local cerebral hypoxia and subsequent permanent neurologic sequealea. Adverse cerebral effects of SE include increased intracranial pressure, cerebral vasodilatation, cerebral edema, and irreversible neuronal cell death. The systemic effects of untreated SE are also quite detrimental and primarily relate to metabolic acidosis resulting from lactate generation from prolonged muscle contraction. Prolonged muscle tonicity often results in myocyte injury with hyperthermia and rhabdomyolysis which can lead to acute renal failure as well as hyperkalemia and ventricular arrhythmias. Metabolic acidosis typically worsens hyperkalemia. Aspiration of gastric contents can result in acute acid-induced respiratory distress syndrome with hypoxic and hypercarbic and respiratory failure.

ETIOLOGY

Although tumors within the cerebral hemispheres are the most common cause of SE in the cancer patient, there are many other possible etiologies that need to be considered in the appropriate setting:

- Metastatic tumor
  - Lung, breast, renal cell, or germ cell carcinoma
  - Melanoma: more epileptogenic than other metastases
- Primary brain tumor
  - Low-grade glioma, oligodendroglioma, glioblastoma multiforme
  - Primary central nervous system lymphoma
- Metabolic derangements
  - Hyponatremia, hypocalcemia, hypomagnesemia
  - Hypoglycemia, hyperglycemia
  - Hypoxia
- Cerebral infarction or hemorrhage
- Radiation therapy: early or delayed
- Central nervous system infection
  - Herpes simplex encephalitis, bacterial meningitis, cerebral abscess

- Chemotherapy
  - L-asparaginase
  - 5-Fluorouracil
  - Busulfan
  - Chlorambucil
  - Ifosfamide
  - Cytarabine
  - Methotrexate
  - Interleukin-2
- Miscellaneous medications
  - Antibiotics: penicillins, imipenem, quinolones
  - Propoxyphene
    - Metabolized to neurotoxin, norpropoxyphene, which may induce seizures in the elderly
  - Meperidine
    - High risk in patients with impaired renal function due to accumulation of metabolite, normeperidine, which lowers seizure threshold. Meperidine should be used with caution in the cancer population
  - Antiemetics: ondansetron, haloperidol, phenothiazines

Symptoms and Signs

Seizure activity may be focal (if activity confined to one lobe) with persevered consciousness or generalized (if activity is bihemispheric) and produce impaired consciousness. Generalized seizures can present with tonic-clonic activity (a so-called "grand mal" seizure) or with an alert but disoriented, unresponsive state as occurs with complex-partial seizure activity. Status epilepticus associated with tonic-clonic seizures is relatively easy to diagnose, but identify more subtle cases of SE due to complex-partial seizures are more difficult to identify (non-convulsive SE). Common symptoms and signs of SE include:

- Impaired consciousness
- Prolonged tonic-clonic muscle movements
- Urinary incontinence
- Syncope
- Muscle rigidity
- Fever
- Tachycardia
- Apnea
- Abnormal reflexes
- Staring, lip-smacking, and automatisms with complex-parital SE

Diagnostic Studies

Since delay of treatment of tonic-clonic SE can result in significant morbidity and mortality, anti-seizure therapy must be commenced in conjunction with diagnostic studies if the cause is not readily apparent. However, useful studies in cases of SE of unclear etiology may include:

- Serum glucose
- Serum chemistries and electrolytes
- Pulse oximetry
- Arterial blood gas analysis
- Toxicology screen
- Computed tomography or magnetic resonance imaging
  - May reveal previously undetected mass lesion, hemorrhage, infarction, or evidence of herpes encephalitis
- Lumbar puncture
  - If CNS infection is suspected
- Electroencephalogram (EEG)
  - Helpful especially in cases of non-convulsive status epilepticus due to complex-partial seizures

TREATMENT

Acute treatment of SE hinges upon rapid airway protection, intravenous access, hemodynamic support, and correction of any reversible precipitating factor such as hypoglycemia. Treatment of SE should not wait until diagnostic studies are complete due to the increased risk of brain injury and organ dysfunction. The intial drug of choice for terminating SE is intravenous lorezepam; diazepam is also effective. Lorezepam is successful in terminating as many as 65% of cases of SE as documented in a recent study. Phenytoin or fosphenytoin are widely utilized to prevent ongoing seizures and are effective at terminating SE and should be given following benzodiazepines. If SE continues despite these measures, phenobarbitol may be successful. However, if SE remains unresponsive, consultation with a critical care neurologist for general anesthesia with propofol or barbiturate coma is indicated. Long-term therapy with an oral anti-epileptic agent is warranted in the absence of a reversible risk factor, and should be directed by a neurologist or oncologist with expertise in managing patients with brain neoplasia.

PROGNOSIS

Untreated, SE can prove fatal as a result of diffuse hypoxic cerebral injury, respiratory failure, or multiple organ dysfunction syndrome. If the patient responds readily to medical therapy and underlying precipitants are corrected, prognosis is heavily dependent on the status of the underlying malignancy. Patients with chemotherapy-resistant, widespread metastatic tumors with multiple brain metastases have a very poor prognosis.

ADDITIONAL READING

Quinn JA, DeAngelis LM. Neurologic emergencies in the cancer patient. *Semin Oncol* 2000;27:311–321.

Marinella MA. Non-convulsive status epilepticus. In: *Frequently Overlooked Diagnoses in Acute Care.* Philadelphia: Hanley and Belfus, 2003.

Sperling MR, Ko J. Seizures and brain tumors. *Semin Oncol* 2006;33:333–341.

Stein DA, Chamberlain MC. Evaluation and management of seizures in the patient with cancer. *Oncology* 1991;5:33–39.

Sul JK, DeAngelis LM. Neurologic complications of cancer chemotherapy. *Semin Oncol* 2006;33:332–342.

Trieman DM, Meyers PD, Walton NY, et al. A comparison of four treatments for generalized convulsive status epilepticus. *N Engl J Med* 1998;339:792–798.

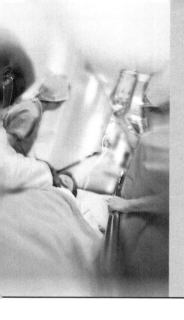

34

Cerebral Infarction and Stroke

DEFINITION

Cerebral infarction, or stroke, results when the brain parenchyma is deprived of oxygen via occlusion of any segment of the cerebral arterial circulation, which leads to ischemic necrosis and subsequent irreversible neurologic dysfunction.

CLINICAL SETTING

The cancer patient may suffer a stroke due to not only traditional risk factors but also due to unique effects of malignant disease and anti-cancer therapies; only these features will be discussed.

PATHOGENESIS

Occlusion of a major artery (e.g., carotid or middle cerebral artery) or smaller branch vessel with an *in situ* thrombus, embolic material, or extrinsic compression, rapidly leads to oxygen deprivation of brain parenchyma and subsequent irreversible neuronal cell death. Cerebral arterial thrombosis can occur within a normal blood vessel or upon a pre-existing plaque or area of endothelial injury. Prior radiation therapy to the neck area is known to accelerate atherosclerosis and increases the risk of subsequent stroke; intracranial vasculopathy can rarely complicate whole brain radiotherapy. Patients with various cancers, especially carcinomas, may develop a hypercoagulable state which can result in thrombotic arterial occlusion. Tumor cells from solid neoplasms as well as hematologic cancers can release myriad procoagulants that can induce arterial or venous thrombosis. Hypercoagulability is reported by most authors as the most common etiology of neoplasia-related cerebral infarction. Another mechanism of acute stroke in the patient with cancer is from an embolic source. Patients with cancer may suffer embolic stroke from a variety of sources including marantic or non-bacterial thrombotic endocarditis which consists of sterile fibrin-rich valvular vegetations in the setting of advanced adenocarcinomas and low-grade disseminated intravascular coagulation (DIC). Embolic stroke can also occur in the setting of a deep venous thrombosis that migrates through a patent foramen ovale or from a left ventricular thrombus in the setting of anthracycline cardiomyopathy. An uncommon, but potentially fatal and yet overlooked cause of embolic stroke, is venous air embolism which is discussed in detail in another chapter. Cardiac myxoma can occasionally present as acute embolic stroke.

Other pathogenic mechanisms of cerebral infarction in the cancer population include widespread thrombotic occlusion of small vessels which can occur in the setting of DIC, thrombotic thrombocytopenic purpura (TTP), or heparin-induced thrombocytopenia (HIT). Small vessel intravascular coagulation may occur with advanced breast cancer and is characterized by arteriolar thrombosis. Diffuse small vessel cerebral infarction can be caused by tumor emboli, paraneoplastic cerebral angiitis (usually related to Hodgkin's lymphoma), or intravascular lymphomatosis, a rare subtype of diffuse large cell lymphoma. Rarely, arterial compression by a primary brain tumor or metastatic focus can result in stroke. Chemotherapy can precipitate endothelial cell damage, induce vasospasm, or derange endogenous clotting factors, all of which can increase the risk of stroke. L-asparaginase is the most well-known etiology of cerebral venous or arterial thrombosis via depletion of endogenous anticoagulant proteins. Infection-related stroke can occur with angiotropic organisms such as *Aspergillus* species which cause direct vascular invasion and thrombosis. Rhinocerebral mucormycosis can occasionally invade cerebral arterioles and result in infarction. Finally, bacterial or fungal endocarditis can result in embolic stroke in the setting of prolonged neutropenia and acute leukemia.

ETIOLOGY

Most cases of cerebral infarction involving the cancer patient result from hypercoagulability with *in situ* thrombosis or embolic phenomena; however, other causes to be considered include:

- *In situ* large vessel thrombosis (e.g., internal carotid or middle cerebral artery)
  - Atherosclerosis
    - Accelerated by prior radiation to head and neck region
  - Hypercoagulable state secondary to adenocarcinoma or glioma
  - Arterial dissection
- Embolic source
  - Atrial fibrillation
  - Left ventricular thrombus in setting of anthracycline cardiomyopathy
  - Marantic endocarditis
  - Bacterial/fungal endocarditis
  - Left atrial myxoma

- ○ Venous air embolism
- ○ Tumor embolism
- ○ Bone marrow embolism
  - Can occur with metastatic tumor to marrow, bone marrow necrosis, sickle cell disease, or pathologic long-bone fracture
- Widespread small vessel intravascular thrombosis
  - ○ Often in setting of hypercoagulable state or thrombotic microangiopathy
    - DIC, TTP, HIT
- Extrinsic vascular compression
  - ○ Primary brain tumor, metastatic tumor, plasmacytoma
- Miscellaneous
  - ○ L-aparaginase, cisplatinum
  - ○ Cerebral angiitis/vasculitis
    - Hodgkin's lymphoma, carcinomas, fungal infections

SYMPTOMS AND SIGNS

The cancer patient who suffers from stroke due to large vessel occlusion or an embolic source presents in a manner similar to the non-cancer patient. However, given the numerous potential etiologies of stroke in the cancer population and the diverse pathogenesis, a variety of symptoms and signs may be present:

- Garbled speech
- Dysarthria
- Facial or extremity weakness
- Ataxia
- Visual complaints
- Parasthesia
- Focal neurologic signs (upper motor neuron in nature)
  - ○ Various cranial nerve findings
  - ○ Expressive or receptive aphasia
  - ○ Hemiparesis
  - ○ Hemiparasthesia
  - ○ Hyperreflexia
  - ○ Babinski sign present
  - ○ Cerebellar signs: ataxia, dysdiadokinesia

DIAGNOSTIC STUDIES

Cerebral infarction should be considered in the cancer patient who develops focal neurologic complaints or findings. Diagnostic studies most useful to diagnose stroke in this population include:

- Computed tomography (CT) of brain
  - ○ Non-contrast enchanced scan initial test of choice to exclude intracerebral hemorrhage
  - ○ Contrast enhancement may help delineate acute stroke from tumor mass

- Computed tomographic angiography (CTA) of neck and cerebral vasculature
  - Emerging method of assessing for arterial thrombosis, dissection, aneurysm formation, emboli, or extrinsic vascular compression from tumor mass
    - Use with caution in setting of renal disease or nephrotoxins
- Magnetic resonance imaging (MRI) of brain
  - Most sensitive imaging test to assess for mass lesion with gadolinium enhancement and acute focal or diffuse cerebral infarction via diffusion-weighted imaging
  - Use gadolinium with caution in setting of renal failure due to risk of nephrogenic fibrosing dermopathy
- Magnetic resonance angiography of neck and cerebral vasculature
  - Useful in conjuction with brain MRI to assess for arterial thrombosis, dissection, aneurysm formation, emboli, or extravascular compression due to tumor mass
- Carotid ultrasound
  - Non-invasive, rapid method to assess for carotid artery occlusion, thrombosis, or dissection
- Echocardiography
  - Useful to detect cardioembolic source of stroke with transesophageal method the preferred procedure due to high sensitivity and specificity
    - Atrial or ventricular thrombus, vegetations due to marantic or infectious endocarditis, patent foramen ovale
- Conventional angiography
  - Invasive and carries risk of stroke and arterial injury
  - May be most useful in cases of diffuse cerebral infarction of unclear etiology
    - Cerebral angiitis/vasculitis, multiple emboli, diffuse intravascular thrombosis, Moyamoya

TREATMENT

Treatment of the cancer patient with an acute stroke poses potential difficulties due to the risk of hemorrhage intrinsic to many malignancies, chemotherapy-related thrombocytopenia, brain metastasis, and limited life-expectancy of many patients. Generally, atherothrombotic stroke in the setting of atherosclerosis should be treated with aspirin and other vascular protective agents (e.g., statins, anti-hypertensives). Patients with atrial fibrillation, a left ventricular thrombus, or a patent foramen ovale and who have no contraindication to anticoagulation should receive warfarin. Patients with marantic endocarditis or DIC may benefit from anti-coagulation, but with risk of severe bleeding. Endocarditis should be treated with prolonged antibiotics, and in certain cases, valvular replacement if the patient can tolerate the procedure. Treatment of more obscure causes of stroke should be collaborated with a neurologist and hematologist/oncologist.

PROGNOSIS

Acute cerebral infarction in the cancer patient can have devastating consequences and is often fatal, especially in cases of middle-cerebral artery occlusion, bihemispheric involvement, or secondary hemorrhage within the infarct. The status of the underlying neoplasm and presence or absence of brain metastasis has major influence on long-term prognosis but, in general, patients with widespread carcinoma and brain metastasis may survive only days or weeks after a significant stroke.

ADDITIONAL READING

Blanchard DG, Ross RS, Dittrich HC. Nonbacterial thrombotic endocarditis. Assessment by transesophageal echocardiograpy. *Chest* 1992;102:954–956.

Chaturvedi S, Ansell J, Recht L. Should cerebral ischemic events in cancer patients be considered a manifestation of hypercoagulability? *Stroke* 1994;25:1215–1218.

Graus F, Rogers LR, Posner JB. Cerebrovascular complications in patients with cancer. *Medicine (Baltimore)* 1985;64:16–35.

O'Neill BP, Dinapoli RP, Ozazaki H. Cerebral infarction as a result of tumor emboli. *Cancer* 1987;60:90–95.

Rogers LR. Cerebrovascular complications in cancer patients. *Neurol Clin N Am* 2003;21:167–192.

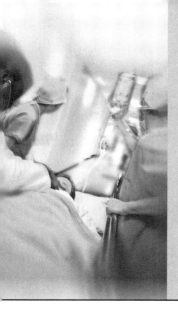

35

Reversible Posterior Leuko-encephalopathy Syndrome

DEFINITION

Reversible posterior leukoencephalopathy syndrome (RPLS) is a clinical-radiologic vascular leakage syndrome characterized by various neurologic symptoms with a predilection for involving the posterior cerebral circulation on diagnostic imaging studies.

CLINICAL SETTING

Although RPLS can occur in the general population, patients with cancer are at risk for development of RPLS in the setting chemotherapy administration, renal failure, and the post-operative state.

PATHOGENESIS

Since the first description of RPLS in 1996 in a group of patients with pre-eclampsia/eclampsia, organ transplantation, and hypertensive encephalopathy, the syndrome has been reported in the oncology population. Regardless of the underlying pathogenic etiology, clinical and radiographic findings of RPLS are similar in most patients, making the diagnosis primarily syndromic. Impaired cerebral autoregulation, especially of the posterior circulation, with vasospasm, breakdown of the blood brain barrier, and capillary leak are felt to be the precipitants of RPLS. Many patients reported in the literature had antecedent severe and uncontrolled hypertension especially those with pre-eclampsia, renal disease, or who were taking chronic anti-rejection medications for an orthotopic renal transplant. Cyclosporine is known to be directly toxic to endothelial cells and induces release of endothelin and thromboxane A2 and may contribute to the development of RPLS. However, cases of RPLS have emerged in the absence of severe hypertension suggesting that the pathogenesis for vascular dysfunction is not solely dependant upon elevated vascular pressures.

The white matter is primarily involved with RPLS and magnetic resonance imaging (MRI) classically reveals vasogenic edema manifested as T2 signal hyperintensity involving the bilateral occipital lobes. The parietal lobes, basal ganglia, brainstem, and cerebellar hemispheres can be involved in some patients. Reasons for RPLS having a predilection for involving the posterior circulation are unclear but may be related to decreased sympathetic innervation in this area rendering this vasculature very sensitive to acute changes in cerebral pressures and blood flow. Additionally, the endothelium in this vascular territory may be more prone to damage from various medications, including immunosuppressives, chemotherapeutic agents, and antineoplastic biologic agents. In any event, endothelial damage leads to breakdown of the blood brain barrier and transudation of plasma and erythrocytes into the surrounding brain tissues which results in acute neurologic dysfunction. Most patients experience clinical recovery with resolution of clinical findings and imaging abnormalities which supports the reversible nature of the vascular leak.

Etiology

The etiologies of RPLS in the cancer patient are expanding, especially with the introduction of newer chemotherapeutic and biologic agents. Some of the most common reported etiologies of RPLS within this population include:

- Severe, uncontrolled hypertension
- Pre-eclampsia/eclampsia
- General anesthesia in setting of cytotoxic drug use
- Acute renal failure
- Immunosuppressive agents
  - Cyclosporine, tacrolimus, interferon alfa
- Chemotherapy and anti-cancer agents
  - Bevacizumab
  - Cisplatinum
  - Cytarabine
  - Doxorubicin
  - Gemcitabine
  - Ifosfamide
  - Methotrexate
  - Oxaliplatin
  - Rituximab
  - Sorafenib

Symptoms and Signs

Onset of RPLS is usually sudden and should be considered in any cancer patient receiving chemotherapy, especially if severe hypertension is present. The most commonly reported clinical manifestations include:

- Headache
- Cortical blindness/visual disturbances
- Seizures
- Confusion
- Vomiting
- Somnulence
- Flat affect
- Hypertension
- Hemiparesis
- Hyperreflexia
- Asterixis

Diagnostic Studies

The diagnosis of RPLS should be suspected in any cancer patient who develops acute neurologic symptoms, especially seizures or visual changes. The most useful diagnostic studies include:

- Computed tomography (CT)
  - Hypodensities and edema in posterior parietal-occipital lobes or cerebellum, but of limited sensitivity
- Magnetic resonance imaging (MRI)
  - Imaging study of choice for RPLS
  - Typical findings include hyperintense white matter signal abnormalities involving the bilateral parieto-occipital regions; the cerebellum, basal ganglia, and frontal lobes can be involved on occasion
    - T2-weighted and fluid-attenuated inversion recovery (FLAIR) images most useful for diagnosis
  - The calcarine and paramedian occipital structures are usually spared, a useful finding that helps to distinguish RPLS from bilateral infarction of the posterior cerebral artery territory

Treatment

Treatment of RPLS is primarily supportive, with removal of any offending agent such as a chemotherapeutic drug. If severe hypertension is present, which can occur with bevacizumab, anti-hypertensive drug therapy should be considered, especially if evidence of encephalopathy exists. Some authors have administered anti-epileptic agents and corticosteroids.

PROGNOSIS

Most patients with RPLS recover without sequelae, although a few patients may suffer from residual neurologic changes. Follow-up MRI typically shows resolution of white matter changes within days to weeks, which typically correlates with clinical improvement.

ADDITIONAL READING

Allen JA, Adlakha A, Bergethon PR. Reversible posterior leukoencephalopathy syndrome after bevacizumab/FOLFIRI regimen for metastatic colon cancer. *Arch Neurol* 2006;63:1475–1478.

Hinchey J, Chaves C, Appignani B, et al. A reversible posterior leukoencephalopathy syndrome. *N Engl J Med* 1996;334:494–500.

Glusker P, Recht L, Lane B. Reversible posterior leukoencephalopathy syndrome and bevacizumab. *N Engl J Med* 2006;354:980–981.

Pinedo DM, Shah-Kahn F, Shah PC. Reversible posterior leukoencephalopathy syndrome associated with oxaliplatin. *J Clin Oncol* 2007;25:5320–5321.

Rajaskehar A, George TL. Gemcitabine-induced reversible posterior leukoencephalopathy syndrome: a case report and review of the literature. *Oncologist* 2007;12:1332–1335.

V

GENITOURINARY
AND
RENAL
COMPLICATIONS

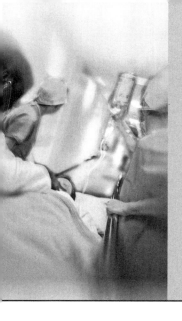

36

Acute Renal Failure

DEFINITION

Acute renal failure (ARF) is defined as an acute decline of the glomerular filtration rate (GFR) that occurs over a period of hours to days.

CLINICAL SETTING

The cancer population is prone to developing ARF in many clinical settings such as chemotherapy administration, vomiting and diarrhea-induced volume depletion, sepsis, and urinary tract obstruction.

PATHOGENESIS

A simplified approach to the pathogenic mechanisms of ARF is the classification into prerenal, intrinsic renal, and postrenal causes. Patients with cancer may develop ARF due to one of these mechanisms or a combination of them. A brief discussion of each pathogenic mechanism will be presented.

Prerenal ARF results from a decrease in the effective arterial circulating volume with subsequent decrease in renal blood flow. If the decrease is severe and prolonged, it leads to renal tubular ischemia. Common mechanisms of decreased renal perfusion in the cancer population include volume depletion due to vomiting or diarrhea, hypotension resulting from dehydration or sepsis, and third-spacing of intravascular volume in the setting of hypoalbuminemia or effusions. The renal tissue can remain viable through preserved perfusion via vascular autoregulation. Afferent arteriolar vasodilation via smooth muscle relaxation due to intrarenal release of nitric oxide and vasodilatory prostaglandins and efferent arteriolar vasoconstriction through angiotensin II maintain glomerular blood-flow unless mean arteriolar pressure remains <60 mmHg for prolonged periods. Non-steroidal drugs inhibit synthesis of vasodilatory prostaglandins and angiotensin-converting enzyme inhibitors inhibit vasconstrictive angiotensin II, both of which can precipitate ARF during prerenal conditions. Compensatory proximal tubular resorption of urinary sodium increases which reduces the amount available to the distal tubule.

Intrinsic ARF is quite common in this patient population and has numerous etiologies. Many of the etiologies are simultaneously present, thereby increasing the risk of renal damage. Intrinsic ARF most commonly results from damage to the renal tubular epithelium (acute tubular necrosis [ATN] but also may result from damage to the glomeruli (glomerulonephritis), interstitium (interstitial nephritis), or major renal vasculature. The most common cause of ARF in cancer patients is ATN which has numerous precipitants, but typically results from prolonged prerenal conditions, hypotension, or nephrotoxic drugs. Altered pre- and post-glomerular hemodynamics, as well as local free-radical generation, contribute to the development of ATN. The renal tubular cells respond to toxic or ischemic insults, with initial dysfunction manifesting as concentrating defects and sodium wasting. Eventually, necrosis of the tubule cells occurs with sloughing into the distal tubular system causing intraluminal micro-obstruction. Although many cases of ARF due to ATN are reversible, some patients develop permanent renal injury and require dialysis. This is especially likely to occur in conditions such as hepatorenal syndrome, vasculitis, glomerulonephritis, or severe multiple myeloma, in which many mechanisms may interplay. Although many chemotherapeutic agents can induce ARF, special mention will be made of cisplatinum nephrotoxicity. The kidneys are the main excretory organ for cisplatinum elimination and, in the presence of a low chloride environment, are prone to toxicity. After cisplatinum enters the tubular cell, hydroxyl radicals bind to nucleophilic sites on DNA and induce cell death via necrosis or apoptosis. Cisplatinum can also induce damage to the loop of Henle which causes renal magnesium and potassium wasting, even without overt ARF.

The final mechanism of ARF is the postrenal variety, which is quite common in patients with abdominal-pelvic malignancies. Obstruction of the ureters is common in patients with retroperitoneal or pelvic adenopathy, large tumor masses, or fibrosis from prior radiation or tumor. Occasionally, ARF can result from luminal obstruction within the ureters from blood clots, fungal masses, uric acid crystals in the setting of tumor lysis syndrome, or drug-related crystallization as in the case with high-dose methotrexate. Endogenous pigments can induce renal injury due to massive hemolysis or rhabdomyolysis. Bladder outlet obstruction is another mechanism of postrenal ARF and may result from invasive cervical, endometrial, or prostate carcinoma. Urethral strictures from prior urethral catheterization or radiation may be implicated in some cases. Whatever the mechanism, postrenal obstruction elevates the intratubular and intraglomerular pressures leading to the reversal of the driving force for glomerular filtration. Then, ARF ensues.

ETIOLOGY

Etiologies of ARF in the cancer patient are best categorized into prerenal, renal, and postrenal mechanisms:

- Prerenal ARF
  - Hypovolemia
    - Gastrointestinal loss
      - Vomiting
      - Diarrhea
      - Nasogastric suctioning
      - Fistulae
      - Drains
    - Renal loss
      - Polyuria due to hypercalcemia
      - Hyperglycemia
      - Mannitol
      - Diabetes insipidus
      - Diuretic therapy
      - Post-obstructive diuresis
    - Other losses
      - Sweating
      - Skin injury
      - Hyperventilation
      - Fever
  - Hypotension
    - Sepsis, volume depletion
  - Reduction of cardiac output
    - Doxorubicin cardiomyopathy (congestive heart failure)
    - Cardiac tamponade
    - Massive pulmonary embolism
  - Capillary leak syndromes
    - Interleukin-2, all-trans retinoic acid (ATRA) syndrome
  - Hepatorenal syndrome
    - Metastatic liver disease
    - Veno-occlusive disease
    - Hepatoma
    - Cirrhosis
  - Third-spacing of fluids
    - Ascites or edema
    - IL-2, ATRA syndrome
    - Hypoalbuminemia
    - Pancreatitis
    - Sepsis

- - - Liver disease
  - ○ Drugs
    - Non-steroidal anti-inflammatory drugs
    - Angiotensin converting enzyme inhibitors
    - Diuretics
- Renal ARF
  - ○ Tubular injury (ATN)
    - Hypotension/shock/sepsis of any cause
    - Dehydration/prolonged volume depletion
    - Hepatorenal syndrome (due to intense vasoconstriction)
    - Tumor lysis syndrome
    - Multiple myeloma/paraproteins
    - Hypercalcemia
    - Hemoglobinuria due to hemolysis
    - Myoglobinuria due to rhabdomyolysis
    - Intravenous contrast dye
    - Chemotherapeutic agents
      - — Cisplatinum
      - — Ifosfamide, cyclophosphamide
    - Miscellaneous agents
      - — NSAIDS
      - — Intravenous contrast
      - — Aminoglycosides
      - — Amphotercin B
      - — Vancomycin
      - — Intravenous immune globulin
  - ○ Glomerular injury
    - Paraneoplastic glomerulosclerosis or membranous nephropathy
      - — Solid tumors (lung, breast, colon, prostate, pancreas)
      - — Lymphomas
    - Proliferative glomerulonephritis
      - — Chronic lymphocytic leukemia, lymphoma, melanoma
      - — Cryoglobulinemia
      - — Solid tumors
    - Vasculitis or thrombotic microangiopathy
      - — Paraneoplastic phenomenon
      - — Mitomycin-C, cisplatinum, gemcitabine, cyclosporine
      - — Thrombotic thrombocytopenic purpura
    - Amyloidosis
  - ○ Interstitial injury (interstitial nephritis)

- Drugs (NSAIDS, beta-lactam antibiotics)
- Autoimmune/paraneoplastic
- Tumor or leukemic infiltration of interstitium
  - ○ Obstruction of main renal artery or vein
    - Renal artery embolism
      - — May complicate atrial fibrillation, marantic or infectious endocarditis, or left ventricular thrombus in setting of cardiomyopathy
    - Renal vein thrombosis: thrombotic or tumor
- Postrenal ARF
  - ○ Ureteral obstruction
    - Extrinsic: tumor mass, lymphadenopathy, fibrosis, hematoma, abscess
    - Intraluminal: uric acid crystals, methotrexate or acyclovir crystals, blood clot, fungus mass, myeloma proteins, papillary necrosis
  - ○ Bladder outlet obstruction
    - Prostate, cervical, uterine carcinoma
    - Radiation fibrosis
    - Blood clot/hemorrhagic cystitis
    - Neurogenic bladder

Symptoms and Signs

Since ARF typically develops over days to a few weeks, classic uremic symptoms are often absent and symptoms and signs are often attributable to the underlying illness. Nonetheless, ARF can cause the following:

- Nausea
- Vomiting
- Weakness
- Thirst
- Anorexia
- Confusion
- Polyuria
- Oliguria or anuria
  - ○ Anuria (<50 ml of urine per 24 hours) indicative of complete obstruction, bilateral cortical necrosis, rapidly progressive glomerulonephritis, or myeloma kidney with cast nephropathy
- Hematuria
- Hemoglobinuria/myoglobinuria
- Tachycardia
- Dry oral mucosa
- Absent axillary sweat
- Hypotension (in cases of prerenal states)

Diagnostic Studies

The diagnois of ARF hinges upon biochemical studies and select imaging studies which are interpreted in context of the clinical setting to narrow the differential diagnosis. The most useful studies include:

- Serum urea nitrogen and creatinine
  - Need to interpret serum creatinine in context of age, gender, and weight
  - High urea nitrogen: creatinine ratio supportive of prerenal ARF
  - Cockroft-Gault formula helpful, but not entirely accurate in acute setting for calculating glomerular filtration rate
- Serum electrolytes
  - Hyperkalemia, hyperphosphatemia, hypocalcemia may be present
  - Elevated anion gap common
- Urinalysis
  - Bland urine sediment in cases of postrenal ARF
  - Muddy brown casts classic finding in cases of ATN
  - Red blood cell casts or dysmorphic erythrocytes diagnostic of glomerulonephritis
  - Urine eosinophils indicative of interstitial nephritis
- Urine sodium
  - Urine sodium <20 mmol/L consistent with prerenal state; contrast induced ATN or pigment nephropathy on occasion associated with low urine sodium
  - Urine Na >40 mmol/L consistent with renal causes of ARF
- Calculation of the fractional excretion of sodium (FeNa)
  - FeNa <1%: prerenal ARF, contrast nephropathy, pigment nephropathy
  - FeNa >1% to 2%: intrinsic renal ARF
- Renal ultrasound
  - Useful to exclude features of urinary tract obstruction such as hydonephrosis or hydroureter
  - Small, hyperechoic kidneys suggest element of chronic renal failure

Treatment

Treatment of the cancer patient with ARF is often challenging due to co-existing etiologies, as well as the need for ongoing anticancer therapy. Discontinuation of precipitating drugs or toxins is important. Also important is rapid exclusion of obstructive uropathy which can often be treated with local decompressive therapy such as urethral catheterization, percutaneous nephrostomy, or ureteral stents. It is very important to provide adequate intravascular volume with crystalloids, correct hyperkalemia, provide nutrition, and treat infection. Dopamine is not effective at preventing or reversing ARF. Indications for renal replacement therapy, such as hemodialysis or continuous renal replacement therapy, include refractory volume overload, severe hyperkalemia, and metabolic acidosis. It is important to avoid nephrotoxins and to adjust the dosage of renally-eliminated drugs.

Prognosis

The prognosis of ARF in the cancer patient depends on the etiology of ARF, the presence of infection or sepsis, and the status of the underlying malignancy. Patients with septic shock and multiple organ dysfunction syndrome have a very poor prognosis. On the contrary, patients with recent onset bladder outlet obstruction may have a favorable prognosis with relief of the obstruction. In a patient with an otherwise incurable or terminal malignancy, allowing the renal failure to progress to uremia may afford the patient a peaceful death.

Additional Reading

Damron M, Ciroldi M, Thiery G, et al. Clinical review: specific aspects of acute renal failure in cancer patients. *Crit Care* 2006;10:211.

Kapoor M, Chan GZ. Malignancy and renal disease. *Crit Care Clin* 2001;17:571–597.

Lameire NH, Flombaum CD, Moreau D, et al. Acute renal failure in cancer patients. *Ann Med* 2005;37;13–25.

Lugones F, Leblanc M. Acute renal failure in cancer patients. In: *Cancer and the Kidney.* Cohen EP, ed. Oxford: Oxford University Press, 2005, pp. 55–91.

Meyer TW, Hostetter TH. Uremia. *N Engl J Med* 2007;357:1316–1325.

Monfardini S. Evaluation of renal function in elderly cancer patients. *Ann Oncol* 2004;15:183–184.

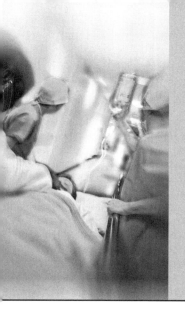

37

Obstructive Uropathy

DEFINITION

Obstructive uropathy (OU) results from obstruction of urine flow from anywhere along the urinary collecting system—typically the renal pelvis to the urethra—and is a common cause of morbidity in the cancer population.

CLINICAL SETTING

Malignancy-associated OU typically occurs in patients with advanced solid tumors involving the abdominopelvic region.

PATHOGENESIS

Obstruction of the urinary collecting system is typically a foreboding sign in the cancer patient. It often occurs in the setting of advanced malignancy, typically following anticancer therapies such as surgery, radiation, and chemotherapy. Most cases of OU occur slowly and result from tumor growth, lymphadenopathy, or radiation-induced fibrosis involving the ureters or bladder outlet. Seventy percent of cases of solid tumor-related OU result from carcinoma of the cervix, bladder, and prostate and cause obstruction by direct tumor encasement of the collecting system. Although uncommon, renal or urothelial cancers can invade the ureteral pelvis causing unilateral OU. Three anatomic regions are quite susceptible to OU. They are the ureteropelvic junction, the area where the ureters cross over the iliac vasculature at the pelvic inlet, and the ureterovesical junction. Ureteral obstruction can occur in cases of intrarenal hemorrhage which can result in an intraluminal blood clot occluding urine flow, in a manner similar to a renal stone. Renal parenchymal infections with fungal organisms can shed fungus balls and also precipitate acute ureteral obstruction. Massive tumor lysis can result in supersaturation of the urine with uric acid, resulting in crystalline obstruction of the ureters.

Whatever the cause of OU, intraluminal pressure within the collecting system increases closer to the obstruction site. As the pressure rises, ureteral peristalsis is reversed and eventually hydroureter and hydronephrosis ensue. This increased intraluminal hydrostatic pressure is transmitted to Bowman's space causing a decline in the glomerular filtration rate. Local release of angiotensin II and thromboxanes may cause renal vasoconstriction contributing to further renal injury. Another element of OU-induced renal failure results from the release of inflammatory mediators and cytokines. Urine stasis predisposes to infection and sepsis and can further augment the renal damage in cases of OU.

Following relief of OU via medical or surgical intervention, a peculiar pathogenic process known as post-obstructive diuresis commonly occurs. There are three mechanisms of this phenomenon, which can lead to significant volume depletion and electrolyte depletion. First, with prolonged obstruction, urea and other endogenous osmotic molecules are retained. If the OU is relieved, these agents induce an osmotic diuresis with ensuing electrolyte loss. This urea-diuresis often resolves within 48 hours with rapid decline in the blood urea nitrogen (BUN) level. Another mechanism of post-obstructive diuresis is sodium diuresis which results from excretion of UO-retained sodium and water. Although volume depletion can occur, this phase usually dissipates within 72 hours. The third mechanism of post-OU diuresis is water diuresis, which results from an acquired nephrogenic diabetes insipidus due to nephron response to antidiuretic hormone (ADH). This phase of diuresis may last for weeks and often requires specific intervention to avoid excess free-water loss and hypernatremia.

ETIOLOGY

The etiologies of OU can be approached clinically based on anatomic areas:

- Renal pelvis obstruction
  - Urothelial carcinoma
  - Renal cell carcinoma
  - Blood clot
  - Fungus ball
- Ureteral obstruction
  - Pelvic malignancies
    - Prostate, cervix, bladder, ovary
  - Metastatic solid tumors
    - Colorectal, breast, gastric
  - Lymphoma/retroperitoneal lymphadenopathy
  - Retroperitoneal sarcoma
  - Retroperitoneal fibrosis
    - Radiation, chemotherapy, surgery
- Bladder outlet obstruction

- Prostate cancer
- Bladder cancer
- Cervical cancer
- Endometrial cancer
- Blood clot (hemorrhagic cystitis)
- Fungus ball
- Urolithiasis
- Urethral obstruction
  - Stricture (radiation, frequent catheterization)
  - Urethral carcinoma
  - Penile carcinoma
  - Priapism

Symptoms and Signs

Most cases of OU occur in patients with advanced solid tumors. Many of the symptoms these patients experience are related to their underlying cancer. However, UO can induce various clinical findings, especially if bilateral ureteral obstuction is present. Some examples are

- Fatigue
- Anorexia
- Weight loss
- Dysguesia
- Pelvic or flank pain
  - In cases of acute ureteral obstruction, such as blood clot, fungus ball, nephrolithiasis, crystalline obstruction from uric acid, or papillary necrosis
- Polyuria
  - May occur with subacute obstruction due to an acquired tubular concentrating defect
- Anuria, if bilateral ureteral or urethral obstruction present
- Hematuria
  - May indicate primary renal or urothelial neoplasm
  - Significant bladder distention resulting from outlet obstruction often causes bladder mucosal ischemia and gross hematuria
- Hesitancy, dysuria, frequency
  - Typical of urethral obstruction
- Fever and chills, if urine infection is present
- Hypotension, if urine infection is present
- Palpable renal mass or swollen kidney, if significant hydronephrosis
- Flank tenderness
- Enlarged prostate
- Rectal mass or palpable mass in rectouterine pouch ("Blumer's shelf")
  - Indicative of metastatic pelvic malignancy
- Tympanitic, tender bladder if bladder outlet obstruction present

DIAGNOSTIC STUDIES

Obstructive uropathy should be considered in any cancer patient with predisposing factors who develops renal failure. As outlined in the chapter on acute renal failure, biochemical studies are abnormal and lead to further diagnostic evaluation, which should include:

- Bilateral renal ultrasonography
  - Non-invasive imaging study of choice to detect hydronephrosis, hydrourepter, bladder distention, or mass lesions compressing the collecting system
- Computed tomography of the abdomen and pelvis
  - Provides anatomic detail of the kidney, ureters, bladder, and surrounding retroperitoneal tissues and lymph node basins for compressive etiologies
  - Intravenous contrast must be used with caution (if at all) to avoid further renal damage
- Intravenous pyelogram (IVP)
  - Provides excellent detail of the entire anatomy of the collecting system from the renal calyces to the bladder
  - Use with caution with serum creatinine >1.5 mg/dl
- Radionuclide scan
  - Nuclear medicine study in which venous administration of radiotracer is used to assess functional contribution of each kidney
  - In patients with hydronephrosis, a delayed excretion of tracer is consistent with anatomic obstruction, whereas prompt excretion of tracer is consistent with a functional dilatation of the collecting system
- Retrograde pyelogram
  - Invasive study in which contrast is injected with ureteral orifices to detect intraluminal obstruction, strictures, or extrinsic compression
- Cystoscopy
  - Invasive procedure which allows visualization of lower urinary tract, as well as retrograde pyelography or stent insertion that can be performed with diagnostic procedure

TREATMENT

Treatment of OU in the cancer patient often involves a concerted effort between the oncologist, urologist, and interventional radiologist. Perhaps the first intervention in a patient with suspected OU is insertion of a Foley catheter to relieve potential bladder outlet or urethral obstruction. Correction of fluid and electrolyte derangements from post-obstructive diuresis and treatment of infection is mandatory. Indeed, infected urine in the presence of obstruction at any level may lead to septic shock. Since ureteral obstruction is a very common cause of OU in the solid tumor patient, restoring flow within the ureters in an expedient fashion is paramount. If the patient can tolerate anesthesia, cystoscopic insertion of ureteral stents is an effective and safe way to relieve obstruction. Another option that may be useful is percutaneous placement of nephrostomy tubes under fluoroscopic guidance. However, patients who undergo either procedure are at risk for tube or stent occlusion and infection, which can be fatal. External beam radiation or chemotherapy in attempt to shrink the tumor mass could be considered in treatment-sensitive neoplasms such as lymphoma, germ cell tumors, or small cell carcinoma. The clinician should also consider the patient's underlying disease status. Patients with terminal cancer and poor performance status may not be best served by an invasive procedure in their remaining time.

PROGNOSIS

Malignant OU is generally a pre-terminal event in patients with advanced solid cancers. In patients with advanced cancer who undergo percutaneous or cytoscopic stent insertion to relieve OU, some authors have noted an average survival time of only 5 months, 50% of which was spent in the hospital.

ADDITIONAL READING

Donat SM, Russo P. Ureteral decompression in advanced nonurologic malignancies. *Ann Surg Oncol* 1996;3:393–399.

Harding JR. Percutaneous antegrade ureteric stent insertion in malignant disease. *J Royal Soc Med* 1993;86:511–513.

Philipneri M, Bastani B. Urinary tract obstruction in cancer patients. In: *Cancer and the Kidney.* Cohen EP, ed. Oxford: Oxford University Press, 2005, pp. 181–199.

Russo P. Urologic emergencies in the cancer patient. *Semin Oncol* 2000;27:284–298.

Shekarriz B, Shekarriz H, Upadhyay J, et al. Outcome of palliative urinary diversion in the treament of advanced malignancies. *Cancer* 1999;85:998–1003.

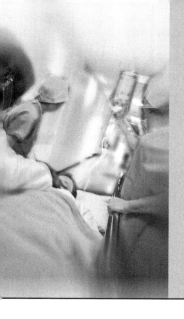

38

Hemorrhagic Cystitis

DEFINITION

Hemorrhagic cystitis (HC) consists of bladder mucosal inflammation and ulceration resulting in gross hematuria and intravesical clot formation.

CLINICAL SETTING

Administration of certain chemotherapeutic agents, such as cyclophosphamide, and infection with urotropic viruses comprise the most common settings in which HC occurs.

PATHOGENESIS

The major causes of HC in cancer patients include chemotherapy, radiation injury, and viral infections of the bladder mucosa, especially in bone marrow transplant and immunosuppressed patients. The most well-known chemotherapeutic agents causing HC are cyclophosphamide and ifosfamide, especially when administered in high doses for lymphoma or bone marrow transplantation. Cyclophosphamide and ifosfamide are hepatically metabolized into their active metabolite, phosphoramide mustard, and the urotoxic substance, acrolein. Acrolein induces hemorrhagic inflammation of the urothelium which can result in severe hemorrhage and clot retention. Radiation therapy for genitourinary, bowel, or pelvic tumors can occasionally result in telangectasias of the bladder mucosa, which can rupture and lead to hemorrhage. Infections with the cytopathic viruses adenovirus, polyomavirus, or cytomegalovirus can lead to hemorrhagic cystitis in patients with hematologic malignancies or recent hematopoietic stem cell transplantation. Thrombocytopenia and coagulopathy may augment HC resulting in massive bleeding and hemorrhagic shock. Bladder outlet obstruction from an organized clot may induce acute urinary retention, anuria, and severe pain.

ETIOLOGY

The most common etiologies of HC in the cancer population include:

- Chemotherapy
  - Cylcophosphamide
  - Ifosfamide
  - Busulfan
- Radiation therapy
- Viral infections
  - Polyoma BK virus
  - Adenovirus
  - Cytomegalovirus
- Graft versus host disease

SYMPTOMS AND SIGNS

Hemorrhagic cystitis should be considered in any patient with risk factors who present with the following:

- Hematuria
- Passage of blood clots
- Dysuria
- Frequency
- Pelvic pain
- Bladder distention

DIAGNOSTIC STUDIES

Diagnosis of HC is mainly clinical and should be suspected if irritative voiding symptoms and hematuria occur in patients with underlying risk factors. However, useful ancillary tests include:

- Urinalysis
  - Reveals hematuria and pyuria
- Complete blood count
  - Anemia is common with significant bleeding
- Renal and pelvic ultrasound
  - Usually normal but may reveal bladder distention or echogenic clot within the bladder

TREATMENT

Treatment of HC involves maintaining urine flow in order to prevent bladder outlet obstruction due to clot retention. Placement of a large-diameter, multi-lumen urethral catheter into the bladder with continuous saline irrigation is important to flush out clots and prevent further clot formation. If severe hematuria persists or irrigation fails to evacuate intravesical clots, cystoscopic clot extraction is necessary. Although correction of thrombocytopenia and coagulopathy is important, diffuse bladder hemorrhage often requires intravesical instillation of a local hemostatic-coagulative agent such as alum or formalin under the guidance of a urologist. Hyperbaric oxygen therapy has been utilized with success in patients with severe HC due to radiation. Life-threatening HC may be halted with transarterial embolization of the vesical arteries. Refractory cases may require urgent cystectomy with permanent diversion, but this carries a substantial morbidity in the cancer population. Recent reports demonstrate the effectiveness of recombinant factor VIIa in cases of treatment-refractory HC, and may spare the need for invasive or surgical procedures.

PROGNOSIS

Patients with chemotherapy-induced HC often have a favorable prognosis with supportive care and aggressive hydration and use of Mesna with subsequent cycles of cyclophosphamide and ifosfamide. Exsanguination causing hemodynamic instability in patients with severe immunosuppression or advanced cancer have a poor prognosis.

ADDITIONAL READING

El-Zimaity M, Saliba R, Chan K, et al. Hemorrhagic cystitis after allogeneic hematopoietic stem cell transplantation: donor type matters. *Blood* 2004; 103:4674–4680.

Leung AYH, Lie AKW, Yuen KY, et al. Clinicopathological features and risk factors of clinically overt haemorrhagic cystitis complicating bone marrow transplantation. *Bone Marrow Transplant* 2002;29:509–513.

Mackie S, Lam T, Rai B, et al. Management of urological hemorrhage and the role of transarterial embolization. *Minerva Med* 2007;98:511–524.

Russo P. Urologic emergencies in the cancer patient. *Semin Oncol* 2000;27:284–298.

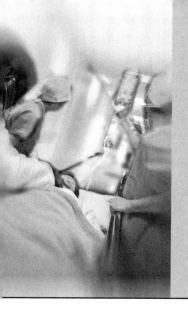

39
Priapism

DEFINTION

Priapism is a persistant, prolonged, and often painful erection that occurs in the absence of sexual stimulation.

CLINCAL SETTING

Priapism in the cancer patient typically occurs in the setting of untreated myeloproliferative disorders or metastatic genitourinary cancers to the penis.

PATHOGENESIS

The penis is composed of two dorsal corpus cavernosa and a single ventral corpus spongiosum. The cavernosa, however, are covered by the rigid tunica albuginea and derive arterial blood flow from the internal pudendal artery. Increased flow into the penis is drained by veins within the corpus cavernosa. When engorged against the tunica albuginea in the setting of hyperviscosity or low-flow, the blood becomes trapped within the cavernosa resulting in priapism. Although only cancer-related priapism will be discussed in this section, a brief pathogenesis of both pathogenic subtypes—so-called high-flow and low-flow priapism—will be discussed. High-flow priapism almost exclusively occurs in the setting of perineal, or straddle-type trauma, whereby laceration of a cavernous artery creates an arteriovenous shunt into the cavernosal bodies resulting in increased arterial inflow. Priapism in the oncology setting is of the low-flow, or ischemic type, in which there is static or absent corporal blood flow, leading to an ischemic and acidotic environment. Typical blood gas analysis of the corpus cavernosa reveals a low pH, low PO_2, and high PCO_2. Any process that diminishes or halts venous outflow from the corpus cavernosa greater than 24 hours can lead to ischemia and infarction of penile tissue. Damage to the cavernosal endothelium and formation of thrombi contributes to ischemic fibrosis and permanent damage to the corpora, thereby inhibiting future erectile function. Predisposing factors inducing sluggish corporal blood flow in the cancer patient include hyperviscosity from paraproteinemia or myeloproliferative disorders, hyperleukocytosis, and hypercoagulable states. All of these induce stasis-related clot formation. Patients with extremely elevated leukocyte counts associated with myeloid leukemias are prone to low-flow priapism. A metastatic deposit within the penile shaft can result in venous compression and priapism resulting from tumor cell infiltration of the corpora or tumor emboli within the vessels.

ETIOLOGY

Patients with solid tumors or hematologic disorders may develop priapism related to their underlying disease or treatment:

- Hyperviscosity syndromes
  - Chronic myelogenous leukemia (CML)
    - Associated with leukocyte counts over 100,000 cells/mm^3 with ensuing leukostasis
  - Polycythemia vera
  - Multiple myeloma
- Amyloidosis
- Sickle cell anemia
- Hypercoagulable states
  - Protein C and S deficiencies, antiphospholipid antibody syndrome, cancer
- Cauda equina syndrome due to spine metastasis
- Brainstem metastasis
- Metastatic tumors to penis
  - Prostate cancer (most common)
  - Bladder cancer
  - Renal cell carcinoma
  - Germ cell tumors
  - Colorectal cancer
  - Lung cancer
- Medications
  - Trazodone
  - Phenothiazines
  - Resperidol
  - Androgens
  - Vancomycin

SYMPTOMS AND SIGNS

Priapism is a relatively easy clinical diagnosis characterized by prolonged (>20 minutes), spontaneous erection. Common clinical findings of priapism in the cancer population include:

- Painful rigid penis
- Anxiety
- Rigidness and swelling of corpus cavernosa
- Softness of glans penis and corpus spongiosum
- Penile nodules if metastasis present

DIAGNOSTIC STUDIES

A basic evaluation in a cancer patient with priapism may include the following:

- Penile ultrasound with Doppler
  - Very sensitive and specific to identify poor venous flow and thrombosis within corpus cavernosa
- Complete blood count
  - Leukocytosis with immature myeloid cells suggests chronic myelogenous leukemia
  - Thrombocytosis suggestive of essential thrombocytosis
  - Erythrocytosis suggestive of polycythemia vera
- Serum viscosity
  - Increased relative to water viscosity in setting of hyperleukocytosis or significant paraproteinemia
- Serum protein electrophoresis
  - If myeloma is suspected
- Hemoglobin electrophoresis, if patient black or Mediterranean
- Computed tomography of the spine or pelvis
  - Some cases of metastasis to sacral spine or area of pelvic vasculature and nerves may induce priapism
  - Prostate, bladder, and renal cell cancers are the most frequent etiologies of malignant priapism and may be identified
- Blood gas analysis of corpus cavernosa aspiration
  - Reveals acidosis, hypercarbia, hypoxia which is indicative of low-flow priapism
- Core needle biopsy of penile shaft
  - Indicated in cases of metastatic disease to penis

TREATMENT

Low-flow priapism is a medical emergency and treatment should not be delayed while awaiting diagnostic studies. Immediate treatment is indicated not only to relieve the severe pain, but also to decrease the risk of permanent ischemic damage to the penis, which may result in permanent deformity and impotence. The most widely recommended procedure is needle aspiration of the corpus cavernosa in order to decrease intra-corporal pressure to enhance spontaneous venous outflow and improve the local acidotic and hypoxic environment. Local injection of a vasoconstrictor such as phenylephrine is frequently successful in achieving detumescence. Refractory cases may require arterial embolization of the pudendal vessels or surgical shunting. Penile metastasis may be treated with radiation therapy or chemotherapy; penectomy may be necessary if refractory priapism is present. Hyperleukocytosis associated with CML requires leukophereis and hydroxyurea for rapid cytoreduction. Patients with sickle cell anemia often respond to hydration, oxygen supplementation, analgesia, and exchange transfusion.

PROGNOSIS

Patients treated within 12 hours of onset of priapism typically regain normal erectile function and suffer no significant sequelae. However, priapism lasting greater than 24-48 hours may result in permanent penile deformity, impotence, and pain. Overall prognosis depends upon the underlying disease and is very favorable in cases of CML treated with imatinib. Metastasis to the penile shaft typically indicates widespread metastatic disease with survival times varying depending on the primary cancer. Some authors indicate a mean survival of 4 months.

ADDITIONAL READING

Chan PTK, Begin LR, Arnold D, et al. Priapism secondary to penile metastasis: a report of two cases and a review of the literature. *J Surg Oncol* 1998;68:51–59.

Czachor JS. Vancomycin and priapism. *N Engl J Med* 1998;338:1701.

Manuel MB, Leak A, Carroll SA. Priapism in the oncology setting. *Clin J Oncol Nurs* 2007;11:23–25.

Ponniah A, Brown CT, Taylor P. Priapism secondary to leukemia: effective management with prompt leukapheresis. *Int J Urol* 2004;11:809–810.

Russo P. Urologic emergencies in the cancer patient. *Semin Oncol* 2000;27:284–298.

Sadeghi-Nejad H, Dogra V, Seftel AD, et al. Priapism. *Radiol Clin N Am* 2004; 42:427–443.

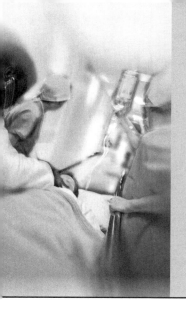

40

Fournier's Gangrene

DEFINITION

Fournier's gangrene (FG) is a life-threatening form of necrotizing fasciitis involving the scrotum, perineum, or abdominal wall resulting in rapidly progressive necrotic tissue loss and sepsis.

CLINICAL SETTING

While FG typically affects patients with poorly controlled diabetes mellitus, patients with malignant disease or acquired immunodeficiency due to cancer treatments are at increased risk for this infection.

PATHOGENESIS

Predisposing factors for FG, include not only poorly controlled diabetes mellitus, but also malignancy, leukemia, chemotherapy, and local tissue trauma. Although FG can occur in the female perineum and genital area, most cases occur in older males with poorly controlled diabetes mellitus and other co-morbidities. This form of necrotizing fasciitis may involve not only the scrotum, but also spread rapidly through the perineum, penis, abdominal wall, and even into the lower extremities. The initial focus of bacterial invasion occurs in the setting of local mucosal or epithelial trauma and may involve the penis, scrotum, perineum, anal area, or the colorectum. Local infection may initially begin as a cellulitic process, perianal abscess, or a colorectal phlegmon/abscess that subsequently tracks through the surrounding tissue. Anaerobes are the predominant organisms involved and include *Clostridia, Bacteroides*, peptostreptococci, *Fusobacterium*, and other microaerophilic streptococcal species. The presence of anaerobes is suggested by the foul-smelling nature of exudates as well as clinical evidence of crepitus and radiographic gas in the perineal soft tissues. Streptococcal species can release exotoxins resulting in toxic shock syndrome and multiple organ dysfunction syndrome (MODS). Facultative anaerobes such as *Klebsiella, E. coli*, and enterococci are also common co-pathogens. A central component of the pathogenesis of FG is the development of synergistic anaerobic bacterial growth in the setting of local tissue hypoxia. Tissue necrosis results from necrotizing inflammation of the subcutaneous tissue and fascia with vascular damage and thrombosis. Histologic findings of FG include vascular thrombosis, subcutaneous fat necrosis, intense neutrophil infiltration, endarteritis, and tissue hemorrhage. Clinical hallmarks of FG include rapid progression of tissue inflammation, severe pain which is often out of proportion to clinical findings, and severe systemic toxicity. The rapid tissue spread results from liberation of bacterial enzymes such as hyaluronidase, streptokinase, and collagenases. Activation of tissue factor potentiates vascular thrombosis and dermal necrosis. Anaerobic organisms may liberate hydrogen and nitrogen which accounts for crepitus and the presence of soft tissue air noted on radiography. Impaired neutrophil chemotaxis resulting from hyperglycemia and neutropenia secondary to hematologic malignancy or chemotherapy are contributing pathogenic mechanisms. The development of systemic inflammatory response syndrome (SIRS) and septic shock results from a cytokine storm with release of interleukins and tumor necrosis factor.

ETIOLOGY

The etiologies and predisposing factors associated with the development of FG in the cancer patient include:

- Diabetes mellitus
  - Often poorly controlled, secondary to corticosteroid use for a variety of oncologic disorders
- Malnutrition
- Alcoholism
- Perirectal abscess
  - May complicate neutropenia during chemotherapy for acute leukemia
- Indwelling urethral catheter trauma
- Urinary tract infection
- Surgical procedures
  - Prostate biopsy
- Perforated colorectal carcinoma
- Acute leukemia (lymphoid and myeloid)
- Chemotherapeutic drugs
- Corticosteroids

Symptoms and Signs

The diagnosis of FG requires a high index of suspicion and should be considered in a male (or rarely female) cancer patient with any of the following:

- Scrotal or perineal pain
- Fever
- Parasthesia or numbness of scrotum
- Tachycardia
- Scrotal swelling
- Erythema and/or ecchymosis of scrotum and perineum
- Crepitus
- Foul-smelling discharge
- Cutaneous necrosis
- Anesthesia of involved skin

Diagnostic Studies

Although the diagnosis of FG can often be made clinically in patients with underlying risk factors, the following diagnostic studies aid in assessing the anatomic degree of involvement as well as providing information regarding overall systemic illness:

- Scrotal ultrasound
  - Rapid and easy to perform at bedside
  - May reveal soft tissue gas, scrotal edema or fluid collection, or altered blood flow on Doppler examination
- Computed tomography of abdomen and pelvis
  - Very sensitive, imaging modality of choice
  - Typically reveals scrotal edema, scrotal effusion, gas within soft tissues, and soft tissue stranding
  - Also helpful in identifying possible focus of FG such as diverticulitis, perforated colorectal cancer, or pelvic area abscess
- Serum chemistries
  - Hyperglycemia, elevated creatinine phosphokinase, evidence of renal failure
- Complete blood count
  - Leukocytosis, thrombocytopenia, anemia
- Blood cultures
- Chest radiograph
  - May reveal evidence of acute respiratory distress syndrome (ARDS)

Treatment

Treatment of FG requires a high index of suspicion and rapid surgical consultation. Patients with FG are often systemically ill and may require admission to an intensive care unit for vasopressors, and occasionally, mechanical ventilation. The cornerstones of management include aggressive surgical debridement of all necrotic tissue and broad-spectrum antibiotics. Some patients may require a suprapubic cystostomy or a diverting colostomy to keep the involved area away from the fecal and urinary stream. Orchiectomy may be required if testicular involvement is present. Antibiotic agents should cover gram-negative bacilli, anaerobes, as well as gram-positive organisms. Patients with acute leukemia have a significant propensity for *Pseudomonas aeruginosa* infection and should be administered agents active against this organism. Meticulous glucose control, post-operative wound care, and nutrition support are mandatory. Some authors recommend hyperbaric oxygen therapy in patients who do not respond to the above measures. Patients with leukemia are difficult to treat due to the universal cytopenias but may be considered for growth factor support.

PROGNOSIS

The prognosis of FG is quite poor with mortality rates of 15% to 50% in various studies. Elderly patients with poorly controlled diabetes and multiple co-morbidities have an especially poor prognosis and often require multiple surgeries and prolonged hospital stays. Patients with active malignancy who are receiving chemotherapy have a dismal prognosis if vasopressors or mechanical ventilation are required.

ADDITIONAL READING

Ash L, Hale J. CT findings of perforated rectal carcinoma presenting as Fournier's gangrene in the emergency department. *Emerg Radiol* 2005;11:295–297.

Brandt MM, Corpron CA, Wahl WL. Necrotizing soft tissue infections: a surgical disease. *Am Surg* 2000;66:967–970.

Chapnick EK, Abter E. Necrotizing soft tissue infections. *Infect Dis Clin N Am* 1996;10:835–842.

Marinella MA. Necrotizing fasciitis. In: *Frequently Overlooked Diagnoses in Acute Care.* Philadelphia: Hanley and Belfus, 2003, pp. 69–73.

Tahmaz L, Erdemir F, Kibar Y, et al. Fournier's gangrene: report of thirty-three cases and a review of the literature. *Int J Urol* 2006;13:960–967.

VI

ENDOCRINE AND METABOLIC COMPLICATIONS

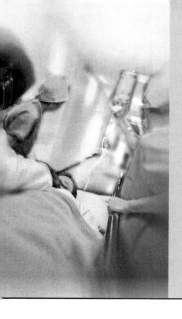

41

Acute Adrenal Insufficiency

DEFINITION

Acute adrenal insufficiency (AAI), or Addisonian crisis, is a life-threatening manifestation of adrenal failure that presents with refractory hypotension or shock.

CLINICAL SETTING

Acute adrenal insufficiency in the cancer patient typically occurs in the setting of widely metastatic malignancy with bilateral adrenal involvement, although certain anticancer agents and infections are occasionally implicated.

PATHOGENESIS

The majority of cancer patients who develop AAI have underlying adrenal dysfunction often associated with non-specific symptoms that may be attributed to cancer or treatment. The majority of cases involve destruction or replacement of the adrenal parenchyma, which will be the focus of this discussion. Typically, more than 90% of the adrenal gland cortex must be lost before symptoms of chronic adrenal failure are manifest. Most cases of AAI complicate subclinical and undiagnosed hypoadrenalism but some patients may present with refractory shock as an initial manifestation of adrenal dysfunction. The adrenal cortex synthesizes cortisol and mineralocorticoids which are vital to various metabolic reactions and hemodynamic stability, respectively. The hypothalamus releases adrenocorticotropic hormone (ACTH) which stimulates the adrenal cortex to produce hormones, notably cortisol. Cortisol is an important hormone for carbohydrate and protein metabolism and regulates central release of ACTH and vasopressin via negative feedback inhibition. If the adrenal cortex is destroyed or replaced with tumor, infectious agents, hemorrhage, granulomata, or amyloid, primary adrenal insufficiency with hypocortisolism and hypoaldosteronism with hemodynamic instability ensues. Hypocortisolism leads to hypoglycemia and decreased systemic vascular resistance, whereas mineralocorticoid deficieny results in hyperkalemia, hyponatremia, hypovolemia, and impaired vascular tone. If there is failure of ACTH release from the brain, secondary adrenal failure is present but since aldosterone secretion by the adrenal is maintained due to local effects of angiotensin II, aldosterone deficiency and hemodynamic collapse are unusual.

Patients with malignancy are especially prone to adrenal dysfunction, which is often subclinical or associated with non-specific symptoms. The adrenal gland enjoys profuse blood perfusion and metastases may lodge in the gland via hematogenous dissemination, although lymphatic metastasis or invasion of the gland by local tumor may destroy tissue. Severe coaguloapathy of any cause can result in massive bilateral adrenal hemorrhage and AAI. Infiltration with infectious organisms, granulomas, or amyloid may also induce AAI. Often, AAI may manifest in a patient with subclincal hypoadrenalism when the patient is under severe physiologic stress (e.g., sepsis, bleeding, surgery, myocardial ischemia, or chemotherapy complications) due to the inability of the diseased cortex to release adequate cortisol.

ETIOLOGY

There are several potential etiologies of AAI in the cancer population. Any patient with systemic malignancy who develops non-specific symptoms should have hypoadrenalism included in the differential diagnosis in order to prevent potentially catastrophic AAI. The most common etiologies in the cancer patient include:

- Chronic use of corticosteroids or megesterol (secondary hypoadrenalism)
- Metastatic malignancy to the adrenal gland
  - Solid tumors
    - Lung, breast, gastric, prostate, urothelial, kidney, pancreas, colon
  - Lymphoma
  - Kaposi's sarcoma
  - Melanoma
- Leukemic infiltration
- Primary adrenal lymphoma
- Hemorrhage
  - Anticoagulation
  - Disseminated intravascular coagulation (DIC)
  - Hemorrhage into necrotic tumor
- Hypotension or shock
- Thrombosis
  - Antiphospholipid antibody syndrome, hypercoagulable states
- Amyloidosis

- Sickle cell anemia
- Adrenal toxic drugs
  - Ketoconazole, aminoglutethamide, mitotane
- Infection
  - Viral
    - Human immunodeficiency virus, cytomegalovirus
  - Granulomatous disease
    - Tuberculosis, histoplasmosis, coccidiomycosis
  - Opportunistic
    - Aspergillosis, mucor

Symptoms and Signs

Subacute or subclinical hypoadrenalism often manifests with non-specific symptoms that are often confused with the patient's underlying neoplasm or cancer treatment. Acute adrenal insufficiency may likewise mimic other acute processes, but should be considered in any cancer patient who develops treatment-refractory hypotension as well as any of the following:

- Weakness
- Anorexia
- Malaise
- Depression or slow thinking
- Weight loss
- Nausea or vomiting
- Diarrhea
- Abdominal pain
- Postural dizziness
- Syncope
- Fever
- Hypotension
  - May be refractory to vasopressors
- Relative bradycardia
- Hyperpigmentation
  - Skin or mucosal surfaces (due to elevation of ACTH)

Diagnostic Studies

Diagnosis of subacute hypoadrenalism or AAI requires a very high index of suspicion in the cancer patient. The most helpful diagnostic studies include:

- Random serum cortisol level
  - May be low, but difficult to interpret without dynamic testing
- Serum ACTH level
  - May be elevated due to loss of negative feedback from hypocortisolism

- Cosyntropin (ACTH) stimulation test
  - Test of choice due to accuracy, ease of performance, and quick turn-around
  - After baseline serum cortisol, 250 mg of intravenous ACTH administered with measurement of cortisol at 30 minutes and 60 minutes
    - Blunted rise (depends on individual laboratory) indicates adrenal gland failure
- Serum biochemistries
  - Hyperkalemia, hyponatremia, metabolic acidosis (with primary adrenal failure only); hypercalcemia
  - Hypoglycemia
- Computed tomography of adrenal glands
  - May reveal adrenal enlargement, hemorrhage, nodularity, or massive tumor infiltration
- Magnetic resonance imaging

TREATMENT

Treatment of AAI must be promptly instituted once the diagnosis is suspected, without awaiting diagnostic tests. Insertion of large-bore venous catheters and infusion of crystalloid and, if necessary, vasopressors is vital. Correction of hyperkalemia or hypercalcemia may not be necessary with treatment of hypocortisolism but, if severe, should be treated in usual fashion. Administration of hydrocortisone by bolus (e.g., 50–100 mg intravenously every 6 hours) or by intravenous infusion (10 mg per hour) is the cornerstone of therapy for AAI. Hydrocortisone will make interpretation of serum cortisol levels difficult but intravenous dexamethazone can be administered without interference. Typically, vasopressors are ineffective without adequate steroid administration. Serum glucose should be monitored carefully with liberal administration of intravenous dextrose as necessary. Once the patient is stable, oral hydrocortisone and fludrocortisone should be commenced indefinitely. Cancer patients with known hypoadrenalism should be counseled to double their daily replacement doses if they develop fever, vomiting, or other acute illness. Larger stress doses of intravenous hydrocortisone are necessary in the setting of severe acute illness, major surgery, or trauma to avoid the precipitation of AAI.

PROGNOSIS

Untreated, AAI can lead to refractory hypotension and shock with cardiovascular collapse and death. The overall prognosis with solid tumor metastasis to the adrenal glands is grim with very short survival times. Patients with lymphomatous involvement may fare better due to the chemosensitivity of this neoplasm.

ADDITIONAL READING

Marinella MA. Schmidt's syndrome presenting during laminectomy. *Heart Lung* 2004;33:412–413.

Marinella MA. Addisonian crisis. In: *Frequently Overlooked Diagnoses in Acute Care.* Philadelphia: Hanley and Belfus, 2003, pp. 17–21.

Oeklers W. Adrenal insufficiency. *N Engl J Med* 1996;335:1206–1212.

Payne DK, Levine SN, Franco DP, et al. Adrenal insufficiency due to metastatic lung carcinoma and shown by abdominal CT scan. *South Med J* 1984;77:1592–1593.

Redman BG, Pazdur R, Zingas AP, et al. Prospective evaluation of adrenal insufficiency in patients with adrenal metastasis. *Cancer* 1987;60:103–107.

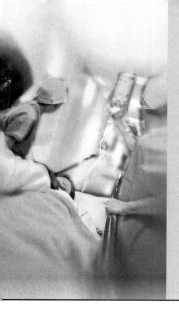

42

Hypoglycemia

DEFINITION

Hypoglycemia results when the serum blood glucose is below normal and may be due to a variety of mechanisms in the cancer patient.

CLINICAL SETTING

Symptomatic hypoglycemia in the cancer patient fulfills Whipple's triad (hypoglycemia, symptoms of hypoglycemia, resolution of symptoms with correction of hypoglycemia) and typically occurs in the setting of advanced metastatic disease and poor oral intake.

PATHOGENESIS

The pathogenesis of hypoglycemia in the oncology population can result from several mechanisms, more than one of which may exist in a single patient. Perhaps the most common pathogenic mechanism of hypoglycemia results from prolonged poor oral intake which results in inadequate glycogen stores. Prolonged malnutrition may also deplete gluconeogenic amino acids which can impair hepatic glucose production. Hepatic infiltration with tumor mass results in destruction of hepatocytes and subsequent hepatic dysfunction with impaired glycogenolysis and gluconeogenesis. Sepsis and infection may also contribute to hypoglycemia. Hypoadrenalism can lead to hypoglycemia due to altered carbohydrate metabolism from cortisol deficiency.

Insulinoma is a rare but classic etiology of hypoglycemia due to production of insulin by tumor cells. Hypoglycemia, known as non-islet cell tumor hypoglycemia

(NICTH), results from release of insulin-like growth factor II (IGF-II) from mesenchymal neoplasms such as fibrosarcoma, hemangiopericytoma, mesothelioma, neurofibroma, and various carcinomas. The mechanism of IGF-II associated hypoglycemia is postulated to result from inhibition of hepatic glucose production and enhancement glucose uptake into skeletal muscle. Lastly, large tumors may act as a "glucose sink" by consuming glucose subsequently inducing hypoglycemia.

ETIOLOGY

Patients with malignancy are at risk for hypoglycemia from multiple etiologies:

- Poor oral intake/malnutrition
- Sepsis
- Renal failure
- Liver failure/cirrhosis
- Adrenal insufficiency
- Medications
  - Insulin, sulfonylureas
  - Quinolones
- Neoplasm
  - Hepatic failure due to extensive metastasis or hepatoma
  - Carcinomas
    - Gastric, breast, renal cell, lung, pancreas
  - Lymphoma/leukemia
  - Mesothelioma
  - Mesenchymal tumors
    - Hemangiopericytoma, fibrosarcoma, leiomyosarcoma

SYMPTOMS AND SIGNS

The diagnosis of hypoglycemia is confirmed clinically by Whipple's triad—documented hypoglycemia, symptoms compatible with hypoglycemia, and resolution of hypoglycemic symptoms with treatment of hypoglycemia. The symptoms of hypoglycemia are divided into neuroglycopenic symptoms and non-neuroglycopenic symptoms which are in large part mediated by counter-regulatory hormones. Hypoglycemia may be overlooked in patients with the inability to communicate the presence of neuroglycopenic symptoms. The most common hypoglycemic symptoms include:

- Fatigue
- Diaphoresis
- Palpitations
- Syncope
- Tachycardia
- Coma
- Focal neurologic deficit (paralysis)

- Neuroglycopenic manifestations
  - Confusion
  - Anxiety
  - Hunger
  - Tremulousness
  - Blurred vision
  - Cortical blindness

DIAGNOSTIC STUDIES

Diagnosis of hypoglycemia in the cancer patient follows a two-step approach: documentation of hypoglycemia followed by determining the etiology of hypoglycemia. Some useful diagnostic studies include:

- Bedside fingerstick glucose
- Serum glucose
- Serum cortisol to exclude hypoadrenalism
- Glucagon stimulation test
  - Rise of serum glucose after 1 mg of glucagon suggests adequate glycogen stores, as is the case with insulinoma or IGF-II secreting tumors
  - No rise in glucose is consistent with severe liver dysfunction due to hepatic replacement with tumor, liver failure, or poor glycogen reserve
- Prolonged fasting to assess for insulinoma
  - Hyperinsulinemia in the setting of hypoglycemia
- Serum studies for NICTH
  - Assay for IGF-II
  - Insulin, C-peptide, and growth hormone levels all suppressed
- Computed tomography
  - May reveal primary tumor such as a sarcoma, insulinoma, or liver metastasis
- Abdominal ultrasound
  - May reveal hepatic tumor replacement

TREATMENT

Hypoglycemia can result in severe neurologic sequelae or even death if treatment is delayed. Therefore, rapid administration of intravenous dextrose (e.g., 50 milliliters of 50% dextrose) is imperative. If intravenous access is unavailable, an injection of glucagon or sublingual glucose gel can be given. Some authors recommend corticosteroids for NICTH, but long-term complications may limit this approach. Treatment of the underlying neoplasm, if possible, may lead to resolution of hypoglycemia, but patients with extensive hepatic metastases may experience refractory hypoglycemia. Patients with insulinoma or a resectable tumor suspected of causing NICTH should be surgically resected. Patients with large tumors not amenable to resection may benefit from cytoreduction with radiotherapy or chemotherapy.

PROGNOSIS

Patients with hypoglycemia due to a resectable, localized neoplasm experience resolution of hypoglycemia with a good long-term prognosis if the tumor is extirpated. However, the prognosis of patients with widely metastatic carcinomas with liver involvement and/or malnutrition have a poor prognosis, with hypoglycemia often being a terminal event.

ADDITIONAL READING

Hoff AO, Vassilopoulou-Sellin R. The role of glucagon administration in the diagnosis and treatment of patients with tumor hypoglycemia. *Cancer* 1998;82: 1585–1592.

Kato A, Bando E, Shinozaki S, et al. Severe hypoglycemia and hypokalemia in association with liver metastases of gastric cancer. *Intern Med* 2004;43:824–828.

Kishi K, Sonomura T, Sato M. Radiotherapy for hypoglycemia associated with large leiomyosarcomas. *Br J Radiol* 1997;70:306–308.

Ma RCW, Lo RSK, Chan JCN, et al. Recurrent hypoglycemia in a patient with metastatic pancreatic carcinoma. *PLoS Med* 2006;3:1255–1257.

Spinazze S, Schrijvers D. Metabolic emergencies. *Crit Rev Hematol Oncol* 2006;58: 79–89.

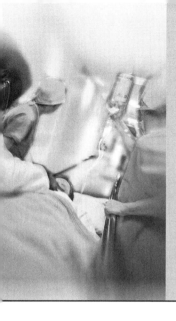

43

Hypercalcemia

DEFINITION

Hypercalcemia is characterized by an increase in serum ionized calcium, and typically total serum calcium, resulting in a variety of adverse physiologic effects.

CLINICAL SETTING

Most patients with malignancy-related hypercalcemia have advanced cancer with a poor prognosis. Some patients with treatable hematopoietic neoplasms may present with symptoms related to hypercalcemia.

PATHOGENESIS

Hypercalcemia associated with malignancy is common, with up to 30% of cancer patients experiencing this complication at some point during their disease. Although immobility, primary hyperparathyroidism, calcium supplements, thiazide diuretics, and other processes may cause hypercalcemia in this population, only the primary mechanisms unique to the cancer patient will be discussed. Overall, the most common etiologies include breast and lung cancer, lymphoma, and multiple myeloma, all of which can induce hypercalcemia by different mechanisms with the end result being increased calcium mobilization from bone and increased renal tubular calcium absorption.

The most common mechanism of hypercalcemia in the cancer population is humoral hypercalcemia of malignancy (HHM) which is mediated by tumoral production of parathyroid hormone-related protein (PTHrP). Localized tumors can cause HHM which typically resolves with eradication of the tumor. PTHrP shares a similar structure to PTH and results in hypercalcemia via increased osteoclastic bone resorption and renal retention of calcium. Squamous cell carcinomas are a common cause of HHM, although other tumor types are associated with this syndrome as well. The next most common mechanism of malignant hypercalcemia is induction of bone osteolysis from skeletal metastasis. Most cases involving this mechanism result from lytic metastases from multiple myeloma or solid tumors, most commonly breast or lung carcinoma. Osteolysis is induced by various autocrine and paracrine mediators released by tumor and inflammatory cells such as PTHrP, tumor necrosis factor (TNF), macrophage inflammatory protein (MIP) 1-α, or receptor activator of nuclear factor-kappa-B ligand (RANKL). The latter two mediators are especially common with multiple myeloma-associated hypercalcemia causing substantial osteoclast activation. Patients with myeloma also are prone to hypercalcemia from decreased glomerular filtration and poor mobility secondary to bone pain.

Lymphomas occasionally produce the active moiety of vitamin D (1,25-dihydroxyvitamin D) which causes enhanced osteoclastic bone resorption and increased intestinal absorption of calcium. The rarest type of hypercalcemia associated with cancer is the ectopic tumor secretion of PTH, which causes hypercalcemia in a manner similar to primary hyperparathyroidism.

ETIOLOGY

Hypercalcemia has a variety of causes in the cancer patient, of which include:

- Humoral hypercalcemia of malignancy (HHM)
  - Squamous cell carcinoma of the lung, esophagus, head and neck, cervix
  - Renal cell carcinoma
  - Ovarian and endometrial carcinoma
  - Breast cancer
- Osteolysis-induced hypercalcemia
  - Breast cancer
  - Multiple myeloma
  - Lymphoma
- Tumor secretion of 1,25-dihydroxyvitamin D
  - Non-Hodgkin's lymphoma
  - Hodgkin's lymphoma
- Ectopic release of PTH
  - Ovarian cancer
- Immobility
- Primary hyperparathyroidism
- Drugs
  - Hydrochlorothiazide
  - Vitamin D preparations
  - Calcium supplements
  - Lithium
  - Shark cartilage
- Granulomatous disease

Symptoms and Signs

Hypercalcemia can be a challenge to diagnose in the cancer patient since symptoms are typically non-specific. However, hypercalcemia should be considered in any patient with malignancy who develops the following:

- Fatigue
- Anorexia
- Nausea/vomiting
- Constipation
- Polydypsia
- Polyuria
  - May result from hypercalcemia-induced diabetes insipidus
- Muscle weakness
- Bone pain
- Hypertension
- Delirium
- Coma

Diagnostic Studies

Diagnosis of hypercalcemia is relatively straightforward once the diagnosis is suspected. The following are the most useful diagnostic studies to diagnose and ascertain the etiology of hypercalcemia:

- Total serum calcium
  - Affected by serum albumin; if hypoalbuminemia is present, ($<$3.5 g/dl), add 0.8 mg/dl to total serum calcium for each 1.0 g/dl the albumin is below 3.5 g/dl
  - Rarely, patients with multiple myeloma may exhibit calcium-binding immunoglobulins that bind serum calcium and falsely elevate total serum calcium
- Ionized serum calcium
  - Most accurate method to assess degree of hypercalcemia
- Serum intact PTH (iPTH)
  - Some authors recommend routinely measuring iPTH since primary hyperparathyroidism is not uncommon in the cancer population
- Serum PTHrP
  - Typically not useful, buy may assist in diagnosis in equivocal cases
- Serum 1,25-dihydroxyvitamin D
  - If lymphoma-related hypercalcemia is suspected
- Serum and urine electrophoresis
  - If multiple myeloma is suspected
- Serum electrolytes and renal function
  - Necessary to exclude derangements of serum sodium, potassium, magnesium, and phosphate
  - Renal failure common with severe hypercalcemia

- Electrocardiogram
  - Shortened QT interval
- Skeletal radiography
  - Useful to screen for blastic or lytic bone lesion
- Bone scan
  - Useful to assess metastatic skeletal burden in the setting of blastic disease

TREATMENT

The first issue to consider is whether treatment is indicated. Patients with widely metastatic terminal cancer may be best served by withholding treatment since hypercalcemia may afford the patient the most humane way to die. Patients with an otherwise favorable prognosis require aggressive volume resuscitation with isotonic saline since volume depletion is universal in the setting of significant hypercalcemia. Patients may require several liters of saline with careful monitoring for volume overload if a history of cardiac disease is present. Volume administration increases the tubular excretion of calcium due to enchanced renal blood flow. Loop diuretics are useful after the patient is volume repleted due to their calcitic effect; however, administration of these drugs in the setting of hypovolvemia only serves to exacerbate the hypercalcemic state. Discontinuation of any calcium products, vitamin D compounds, or thiazide diuretics is important. Patients with hypercalcemic crisis manifested as coma may benefit from calcitonin due to the rapid onset of action, although tachyphylaxis is common after 2 days of use. Corticosteroids are useful with multiple myeloma or if an elevated 1,25-dihydroxy-vitamin D from lymphoma is suspected. Hypophosphatemia should be corrected with oral salts with careful monitoring for hyperphosphatemia and hypocalcemia. The mainstay of treatment for malignancy-related hypercalcemia are the bisphosphonates, pamidronate and zoledronic acid. These intravenous agents are effective in the majority of cases of hypercalcemia and act by inhibiting osteoclast bone resorption. The onset of action is approximately 2 days with a duration of activity of 2 to 3 weeks, in most cases. Since these drugs can adversely affect kidney function and serum electrolytes, dose adjustment and monitoring of serum creatinine and metabolic parameters is important. Dialytic therapy may be useful if volume overload is a concern or if life-threatening hypercalcemia fails to respond to the previously mentioned treatments. Mithramycin and gallium nitrate are rarely utilized due to the development of the bisphosphonates, but may be useful in select patients.

PROGNOSIS

Hypercalcemia is often a pre-terminal event, especially in patients with metastatic solid tumors (e.g., breast, lung) with 50% of such patients succumbing within 30 days. Patients with myeloma or lymphoma typically have a better prognosis and may enjoy prolonged survival if the underlying disease responds to treatment.

ADDITIONAL READING

Flombaum CD. Metabolic emergencies in the cancer patient. *Semin Oncol* 2000;27:322–334.

John R, Oleesky K, Issa B, et al. Pseudo-hypercalcemia in two patients with IgM paraproteinemia. *Ann Clin Biochem* 1997;34:694–696.

Oyajobi BO. Multiple myeloma/hypercalcemia. *Arthitis Res Ther* 2007;9:S1–6.

Spinazze S, Schrijvers D. Metabolic emergencies. *Crit Rev Hematol Oncol* 2006;58:79–89.

Stewart AF. Hypercalcemia associated with cancer. *N Engl J Med* 2005;352:373–379.

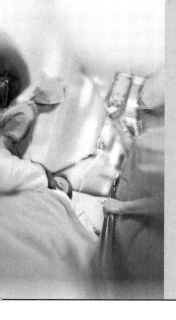

44
Hyponatremia

DEFINITION

Hyponatremia is defined as a decrease in serum sodium ($<$130 mEq/L) due to alterations in total body water balance which invariably results in hypo-osmolality.

CLINICAL SETTING

Hyponatremia is by far the most common electrolyte disorder in patients with solid tumors and hematopoietic malignancies. Hyponatremia has multiple possible etiologies such as hypovolemic, euvolemic, and hypervolemic states.

PATHOGENESIS

Sodium is the most prevalent extracellular cation and is the major determinant of serum osmolality. Therefore, reductions in serum sodium are a surrogate marker for hypo-osmolality. An exception to this general rule is the concept of pseudohyponatremia which occurs when an inappropriate osmotic substance is present in the serum, resulting in an appropriate decrease in sodium to maintain normal serum osmolality. Pseudohyponatremia most commonly occurs in the setting of hyperglycemia, but can also complicate severe hyperlipidemia or hyperproteinemic states such as multiple myeloma or Waldenstrom's macroglobulinemia.

  True hyponatremia and hypo-osmolality reflects an excess of free water in the extracellular compartment. Normally, water intake is prompted by thirst and excretion is mediated by anti-diuretic hormone (ADH). As serum osmolality increases, thirst is triggered and ADH is secreted by hypothalamic neurons which targets the renal collecting ducts to absorb water. There are numerous appropriate stimuli for ADH release in the cancer population including pain, nausea, vomiting, surgical procedures, narcotic analgesics, anxiety, volume depletion, and hypotension. In fact, decreased tissue perfusion is a very potent stimulus for ADH release via stimulation of arterial baroreceptors that sense decreases in effective circulating volume. The most common causes of decreased vascular volume are edematous states (e.g., due to docetaxel, nephrosis, congestive heart failure, or cirrhosis) and true loss of water and sodium such as occurs with vomiting, diarrhea, or salt-wasting nephropathy. The latter may complicate cisplatinum administration, adrenal insufficiency, or the cerebral salt-wasting syndrome resulting from intracranial surgery, mass lesions, or hemorrhage. True volume depletion results in oliguria and renal tubular retention of sodium, causing a decrease in serum sodium elimination, which is a useful diagnostic feature of hypovolemic hyponatremia. Patients with salt-wasting nephropathy, however, manifest clinical evidence of volume depletion but elevated levels of urine sodium ($>$40 mEq/L) in contrast to extra-renal sodium losses in which the urine sodium is decreased ($<$20 mEq/L).

Hyponatremia associated with hypo-osmolality results from excessive water intake or decreased water elimination. If water intake is excessive, the kidney attempts to excrete a maximally dilute urine with urine osmolality in the range of 100 mOsm/L. However, if the urine osmolality is high in a cancer patient with hyponatremia, a defect in water excretion from inappropriate ADH release is most often present, a condition known as the syndrome of inappropriate anti-diuretic hormone (SIADH) secretion. The classic features of SIADH are clinical euvolemia, hypo-osmolality, and inappropriately high urine sodium and osmolality. The pathogenic characteristic of SIADH-induced hyponatremia is excess water resorption and renal sodium loss. This water resorption is reflected by hypouricemia and low blood urea nitrogen. There are many etiologies of SIADH in the cancer patient, but certain tumor cells (notably small cell carcinomas) secrete ADH. In fact, any noxious stimulus involving the central nervous system or lungs can result in ADH release and SIADH. Additionally, many drugs utilized in oncology are associated with the development of SIADH.

The main danger of severe hyponatremia is the development of cerebral edema, especially if hyponatremia is profound or serum sodium levels decline rapidly. Seizures and coma are indicative of cerebral edema and life-threatening hyponatremia.

ETIOLOGY

The etiologies of hyponatremia in the cancer patient are protean and a simplified approach to determining the cause is characterizing hyponatremia by the volume status:

- Hypovolemic hyponatremia (associated with extra-renal or renal fluid and/or sodium losses)
  - Vomiting
  - Diarrhea
  - Nasogastric suctioning
  - Enteric fistulae

- ○ Sweating
- ○ Diuretics
- ○ Salt-wasting nephropathy
  - Cisplatinum administration
  - Cerebral salt wasting due to intracranial surgery or pathology
  - Adrenal insufficiency
- Hypervolemic hyponatremia (associated with edematous states)
  - ○ Hypoalbuminemia and excess intravenous fluids
  - ○ Congestive heart failure
  - ○ Cirrhotic liver disease
  - ○ Malignant ascites
  - ○ Severe pancreatitis or ileus with third-spacing
  - ○ Excessive hypotonic fluid administration
  - ○ Anti-cancer drugs
    - Docetaxel
    - Gemcitabine
    - Interleukin (IL)-2
- Euvolemic hyponatremia (SIADH)
  - ○ Neoplasms
    - Small cell carcinoma
      - — Accounts for 75% of tumor-induced SIADH; occurs in 10% of patients with small cell carcinomas
    - Other carcinomas (breast, ovarian, pancreatic, lung, prostate, bladder)
    - Lymphoma
    - Mesothelioma
    - Sarcoma
    - Brain tumors
    - Leukemia
  - ○ Pulmonary disease
  - ○ Central nervous system insults
  - ○ Chemotherapy-induced nausea in setting of hydration
  - ○ Pain and surgery
  - ○ Chemotherapeutic agents
    - Vincristine, vinorelbine, vinblastine, cyclophosphamide, ifosfamide, melphalan, chlorambucil, cisplatinum
  - ○ Miscellaneous drugs
    - Morphine sulphate/narcotics, selective serotonin reuptake inhibitors, carbemazepine, general anesthesia

Symptoms and Signs

Mild hyponatremia and slowly-evolving hyponatremia are often symptomatic. Although severe hyponatremia (<120 mEq/L) is typically associated with neurologic symptoms and signs, a rapid decline in serum sodium is perhaps the main determinant of the adverse clinical effects of hyponatremia. Common symptoms and signs include:

- Nausea/vomiting
- Fatigue
- Anorexia
- Headache
- Dizziness
- Confusion
- Hallucinations
- Seizures
- Coma
- Tachycardia, dry mucous membranes, hypotension, and oliguria with hypo-volemic hyponatremia
- Edema and pulmonary rales with hypervolemic hyponatremia

DIAGNOSTIC STUDIES

Since hyponatremia presents with non-specific clinical findings, a thoughtful di-agnostic evaluation is important, especially in the cancer patient. The following studies are most helpful in the diagnosis of hyponatremia:

- Orthostatic vital signs
  - Hypotension and tachycardia are consistent with hypovolemic hypona-tremia due to extra-renal losses, sodium-wasting nephropathy, or cerebral salt wasting
- Serum sodium level
  - Failure of serum sodium to correct with isotonic saline suggests SIADH
- Serum osmolality
  - If normal (>280 mosm/kg), pseudohyponatremia is present
  - Hypo-osmolality universal with hyponatremia of any variety
- Urine sodium level
  - Urine sodium <20 meq/L compatible with hypovolemic hyponatremia due to extra-renal losses
  - Urine sodium >40 meq/L in the setting of euvolemia is compatible with SIADH
  - Urine sodium >40 meq/L in the setting of hypovolemia is compatible with sodium-wasting nephropathy or cerebral salt wasting
- Urine osmolarity
  - Urine osmolarity <100–150 mosm/L in the setting of hyponatremia suggestive of water intoxication (due to hypotonic intravenous fluids or psychogenic polydypsia)
  - Urine osmolality greater than serum osmolality in the setting of hypona-tremia is compatible with SIADH
- Serum uric acid
  - Hypouricemia common with SIADH due to increased urate clearance

- The following may be useful in selected patients if SIADH is present
  - Serum thyroid stimulating hormone and cortisol
    - Since hypothyroidism and hypoadrenalism can induce renal sodium loss, normal levels are needed to diagnose SIADH
  - Cerebral imaging studies to exclude central nervous system disease
  - Chest radiography or computed tomography to exclude pulmonary disease

TREATMENT

The treatment of hyponatremia hinges upon the patient's clinical volume status. Hypovolemic patients, due to vomiting, diarrhea, or nasogastric suction, require administration of isotonic saline supplemented with other electrolytes as necessary. Patients with hypervolemic hyponatremia due to heart failure, nephrosis, or cirrhosis typically require parenteral loop diuretics. Patients with profound or rapidly occurring hyponatremia who present with seizures or coma require careful administration of 3% saline solution, often with loop diuretics to avoid fluid overload. Formulas for calculating total body sodium and fluid deficits are available, but are beyond the scope of this text. Care should be taken to not increase the serum sodium more rapidly than 0.5 meq/L per hour or more than 12 meq/L in a 12-hour period to avoid the osmotic demyelination syndrome, which can be fatal. Regular monitoring of serum sodium is vital during initial correction of hyponatremia. Patients with SIADH are most easily treated with fluid restriction (e.g., 1000–1200 cc of fluid per 24-hour period). Loop diuretics may be necessary in some patients with SIADH. Demeclocycline, a tetracycline analogue that decreases ADH action on the renal tubules inducing nephrogenic diabetes insipidus, may be helpful for chronic SIADH in patients with small cell lung cancer or other malignancies. A recently released vasopressin-antagonist, conivaptan, may benefit some patients with severe or treatment-refractory SIADH. Treatment of small cell or other cancers with chemotherapy often resolves SIADH if the tumor is eradicated.

PROGNOSIS

Severe, rapidly developing hyponatremia can be life-threatening if cerebral edema, seizures, or coma develop. Generally, the prognosis of hyponatremia in the cancer patient is favorable, with the most important determinant being the status and treatment response of the underlying malignancy.

ADDITIONAL READING

Ellison DH, Berl T. The syndrome of inappropriate antidiuresis. *N Engl J Med* 2007; 356:2064–2072.

Flombaum CD. Metabolic emergencies in the cancer patient. *Semin Oncol* 2000; 27:322–334.

Passamonte PM. Hypouricemia, inappropriate secretion of anti-diuretic hormone and small cell carcinoma of the lung. *Arch Intern Med* 1984;144:1569–1570.

Apinazze S, Schrijvers D. Metabolic emergencies. *Crit Rev Hematol Oncol* 2006; 58:79–89.

Trump DL. Serious hyponatremia in patients with cancer: management with demeclocycline. *Cancer* 1981;47:2908–2912.

Vanhees SL, Parideans R, Vansteenkiste JF. Syndrome of inappropriate antidiuretic hormone associated with chemotherapy-induced tumor lysis in small cell lung cancer: case report and literature review. *Ann Oncol* 2000;11:1061–1065.

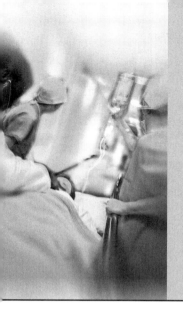

45

Tumor Lysis Syndrome

DEFINITION

Tumor lysis (TLS) syndrome results from the rapid release of intracellular constituents into the bloodstream either spontaneously or during chemotherapy or radiotherapy of certain rapidly growing solid tumors or hematopoietic malignancies.

CLINICAL SETTING

The TLS typically occurs in the setting of chemotherapy-sensitive lymphomas, leukemias, and certain solid tumors, typically small cell lung cancer. Some neoplasms with rapid cell growth may develop spontaneous TLS in the absence of anticancer therapy, and are at especially high risk of treatment-related complications.

PATHOGENESIS

When malignancies with a short doubling time and high growth fraction receive chemotherapy or radiotherapy, a significant amout of tumor cells are killed resulting in release of various intracellular products that may induce metabolic derangements. The classic neoplasm highly associated with TLS is Burkitt's lymphoma, but other malignanices can cause TLS and will be discussed in the following text. The most significant cellular constituents include uric acid, potassium, and phosphates with hyperuricemia, hyperkalemia, and hyperphosphatemia, respectively, developing especially in patients with underlying renal dysfunction due to decreased excretion. Hypocalcemia is also common and results from hyperphosphatemia-inducing calcium-phosphate precipitation in various tissues. Calcium-phosphate precipitation within the renal parenchyma as well as tubular toxicity may play a role in TLS-associated acute renal failure (ARF), which is the major cause of morbidity and mortality. The primary pathogenic mechanism of TLS-associated ARF from intratubular precipitation of uric acid, resulting in acute tubular necrosis. Occasionally, uric acid stones may form and obstruct the collecting system resulting in acute obstructive uropathy. With cell lysis, purines are released and catabolized to hypoxanthine then xanthine, and, finally, uric acid by the enzyme xanthine oxidase. Allopurinol inhibits xanthine oxidase and remains an important part of treating TLS. Since allopurinol blocks xanthine metabolism into uric acid, elevated serum xanthine levels can result in intratubular deposition of xanthine crystals, further contributing to renal dysfunction. Uric acid is poorly soluble in an acidic urine but urinary alkalinization increases solulability. Hyperkalemia is common and results from intracellular potassium release as well as acute renal failure. Hyperkalemia can be fatal due to the arrhythmogenic effects.

ETIOLOGY

Tumor lysis syndrome can occur spontaneously in patients with significant tumor burden with baseline increases in creatinine, uric acid, and lactate dehydrogenase (LDH) being the key risk factors. However, most cases complicate chemotherapy administration to patients with sensitive neoplasms such as:

- Burkitt's lymphoma
- Diffuse large cell lymphoma
- Acute lymphoblastic leukemia
- Acute myeloid leukemia
- Chronic lymphocytic leukemia
- Chronic myelogenous leukemia with blast crisis
- Solid tumors
  - Extensive-stage small cell carcinoma with liver involvement most common
  - Germ cell neoplasms, breast cancer, gastric cancer, ovarian cancer

SYMPTOMS AND SIGNS

Symptoms and signs directly attributable to TLS are difficult to identify since the underlying neoplasm and treatment regimens may produce findings that overlap with TLS. Generally, clinical manifestations of TLS include:

- Nausea/vomiting
- Lethargy
- Tetany and muscle weakness secondary to hypocalcemia
- Palpitations
- Flank pain due to uric acid nephrolithiasis
- Edema
- Seizures
- Carpopedal spasm, Trousseau's sign, Chvostek's sign if hypocalcemia is severe

DIAGNOSTIC STUDIES

The most important element in the diagnosis and management is to anticipate patients at high risk for TLS. The following studies should be obtained in any patient suspected of developing TLS:

- Serum electrolytes and renal function
  - Hyperphosphatemia
  - Hyperkalemia
  - Hypocalcemia
  - Elevated anion gap
- Lactate dehydrogenase
  - Increases with tumor cell destruction
- Serum uric acid
  - Hyperuricemia is the hallmark of TLS
- Urinalysis
  - May reveal urate crystals or muddy granular casts in the setting of ATN
- Electrocardiogram
  - May reveal peaked T waves and widening of the QRS complex if hyperkalemia is severe (>6 meq/L)
  - Prolongation of the QT interval may be present if hypocalcemia is severe

TREATMENT

The most important element in the management of TLS is anticipating patients at high risk of developing this syndrome with chemotherapy in order to institute prophylactic measures to prevent morbidity and mortality. Typical prophylactic measures include vigorous hydration with crystalloids, urinary alkalinization with bicarbonate compounds, and allopurinol to prevent uric acid formation. However, allopurinol may take a few days to maximally inhibit urate formation, which may pose a problem in patients who require urgent chemotherapy. Caution must be exercised if mercaptopurine or azathioprine are concurrently administered since allopurinol interferes with metabolism of these agents. A new treatment option to prevent or treat hyperuricemia in a rapid manner is the recombinant enzyme rasburicase which immediately catalyzes uric acid into the soluble renally-excreted non-toxic metabolite, allantoin. Rasburicase is especially effective in treating hyperuricemia in patients with overt TLS since it enhances catabolism of existing uric acid, unlike allopurinol. Rasburicase should be avoided in patients with glucose-6-phosphate dehydrogenase deficiency.

PROGNOSIS

The prognosis of TLS largely depends on the status of the underlying neoplasm. Hyperkalemia is the most significant cause of death early in the course of TLS as the result of ventricular arrhythmias. Patients who develop ARF are at increased risk of bleeding and infection, especially if hemodialysis is required, which adversely effects prognosis in many patients.

ADDITIONAL READING

Cairo MS, Bishop M. Tumour lysis syndrome: new therapeutic strategies and classification. *Br J Haematol* 2004;127:3–11.

Cammalleri L, Malaguarnera M. Rasburicase represents a new tool for hyperuricemia in tumor lysis syndrome and in gout. *Int J Med Sci* 2007;4:83–93.

Flombaum CD. Metabolic emergencies in the cancer patient. *Semin Oncol* 2000; 27:322–334.

Marinella MA. Fatal tumor lysis syndrome and gastric hemorrhage associated with metastatic small cell lung carcinoma. *Med Pediatr Oncol* 1999;32:464–465.

Sallan S. Management of acute tumor lysis syndrome. *Semin Oncol* 2001;28:9–18.

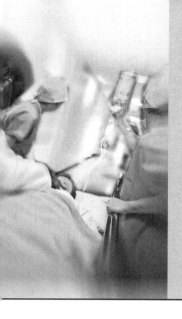

46

Refeeding
Syndrome

DEFINITION

The refeeding syndrome (RFS) is a common, yet under-recognized metabolic disorder characterized by hypophosphatemia and, commonly, hypokalemia, hypomagnesemia, fluid retention, and hyperglycemia occurring in malnourished patients upon reinstitution of oral, enteral, or intravenous nutrition.

CLINICAL SETTING

Within the cancer population, RFS typically occurs in the setting of prolonged vomiting, diarrhea, and anorexia due to underlying malignancy or various anti-cancer therapies such as chemotherapy and surgery.

PATHOGENESIS

The RFS is a common metabolic syndrome typically occurring in acutely ill hospitalized patients. It is characterized by the development of hypophosphatemia and, commonly, hypomagnesemia, hypokalemia, hyperglycemia, and fluid retention upon reinstitution of nutrition or administration of glucose solutions. This syndrome, which is potentially fatal due to cardiac arrhythmia, was first described in starved World War II prisoners of war and Leningrad occupants after the acute institution of nutrition. The RFS was also noted to commonly complicate refeeding of patients with anorexia nervosa when administered aggressive nutritional intervention. Risk factors for RFS are outlined in the following text, but the common theme in the cancer patient is acute illness, poor oral intake, vomiting, and diarrhea.

Phosphate is the most abundant intracellular anion and possesses numerous vital cellular functions in virtually all organ systems. With subacute or prolonged poor oral intake, depletion of total-body phosphate occurs, and can be compounded by losses in the vomitus, stool, or nasogastric effluent. Acute transcellular shift is the primary mechanism for severe hypophosphatemia which occurs following administration of glucose-containing fluids, tube feedings, parenteral nutrition, or even oral feedings in the setting of malnutrition or recent poor intake. Glucose loading and the hyperinsulinemia that accompanies it, lead to acute transcellular shift of phosphate to the intracellular compartment, further lowering serum levels. Hypophosphatemia also results from increased glycolysis and cell growth from nutrient-induced anabolism, which requires increased formation of high-energy phosphate bonds. Phosphate is a vital component of nucleic acids, nucleoproteins, phospholipids, and various enzymatic systems such as adenosine triphosphate (ATP), creatine kinase (CK) and 2,3-diphosphoglycerate (2,3-DPG). As a result, hypophosphatemia can lead to diverse organ and cellular dysfunction due to the central role in these structural proteins and enzymes. Clinically, cardio-respiratory complications such as ventricular arrhythmias and respiratory failure are the most life-threatening features of RFS. Depletion of ATP leads to impaired cardiomyocyte function with cardiac instability and failure, as well as diaphragmatic muscle weakness that can result in acute respiratory failure. Depletion of 2,3-DPG results in a shift of the oxygen-dissociation curve to the left, impairing oxygen offloading to the tissues. Hypophosphatemia can also result in hemolysis, impaired neutrophil chemotaxis, and rhabdomyolysis which can result in anemia, infection, and acute renal failure, respectively. Thrombocytopenia may rarely complicate severe hypophosphatemia. In addition to hypophosphatemia, administration of glucose or nutrition therapy often leads to hypokalemia and hypomagnesemia which may result in cardiac and neurologic dysfunction. Patients with RFS are also at risk for acute thiamine depletion due to increased oxidative-reduction demands with carbohydrate administration. Thiamine deficiency can lead to neurologic dysfunction, acute high-output cardiac failure, and metabolic acidosis. Fluid retention and central volume overload from hyperinsulinemia and hyperglycemia can adversely affect cardiac function.

Patients with advanced malignancy are often anorexic and exhibit poor oral intake from a variety of etiologies. Superimposed vomiting and diarrhea can further deplete serum electrolytes, which is only augmented if glucose solutions, tube feedings or total parenteral nutrition (TPN) are administered. Circulating cytokines from tumor cells and sepsis can also exacerbate RFS-related hypophosphatemia.

ETIOLOGY

The etiologies and risk factors for RFS and hypophosphatemia in the cancer population are many, of which include:

- Poor oral intake
  - Anorexia from underlying neoplasm
  - Anorexia from chemotherapy or radiation
  - Oral pain from stomatitis or oral infection

- Vomiting
  - Chemotherapy-related (e.g., cisplatinum, cyclophosphamide)
  - Hyponatremia (e.g., SIADH, volume depletion)
  - Increased intracranial pressure due to brain metastasis
  - Malignant gastric outlet obstruction or small bowel obstruction
  - Abdominal carcinomatosis
- Diarrhea
  - Chemotherapy-induced (e.g., cytosine arabinoside)
  - *Clostridium difficile* colitis
- Old age
- Sepsis
- Abdominal surgery
- Nasogastric suction
- Chemotherapy
- Total parenteral nutrition
- Glucose-containing fluids
- Enteral feeding
- Uncontrolled diabetes mellitus

Symptoms and Signs

Diagnosis of RFS may be difficult since many of the clinical manifestations are not specific to this disorder and may be attributed to other ongoing processes or the cancer itself. In fact, symptoms and signs due to RFS typically result from severe electrolyte depletion and, because of this, RFS should be considered in the at-risk patient with any of the following:

- Fatigue
  - Typically due to electrolyte depletion and starvation
- Palpitations
  - May indicate hypokalemia or hypomagnesemia-induced arrhythmia
- Dizziness
- Syncope
  - May complicate ventricular arrhythmia or Torsades de pointes due to hypokalemia or hypomagnesemia
- Ophthalmoplegia
  - Indicative of Wernicke's encephalopathy (ophthalmoplegia, ataxia, delirium) from thiamine deficiency
- Myalgia/muscle pain
  - Secondary to rhabdomyolysis resulting from hypophosphatemia or hypokalemia
- Dark urine
  - May indicate myoglobinuria from rhabdomyolysis or hemoglobinuria due to hypophosphatemic-hemolysis

- Dyspnea
  - May result from acute cardiac failure or diaphragmatic muscle weakness due to severe hypophosphatemia
- Parasthesia
- Tetany
  - May result from severe hypomagnesemia
- Seizures
- Edema
- Muscle weakness
- Cardiac gallop (S3)
  - Indicates acute cardiomyopathy resulting from hypophosphatemia or wet beri-beri from thiamine deficiency

DIAGNOSTIC STUDIES

Diagnosis of the RFS requires a very high index of suspicion due to the lack of specific clinical findings. The clinician must anticipate the development of RFS in the at-risk cancer patient and consider obtaining the following studies:

- Serum chemistries
  - Hypophosphatemia, hypokalemia, hypomagnesemia
  - Hyperglycemia
  - Elevated CK or myoglobin
- Complete blood count
  - Anemia, thrombocytopenia
- Urinalysis
  - Myoglobinuria if rhabdomyolysis is present
- Electrocardiogram
  - Prolongation of the QT interval secondary to hypokalemia or hypomagnesemia
- Echocardiogram
  - Systolic dysfunction may be present in cases of severe hypophosphatemia or beri-beri due to thiamine deficiency

TREATMENT

Anticipation of RFS should prompt monitoring of serum electrolytes within 24 hours of glucose or nutrition administration. Patients at high risk should be administered prophylactic oral phosphate (e.g., potassium or sodium phosphate), potassium (e.g., potassium phosphate or chloride), or magnesium (e.g., magnesium oxide) supplements to avoid a precipitous decline in serum levels, especially if commencing TPN or tube feedings. Patients unable to tolerate oral medications can have electrolyte solutions added to their intravenous fluids. Treatment of established hypophosphatemia is especially important when serum levels are below 1.0 mmol/L. In this case, intravenous potassium or sodium phosphate should be administered in a dose of 0.08 mmol/kg or as a 20 mmol infusion. Careful monitoring of serum phosphate, calcium, sodium, and potassium is important during intravenous administration to avoid over replacement. The choice of phosphate salt depends on whether hypokalemia or hyponatremia is present. Additionally, magnesium sulfate infusions are commonly required to treat hypomagnesemia, which can lead to refractory hypokalemia or, less commonly, hypocalcemia. Administration of thiamine and other water-soluble B-complex vitamins is important since these factors are involved with carbohydrate metabolism.

PROGNOSIS

If unrecognized, RFS can result in sudden death due to cardiac arrhythmia, although this is uncommon if electrolytes are closely monitored. With adequate electrolyte replacement, most patients with RFS improve, but the long-term prognosis depends on the status of the underlying malignancy.

ADDITIONAL READING

Marinella MA. Refeeding syndrome in cancer patients. *Int J Clin Pract* 2008; 62:460–465.

Marinella MA. Refeeding syndrome and hypophosphatemia. *J Intensive Care Med* 2005;20:155–159.

Marinella MA. The refeeding syndrome and hypophosphatemia. *Nutr Rev* 2003; 61:320–323.

Marinella MA. Refeeding syndrome. In: *Frequently Overlooked Diagnoses in Acute Care.* Philadelphia: Hanley and Belfus, 2003, 79–83.

Marinella MA, Burdette SD. Hypokalemia-induced QT interval prolongation. *J Emerg Med* 2000;19:375–376.

Subramanian R, Khador R. Severe hypophosphatemia: pathophysiologic implications, clinical presentations, and treatment. *Medicine (Baltimore)* 2000;79:1–8.

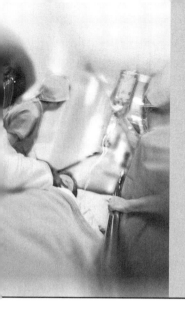

47

Diabetes Insipidus

DEFINITION

Diabetes insipidus (DI) is characterized by the copious output of dilute urine and may result from decreased or absent secretion of antidiuretic hormone (ADH) [central DI] or resistance of the renal tubules to ADH (nephrogenic DI).

CLINICAL SETTING

The cancer patient who develops DI often suffers from hypothalamic-pituitary metastasis from a solid neoplasm, although neurosurgical procedures and renal pathology are also relatively common etiologies of DI in this population.

PATHOGENESIS

The hallmark of DI is the inability to conserve free water that results from absence of ADH or renal tubular insensitivity to ADH. Vasopressin, or ADH, is synthesized in the hypothalamus and is transported along a neural plexus to the the posterior pituitary gland where it is stored and released in response to a decreased effective circulating arterial volume or an increase in serum osmolality. When plasma osmolality exceeds a threshold of approximately 295 mosm/kg, the thirst mechanism is triggered which causes the individual to seek water. Patients with central DI produce scant or no ADH, therefore the renal collecting duct is unable to resorb water which results in excretion of large amounts of very dilute urine and polyuria. Normally, patients with adequate access to water do not have pathologic increases in serum osmolality or sodium. Patients with confusion, dementia, critical illness, or those receiving narcotics or mechanical ventilation may not be able to seek out free water and thus may be at risk for life-threatening hypernatremia and hypovolemic shock. There are several potential etiologies of central DI in the oncology population, which will be discussed in the following text. Generally, however, any insult to the hypothalamus or pituitary due to neoplasm, surgery, or hemorrhage can damage the cells that produce ADH or interrupt the neurogenic transport mechanism to the posterior pituitary, ultimately culminating in central DI. Interestingly, metastatic tumors have a propensity for the posterior pituitary since this part of the gland receives blood supply from the systemic arterial circulation. Also, the posterior pituitary lies in proximity to the dura mater explaining invasion from contiguous tumor in local bone. Rare cases of central DI have been reported with acute myeloid leukemia associated with cytogenetic abnormalities of chromosomes 7 or 3q21q26, although the pathogenic mechanisms remain to be fully elucidated.

Nephrogenic DI occurs in the presence of normal hypothalamic-pituitary secretion of ADH when the collecting ducts in the kidney are unresponsive to the action of ADH due to renal or genitourinary pathology or certain medications. Acquired nephrogenic DI affects cancer patients by many pathogenic mechanisms. Hypokalemia due to diuretic therapy, chemotherapy-induced vomiting or diarrhea, or nasogastric suction can result in nephrogenic DI due to an acquired concentrating defect that is reversible with potassium replacement. Hypercalcemia is common in the cancer population and can induce nephrogenic DI via interstitial calcification and fibrosis which disrupts the renal concentrating mechanism. Chronic urinary tract obstruction can result in nephrogenic DI by a similar mechanism. The most relevant etiologies of drug-induced nephrogenic DI in the cancer population include demeclocycline, a tetracycline analogue used for the treatment of chronic SIADH, and amphotericin B, a nephrotoxic antifungal commonly utilized in leukemic patients with life-threatening fungal infections.

ETIOLOGY

Diabetes insipidus has many potential etiologies in the cancer patient and is best approached by considering central DI and nephrogenic DI separately:

- Central DI
  - Metastatic deposit to the hypothalamus or posterior pituitary
    - Breast and lung cancer most common etiologies of metastatic-induced central DI
    - Carcinomas of the stomach, colon, small bowel, pancreas, prostate, kidney, and thyroid on occasion
    - Melanoma
    - Lymphoma
  - Primary brain tumor with local invasion
    - Craniopharyngioma
    - Astrocytoma

- Oligodendroglioma
- Meningioma
- Acute myelogenous leukemia
  - Associated with chromosomal abnormalities involving 3q21q26 or monosomy 7
  - Leukemic infiltration of hypothalamus or posterior pituitary
- Pituitary surgery
- Severe hypotension with ischemic damage
- Intracerebral hemorrhage
  - In the cancer patient etiologies include hemorrhagic brain metastasis, disseminated intravascular coagulation (DIC), severe thrombocytopenia, acute promyelocytic leukemia, or L-asparaginase
- Radiation therapy of brain parenchyma
- Bacterial or fungal meningitis
- Viral encephalitis
- Nephrogenic DI
  - Hypokalemia
  - Hypercalcemia
  - Urinary tract obstruction/hydronephrosis
  - Chronic renal failure
  - Polycytic kidney disease
  - Drugs
    - Cisplatinum
    - Amphotericin B, gentamicin, demeclocycline
    - Lithium
    - Methoxyflurane

Symptoms and Signs

Many patients may not volunteer symptoms of thirst and increased urine output unless directly questioned. Perhaps most importantly, the clinician should monitor urine output in the hospitalized patient, especially in patients with altered mental status. Symptoms and signs directly attributable to DI of any etiology include:

- Polyuria
  - More than 3 liters of urine output in a 24-hour period, although some patients can urinate more than 10 liters daily
  - Urine is very dilute and colorless
- Thirst
- Polydypsia
- Weight loss
- Anorexia
- Weakness
- Dizziness
- Confusion, somnolence, coma, or seizures, if hypernatremia occurs

DIAGNOSTIC STUDIES

The diagnosis of DI requires a very high index of suspicion and should be suspected in any cancer patient with excessive thirst, polydypsia, polyuria, or hypernatremia. The most useful diagnostic studies include:

- Serum electrolytes
  - May be normal, but hypernatremia present if free-water deficit supervenes
  - Hypokalemia or hypomagnesemia may occur with chronic DI due to medullary wash-out of electrolytes
  - Hypercalcemia can be etiology of nephrogenic DI
- Water deprivation test
  - Diagnostic test of choice in equivocal cases of DI which entails withholding all fluid intake until sufficient volume depletion serves as stimulus for ADH secretion; needs to be performed in the hospital under meticulous monitoring of weight, electrolytes, and vital signs, as severe hypernatremia and hypovolemic shock can result
    - During water deprivation, hourly measurements of body weight, serum osmolality, and urine osmolality performed until three consecutive measurements of osmolality plateau and/or a 5% body weight decline occurs
    - This is followed by administration of 1 mg of intravenous or 10 units of intranasal 1-deamino-8-d-arginine vasopressin (DDAVP)
      - In central DI, urine osmolality increases by more than 50% and indicates a favorable response to pharmacologic replacement with DDAVP
      - In nephrogenic DI, the urine osmolality shows little increase with DDAVP, typically less than 50%
- Urine osmolality
  - Urine osmolality <200 mosm/kg in setting of polyuria supports diagnosis of central or nephrogenic DI
- Magnetic resonance imaging hypothalamus and pituitary gland
  - May reveal tumor deposit or infiltration

TREATMENT

Treatment of DI in the setting of acute illness with associated hypernatremia and volume depletion requires administration of isotonic fluids initially to restore intravascular volume, followed by hypotonic fluids once the patient is hemodynamically stable. Treatment of precipitating causes such as hypokalemia, hypercalcemia, urinary obstruction, or malignancy is also important. If central DI is present, administration of 10 mg of intranasal DDAVP at bedtime (typically one squirt) is quite effective. An additional dose can be given if necessary. Chlorpropramide, carbemazepine, or clofibrate are alternatives if DDAVP is not available or intolerable. Nephrogenic DI does not respond to DDAVP but may respond to thiazide diuretics by decreasing distal tubular absorption of sodium and chloride which allows the proximal tubules to absorb more sodium and water thereby decreasing renal free-water loss.

PROGNOSIS

The critically ill cancer patient with DI who develops severe hypernatremia has a poor prognosis, especially if multi-organ dysfunction or widespread metastatic disease is present. If central DI is not recognized and treated, patients may develop severe hypernatremia with neurologic injury as well as refractory hypovolemic shock, which can be fatal. Long-term survival has been reported in patients with central DI due to chemotherapy-sensitive metastatic neoplasms such as breast cancer with concurrent DDAVP replacement and treatment of the cancer with chemotherapy and/or radiation.

ADDITIONAL READING

Keung YK, Buss D, Powell BL, et al. Central diabetes insipidus and inv(3)(q21q26) and monosomy 7 in acute myeloid leukemia. *Cancer Genet Cytogenet*

Komninos J, Vlassopoulou V, Protopapa D, et al. Tumors metastatic to the pituitary gland: case report and literature review. *J Clin Endocrinol Metab* 2004; 89:574–580.

Makaryus AN, McFarlane SI. Diabetes insipidus: diagnosis and treatment of a complex disease. *Cleve Clin J Med* 2006;73:65–71.

Robertson GL. Antidiuretic hormone: normal and disordered function. *Endocrinol Metabl Clin N Am* 2001;30:671–694.

ten Bokkel Huinink D, Veltman GAM, Huizinga TWJ, et al. Diabetes insipidus in metastatic cancer: two case reports with review of the literature. *Ann Oncol* 2000;11:891–895.

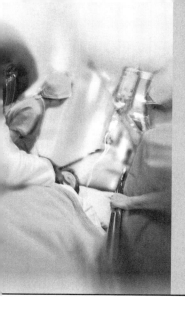

48

Lactic Acidosis

DEFINITION

Lactic acidosis (LA) occurs when lactic acid is pathologically generated resulting in metabolic acidosis and, if severe, shock and death. Two types of LA exist: type A which occurs with severe tissue hypoxia and type B when associated with other diseases, including malignancy, in the absence of hemodynamic embarrassment.

CLINICAL SETTING

Lactic acidosis occurring in the cancer patient typically complicates severe hypoxia and septic shock (type A), although type B LA can occur in the setting of widespread liver metastases or as a unique complication of hematopoietic neoplasms.

PATHOGENESIS

Lactic acid represents the reduced form of pyruvic acid that is generated from the metabolism of glucose during glycolysis. In the presence of adequate tissue oxygenization, the majority of pyruvic acid is metabolized within mitochondria to carbon dioxide and water. However, in the setting of severe tissue hypoxia that often complicates various shock syndromes (e.g., cardiogenic, septic, hemorrhagic shock), the majority of pyruvic acid is converted into LA resulting in a high anion gap metabolic acidosis (type A LA). Other pathogenic mechanisms of type A LA include poor tissue oxygenation from profound anemia or mitochondrial respiratory chain paralysis due to carbon monoxide or cyanide. Type B LA occurs in the absence of overt tissue hypoxia and has been associated with myriad disorders such as diabetes mellitus, renal or liver failure, various drugs, as well as solid tumors and hematopoetic cancers. With regards to type B LA associated with malignancy, a significant number of cases have been reported in the setting of extensive hepatic metastases which is thought to impair LA disposal resulting in significant accumulation and subsequent acidosis. Renal failure may contribute to elevated LA levels due to decreased elimination. Another mechanism of malignancy-associated type B LA is the conversion of glucose to lactic acid by tumor cells exhibiting a high rate of glycolysis (such as hematopoietic neoplasms). Some tumor cells have been demonstrated to express hexokinase which results in increased rates of glycolysis and increased glucose shunting to LA generation. Tumor necrosis factor (TNF) released by the tumor, as well as thiamine deficiency, impairs function of pyruvate dehydrogenase resulting in increased anaerobic metabolism and lactate generation. Methotrexate may induce type B LA by competing with thiamine metabolism and reducing thiamine availability thereby precipitating LA. Resolution of LA with chemotherapy and reappearance of LA with disease recurrence has been observed in several patients with various leukemias and lymphomas. Supportive of neoplastic cellular production of LA is the normalization of serum lactate with chemotherapy in some patients. A final mechanism of LA is so-called D-lactic acidosis which typically occurs in patients with high-grade bowel obstruction or who have had a prior intestinal bypass procedure. The mechanism of D-lactic acidosis is intestinal bacterial production of D-lactate that is absorbed into the bloodstream but not metabolized by the enzyme L-lactate dehydrogenase normally present in the liver.

ETIOLOGY

The etiologies of LA in the cancer patient can be approached by considering those cases due to type A or type B pathogenesis:

- Type A
  - Shock states: septic, cardiogenic, hemorrhagic, hypovolemic, obstructive, or anaphylactic shock
  - Severe anemia
- Type B
  - Acute lymphoblastic or myelogenous leukemia
  - Non-Hodgkin's lymphoma
    - Can occur with any subtype, but more commonly complicates high-grade lymphomas such as Burkitt's or diffuse large cell
  - Chronic lymphocytic leukemia
  - Metastatic breast cancer
  - Extensive stage small cell lung cancer
  - Liver or renal failure
  - Human immunodeficiency virus infection
  - Drugs
    - Metformin
    - Aspirin

- Isoniazid
- Nucleoside reverse transcriptase inhibitors

SYMPTOMS AND SIGNS

Diagnosis of type B LA requires a high index of suspicion and should be considered in any cancer patient with metabolic acidosis and increased serum lactate but without evidence of hypoxia or shock (e.g., type A LA). Symptoms and signs are non-specific but include:

- Confusion/delirium
- Hyperventilation
- Nausea/vomiting
- Anorexia
- Tachypnea
- Seizures
- Coma

DIAGNOSTIC STUDIES

Diagnosis of LA requires first identifying the presence of metabolic acidosis, with subsequent laboratory studies as indicated:

- Serum electrolytes
  - Increased anion gap metabolic acidosis and hypobicarbonatemia
  - Occasional patients can have a normal anion gap despite LA
- Arterial blood lactate level
- Arterial blood gases
  - Typically reveals metabolic acidosis with respiratory compensation and normal PO_2
- Complete blood count
  - Useful if acute leukemia is suspected as etiology of type B LA
- Lactate dehydrogenase
  - May be significantly increased due to tumor burden or hepatic metastases
- Computed tomographic scanning
  - If metastatic malignancy is suspected with attention to lungs and liver
- Mammography in female with unexplained lactic acidosis may reveal breast cancer

TREATMENT

Treatment of type A LA generally entails providing adequate oxygenation, hemo-dynamic support, and correction of severe anemia. These are all measures aimed at increasing tissue perfusion and oxygenation. Type B LA due to leukemia or lymphoma should be treated with chemotherapy. Treatment of metastatic tumors that are chemotherapy-sensitive such as small cell lung cancer or breast cancer should be considered. Some authors recommend thiamine administration for type B LA associated with malignancy, although data is limited. If acidosis is severe, intravenous sodium bicarbonate may be necessary before the source of lactate production is controlled by anti-cancer therapy.

PROGNOSIS

Type A LA due to refractory septic or cardiogenic shock carries a high mortality rate in the cancer patient. Type B LA due to acute leukemia or lymphoma is frequently fatal, although some patients may respond to aggressive chemotherapy.

ADDITIONAL READING

Field M, Block JB, Levin R, et al. Significance of blood lactate elevations among patients with acute leukemia and other neoplastic disorders. *Am J Med* 1966; 40:528–535.

Friedenberg AS, Brandoff DE, Schiffman FJ. Type B lactic acidosis as a severe metabolic complication in lymphoma and leukemia. A case series from a single institution and literature review. *Medicine (Baltimore)* 2007;86:225–232.

Luft D, Deichsel G, Schmulling RM, et al. Definition of clinically relevant lactic acidosis in patients with internal diseases. *Am J Clin Pathol* 1983;80:484–489.

Schulier JP, Nicasie C, Klasteresky J. Lactic acidosis. A metabolic complication of extensive metastatic disease. *Eur J Cancer Clin Oncol* 1983;19:597–601.

Warner E. *Type B lactic acidosis and metastatic breast cancer. 1992;24:75–79.*

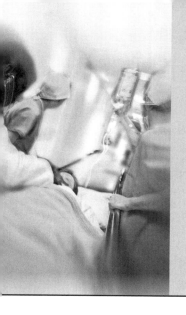

49

Hyper-ammonemia

DEFINITION

Hyperammonemia (HA) in the cancer population is a complex phenomenon defined by elevated serum ammonia levels leading to metabolic encephalopathy and, if not recognized and treated, cerebral edema and death.

CLINICAL SETTING

Although HA in the cancer patient can occur in the setting of severe hepatic dysfunction from underlying cirrhosis or extensive hepatic metastases, it may also develop as a unique complication in patients with hematopoietic malignancies or from the administration of certain medications.

PATHOGENESIS

Ammonia is primarily produced within the gut, with muscle and kidney contributing small amounts to the total body load. Within the gut lumen, ammonia is generated by protein digestion and by certain bacterial species. Severe infections in the neutropenic patient with hematopoietic malignancy may result in HA due to organisms that possess urease or other ammonia-generating enzymes. Ammonia is produced from glutamine within the proximal renal tubules and functions to maintain acid-base homeostasis. Ammonia can also be generated within skeletal muscle during prolonged seizure activity that may occur in the patient with brain tumors or metastasis. The metabolism of endogenously synthesized ammonia occurs within the liver through entry into the urea cycle where it is ultimately metabolized to urea for renal excretion. The urea cycle is a complex cycle consisting of various enzymes including carbamyl phosphate synthetase, arginosuccinate synthetase, and arginase. When the ability of the liver is severely impaired due to underlying cirrhosis or extensive parenchymal neoplasia, increased ammonia generation from any mechanism leads to elevated serum levels and pathologic HA. Gastrointestinal bleeding increases gut ammonia load, which may result in HA in patients with underlying liver dysfunction. Leukemia and myeloma cells may also synthesize ammonia in quantities high enough to cause HA.

The most significant pathophysiologic derangement of HA is cerebral dysfunction resulting from cerebral edema. When ammonia levels increase within the brain, astrocytes metabolize ammonia to glutamine resulting in increased intracellular osmolarity and neuronal swelling and cell death. The injured and swollen astrocytes subsequently release inflammatory cytokines such as tumor necrosis factor (TNF) and interleukins-1 and -6 causing further neuronal cell dysfunction and astrocyte loss via apoptosis. Additionally, elevated astrocyte ammonia levels paralyze Kreb's cycle function resulting in impaired cellular energetics. Increased cerebral blood flow contributes to cerebral edema and when ammonia levels exceed 200 μmol/L, seizures and brain herniation may ensue.

Two unique mechanisms of HA in the cancer patient include administration of the chemotherapeutic agents L-asparaginase and 5-fluorouracil, although high doses of chemotherapy utilized in preparation for hematopoietic stem cell transplantation have also been implicated. The mechanism of chemotherapy-associated HA is unknown but may result from inhibition of enzymes within the urea cycle or increased ammonia production from tissue breakdown and mucositis.

ETIOLOGY

The etiologies of HA in the cancer patient can be considered in the context of whether severe liver disease is present or whether another mechanism is responsible:

- Hepatic parenchymal dysfunction
  - Cirrhotic liver disease
  - Extensive tumor replacement with primary or metastatic neoplasm
- Gastrointestinal hemorrhage (especially if liver dysfunction is present)
- Infection in setting of hematologic malignancy and neutropenia
- Seizures or *status epilepticus*
- Increased protein loading
  - Total parenteral nutrition
  - Tube feedings
- Hematopoietic stem cell transplantation with high-dose chemotherapy
- Hematopoietic neoplasms
  - Acute leukemia
  - Chronic myelomonocytic leukemia
  - Multiple myeloma
- Drugs
  - Valproic acid
  - High-dose corticosteroids

- ○ Chemotherapeutic agents
  - ▪ L-asparaginase, 5-fluorouracil

Symptoms and Signs

The diagnosis of HA requires a high index of suspicion, as symptoms and signs are not specific and can easily be attributed to other diverse causes in this population. The most common clinical findings include:

- Confusion
- Lethargy
- Vomiting
- Hyperventilation (compensatory response to HA)
- Ataxia
- Seizures
- Tachypnea
- Asterixis
- Dysmetria
- Hyperreflexia/clonus
- Coma

Diagnostic Studies

Diagnosis of HA requires laboratory confirmation, with ancillary studies as indicated. Those ancillary studies include:

- Serum ammonia (arterial source optimal)
  - ○ Levels above 200 µnol/L constitute a true emergency due to risk of cerebral herniation
- Arterial blood gas
  - ○ Typically reveals compensatory respiratory alkalosis
  - ○ Metabolic acidosis may complicate some cases
- Liver function tests
  - ○ May indicate underlying hepatic dysfunction, but typically normal in other cases
- Coagulation studies
  - ○ May indicate underlying liver dysfunction
- Complete blood count
  - ○ Helpful if hematopoietic malignancy is suspected
- Serum protein electrophoresis if myeloma suspected

Treatment

Treatment of HA requires general and specific measures which depend on the etiology. General supportive measures such as protein restriction and airway protection with intubation and mechanical ventilation may be necessary if the patient is comatose or agitated. If increased intracranial pressure with cerebral edema or impending herniation is present, administration of mannitol and induced hyperventilation should be considered, as well as neurosurgical consultation for possible insertion of an intracranial pressure monitor or surgical decompression. Induced hypothermia has been advocated by some authors as it has been shown to decrease free radical production, decrease astrocyte swelling, and improve cerebral blood flow parameters. Prophylactic anti-seizure medications may be considered in severe cases. Administration of lactulose orally or via a nasogastric tube may aid in decreasing the bacterial load of ammonia, but may not be helpful in cases of HA resulting from hematopoietic malignancies or chemotherapy. Hemodialysis or continuous venovenous hemofiltration (CVVH) has been suggested for non-liver failure associated cases of HA. Intravenous L-carnitine has been utilized in the setting of HA complicating hematopoietic stem cell transplantion because of the favorable effects on mitochondrial respiration and increased ureagenesis. Hyperammonemia due to multiple myeloma has been successfully treated with chemotherapy.

PROGNOSIS

Severe HA with cerebral edema and herniation carries a high mortality rate because of tonsillar herniation and cardiorespiratory arrest. Patients who develop HA following hematopoietic stem cell transplantation have a reported mortality of 70% to 80%. Patients with HA resulting from severe liver impairment due to extensive metastatic disease have an extremely high mortality rate. However, if mild to moderate HA develops as a consequence of chemotherapy or a chemotherapy-sensitive hematopoietic cancer, recovery often ensues with discontinuation of the offending drug or treatment of the primary disease, respectively.

ADDITIONAL READING

Clay AS, Hainline BE. Hyperammonemia in the ICU. *Chest* 2007;132: 1368–1378.

Frere P, Canivet JL, Gennigens C, et al. Hyperammonemia after high-dose chemotherapy and stem cell transplantation. *Bone Marrow Transplant* 2000; 26:343–345.

Kim YA, Chung HC, Choi HJ, et al. Intermediate dose 5-fluorouracil-induced encephalopathy. *Jpn J Clin Oncol* 2006;36:55–59.

Mitchell RB, Wagner JE, Karp JE, et al. Syndrome of idiopathic hyperammonemia after high-dose chemotherapy. *Am J Med* 1988;85:662–667.

Shah AS, Shetty N, Jaiswal S, et al. Hyperammonemia: an unusual presenting feature of multiple myeloma. *Indian J Med Sci* 2005;59:24–27.

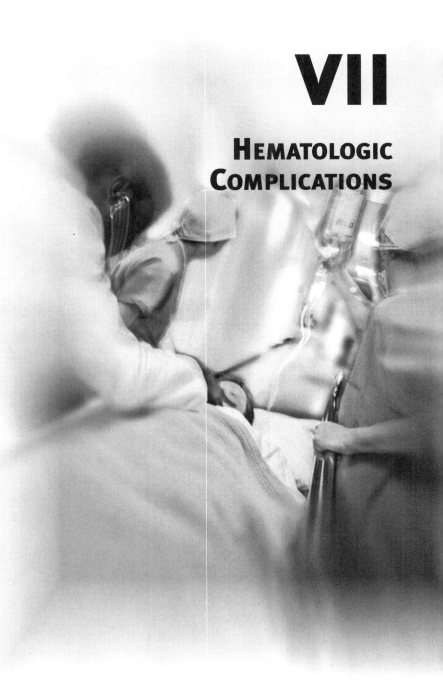

VII

HEMATOLOGIC COMPLICATIONS

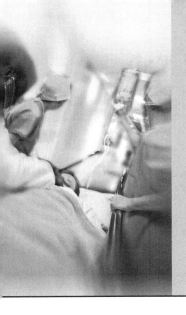

50

Disseminated Intravascular Coagulation

DEFINITION

Disseminated intravascular coagulation (DIC) is a clinical syndrome that may complicate a variety of disorders. It is characterized by widespread activation of the coagulation cascade resulting in the intravascular deposition of fibrin, with subsequent occlusion of small and medium size blood vessels. Simultaneous consumption of clotting factors and platelets may result in a bleeding diathesis.

CLINICAL SETTING

The presence of DIC virtually always accompanies an underlying infectious, traumatic, inflammatory, or neoplastic process, all of which have the ability to activate the coagulation cascade by various cytokines.

PATHOGENESIS

The pathogenesis of DIC is complex, and an in-depth discussion is beyond the scope of this text; however, salient pathogenic features as related to the cancer patient will be discussed. Although the end result of DIC is ischemic damage to various organs resulting from microvascular thrombi or, less commonly, diffuse hemorrhage resulting from consumption of various procoagulant proteins and activation of fibrinolysis, the pathogenesis of DIC is similar regardless of the etiology. Triggering events of DIC such as sepsis, obstetrical catastrophes, multiple trauma, transfusion reactions, or malignancy result in the release of various cytokines including tumor necrosis factor (TNF), interleukin (IL)-1, and IL-6, as well as tissue factor, which serve as initiators of the endogenous coagulation cascade. The generation of thrombin, and subsequently fibrin, plays a central role in the pathogenesis of DIC.

Thrombin generation is typically related to the activation of the extrinsic coagulation pathway from an interaction between tissue factor and factor VIIa, which eventually leads to the generation of thrombin and fibrin via the common coagulation pathway. Simultaneous expression of endogenous anticoagulation mediators and impaired fibrinolysis also contribute to the phenotype of DIC. The source of tissue factor often results from exposure to neoplastic cells, obstetrical fluids and tissues, fat emboli from long bone fracture, or mononuclear cell expression of tissue factor in response to pro-inflammatory cytokines. Various triggers of cytokine production such as tissue trauma, infection, and neoplastic cells, are key to the development of DIC, with IL-6 playing a central role. Sepsis and bacterial infection remain the most common etiology of DIC in the cancer population, and most often occur in response to Gram-negative infection, although Gram-positive, viral, and fungal organisms may act as precipitants in many cases. Cell membrane components of microorganisms, such as lipopolysaccharide or endotoxin, or the release of bacterial exotoxins induce activation of the cytokine network, culminating in coagulation activation as previously described. Solid tumors and hematologic malignancies can also precipitate DIC, with as many as 15% of patients with metastatic cancer exhibiting evidence of DIC. Tissue factor on exposed tumor cells or a cancer procoagulant may serve as triggers for thrombin generation in cases of solid tumors. A unique type of DIC is often encountered in patients with acute promyelocytic leukemia due to the intracellular granules that stimulate fibrinolysis, which may lead to fatal bleeding, although some patients may suffer from thrombosis.

Whether the clinical phenotype of DIC is end-organ ischemia (e.g., brain, heart, kidney, gastrointestinal tract) or diffuse bleeding depends on whether widespread activation of coagulation or fibrinolysis is predominant, although both mechanisms may be present. Most cases of DIC encountered in practice follow a thrombotic-ischemic phenotype, although a bleeding diasthesis should be suspected with bleeding from mucosal or venipuncture sites. All of the major anticoagulant proteins are affected including the most vital anticoagulant antithrombin III, which is often severely depleted. Dysfunction of the protein C system also is important in the pathogenesis of DIC with depressed levels of activated protein C (which may have therapeutic implications) and free protein S contributing to the thrombotic response. Activated protein C is an endogenous protein which enhances fibrinolysis and inhibits inflammation and vascular thrombosis. It is a key modulator of the coagualation and inflammatory events present in severe sepsis. Protein C is the precursor to activated protein C and reduced levels correlate with increased risk of death in patients with sepsis. Elevated plasma levels of plasminogen-activator inhibitor type 1 (PAI-1), which leads to impaired fibrinolysis and fibrin degradation, also contributes to the thrombotic tendency. Given the significant load of fibrin within the vasculature, endogenous plasmin results in generation of fibrin degradation products (FDPs), the presence of which are diagnostically useful. Thrombocytopenia is common in DIC and results from platelet consumption within the microvasculature and may contribute to bleeding. A unique form of severe

DIC known as *purpura fulminans* may complicate widespread carcinoma or septic shock. It is characterized by massive cutaneous hemorrhage with necrosis of the acral areas or limbs, and carries a very high mortality rate. Some patients may experience adrenal failure and shock due to ischemic infarction or adrenal parenchymal hemorrhage.

Etiology

The development of DIC virtually always occurs in the setting of a significant systemic process and is not a diagnosis in-and-of-itself. The cancer population possesses many risks for development of DIC, of which include:

- Infection/sepsis
  - Bacterial: Gram-positive or -negative bacteria
  - Asplenism resulting from splenectomy, splenic irradiation, or malignancy
    - *S. pneumoniae, N. meningiditis, H. influenza, Babesia microti, Vibrio vulnificus, Capnocytophaga* species
  - Viruses
  - Fungal organisms
- Malignancy
  - Adenocarcinoma
    - Prostate, pancreas, lung, ovary, gastric, colorectal
  - Myeloproliferative disorders
  - Brain tumors/gliomas
  - Acute myelogenous and acute promyelocytic leukemia
- L-asparaginase
- Major transfusion reaction with ABO incompatible blood group
- Fat or marrow embolism
  - May occur in the setting of pathologic long bone fracture
- Severe acute pancreatitis
  - May occur due to biliary obstruction, pancreatic metastasis, or chemotherapy

Symptoms and Signs

Many patients with malignancy may exhibit laboratory evidence of low-grade DIC and be asymptomatic. Typically, severe DIC is accompanied by myriad symptoms and signs depending on whether a thrombotic tendency (more common) or a hemorrhagic diasthesis is present and which organ systems are affected. Some of those symptoms and signs are:

- Fever
- Confusion
- Ecchymosis
- Mucosal bleeding
  - Epistaxis, gingival bleeding, hematemesis, melena, hematochezia, hematuria

- Bleeding from venipuncture sites or incisions
- Confusion
- Tachycardia
- Tachypnea
- Hypotension
- Digital gangrene or cutaneous necrotic lesions
  - In cases of *purpura fulminans*
- Symptoms and signs of venous thrombosis
  - Extremity swelling or dyspnea if extremity thrombosis or pulmonary embolism present
  - Headache if cerebral venous thrombosis present
- Symptoms and signs of arterial thrombosis
  - Focal weakness or parasthesia due to cerebral arterial thrombosis or embolism from marantic endocarditis
  - Acute arterial insufficiency of lower extremity with pain, parasthesia and pallor
  - Acute mesenteric ischemia with bowel infarction with severe abdominal pain and shock

DIAGNOSTIC STUDIES

The diagnosis of DIC requires a high index of suspicion and requires careful laboratory assessment since it may be confused with other hematologic disorders such as thrombotic thrombocytopenic purpura (TTP) and since there is no single diagnostic test. The diagnosis of DIC requires a compatible presentation occurring in a patient with an established clinical condition associated with DIC. The following laboratory studies are most helpful:

- Complete blood count
  - Thrombocytopenia
  - Anemia, often microangiopathic
  - Leukocytosis
- Peripheral blood smear
  - Typically reveals paucity of platelets as well as schistocytes and/or reticulocytes, although schistocytes not necessary to make the diagnosis of DIC
- Coagulation panel and associated factors
  - Prolonged prothrombin time (PT) and partial thromboplastin time (PTT)
  - Presence of FDPs and D-dimer
  - Hypofibrinogenemia
    - May be in normal range since fibrinogen is an acute-phase reactant
  - Low levels of antithrombin III, protein C, and the endotheial-derived clotting protein, factor VIII
- Organ biopsy (if diagnosis unclear)
  - Skin or renal biopsy often reveals intravascular, bland thrombi
- Specialized assays for soluble fibrin, fibrinopeptide A, or prothrombin activation fragments (not widely available)

TREATMENT

The overriding therapeutic principle of DIC is treatment of the underlying disorder. For example, treatment of sepsis/infection with abscess drainage or antibiotic therapy and chemotherapy for cases of malignancy. Treatment of DIC associated with acute promyelocytic leukemia requires therapy with all-trans retinoic acid (ATRA) and cytotoxic chemotherapy. Indeed, treatment of DIC and the coagulation derangements without targeting the precipitating illness is a futile endeavor. Patients with laboratory-only evidence of DIC do not require specific therapy. Patients who present with diffuse hemorrhage require platelet transfusions for severe thrombocytopenia and correction of coagulopathy with fresh frozen plasma and/or cryoprecipitate. Refractory, life-threatening hemorrhage not responding to transfusion therapy has been successfully treated with recombinant factor VIIa. Administration of low-dose infusional unfractionated heparin has been advocated by some authors in cases of *purpura fulminans* or significant end-organ ischemia since heparin binds antithrombin III thereby interrupting thrombin formation and fibrin deposition. However, despite this theoretical principle, caution must be exercised to avoid potentially fatal bleeding. Drotrecogin alfa (recombinant human activated protein C) by prolonged continuous infusion has been demonstrated to reduce mortality in patients with severe sepsis but may be problematic in cancer patients who are prone to bleeding from underlying illness, coagulopathy, thrombocytopenia, or chemotherapy.

PROGNOSIS

The prognosis of DIC varies depending on whether it is subclinical or fulminant. Prognosis of patients with only laboratory evidence of DIC depends upon the status and response to treatment of the underlying cancer. Patients with acute promyelocytic leukemia and DIC are at risk for fatal cerebral hemorrhage which remains the most common cause of early death with this disease. The prognosis of fulminant DIC or *purpura fulminans* associated with septic shock is very poor in patients with malignancy.

ADDITIONAL READING

Bernard GR, Vincetnt JL, Laterre PF, et al. Effficacy and safety of recombinant human activated protein C for severe sepsis. *N Engl J Med* 2001;344:699–709.

Davis MDP, Dy KM, Nelson S. Presentation and outcome of purpura fulminans associated with peripheral gangrene in 12 patients at the Mayo Clinic. *J Am Acad Dermatol* 2007;57:944–956.

Frewin R, Henson A, Provan D. ABC of clinical haematology: Haematological emergencies. *BMJ* 1997;314:1333–1336.

Levi M, Ten Cate H. Disseminated intravascular coagulation. *N Engl J Med* 1999;341:586–592.

Nolan J, Sinclair R. Review and management of purpura fulminans and two case reports. *Br J Anaesth* 2001;86:581–586.

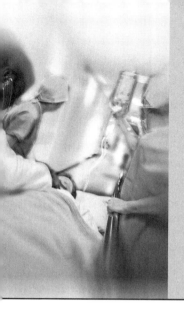

51

Thrombotic Thrombo- cytopenic Purpura

DEFINITION

Thrombotic thrombocytopenic purpura (TTP) is a thrombotic microangiopathy characterized by microangiopathic hemolytic anemia (MAHA) and thrombocytopenia with widespread microvascular thrombi leading to ischemic damage of various organ systems.

CLINICAL SETTING

The cancer population may develop TTP from a variety of mechanisms but most often occurs in the setting of certain chemotherapeutic agents or disseminated malignancy.

PATHOGENESIS

The pathogenesis of TTP is complex and only the acquired form will be discussed in this text as it relates to the oncology population. The classic pentad of clinical findings of TTP consists of MAHA, thrombocytopenia, fever, renal abnormalities, and neurologic dysfunction, which result from widespread microvascular thrombosis, organ ischemia, and cytokine activation. The microthrombi consist of little or no fibrin (as opposed to DIC) and consist of platelet aggregates and large amounts of von Willebrand factor. The formation of microvascular thrombi results from the interaction of large amounts of von Willebrand factor that reacts with circulating platelets resulting in the formation of disseminated platelet-rich thrombi. These thrombi occlude the microvasculature or various organs, including the brain, intestinal tract, and kidneys, and give rise to the protean manifestations of TTP such as stroke, mesenteric infarction, and renal failure, respectively. Acquired TTP is typically mediated by deficiency of a von Willebrand factor-cleaving protease known as ADAMTS-13 (an acronym for "a disintegrin-like and metalloprotease with thrombospondin type 1 motif, member 13"). This ADAMTS-13 protease normally cleaves the newly synthesized large von Willebrand factor multimers that are secreted by the vascular endotheial cells. If acquired deficiency of ADAMTS-13 develops, which may be idiopathic or associated with cancer or various cancer treatments, then the large multimers are not cleaved, resulting in increased levels of abnormally large circulating multimers that have a propensity to bind to the platelet glycoprotein Ib-IX-V receptors for von Willebrand factor and form microthrombi characteristic of TTP. Other mechanisms for development of TTP in malignancy include damage to the endothelium which enhances the release of large von Willebrand factor. Patients with disseminated malignancies may exhibit circulating large multimers or have decreased ADAMTS-13 activity.

Microthrombi occlude small vessels leading to ischemic necrosis of various organs including brain, myocardium, kidney, pancreas, adrenal glands, and the gastrointestinal tract. Because of this, life-threatening complications of cerebral infarction, myocardial infarction, renal failure, pancreatitis, acute adrenal failure, or gastrointestinal perforation can occur. Tissue ischemia and necrosis results in the release of lactate dehydrogenase (LDH) into the bloodstream, which often reaches very high levels and is useful for diagnosis of TTP. Microangiopathic hemolytic anemia results from damage to the erythrocyte during passage through the fibrin-occluded microvasculature. Thrombocytopenia results from the entrapment of platelets within the von Willebrand multimer complexes, although on rare occasion, disseminated intravascular coagulation (DIC) can occur when severe tissue injury is present.

ETIOLOGY

The etiology of TTP in the cancer patient may be idiopathic but is often related to the underlying disease or treatment. Some of the reported etiologies of TTP in the oncologic population include:

- Malignancy
  - Metastatic adenocarcinoma (most often gastric or prostate), hematopoietic cancers
- Allogenic bone marrow transplantation
  - May be related to endothelial damage from high-dose conditioning chemotherapy or total body irradiation
- Solid organ transplantation
  - Especially with use of cyclosporine or tacrolimus
- Total body irradiation
- Infection with *E. coli* 0157:H7
- Surgical procedures/post-operative state

- Chemotherapeutic and anti-cancer agents
  - Mitomycin-C, cisplatinum, gemcitabine, bleomycin, pentostatin
  - Bevacizumab
- Miscellaneous drugs
  - Quinine (may include tonic water), ticlopidine, clopidigrel

Symptoms and Signs

The clinical manifestations of TTP are often protean and related to underlying organ dysfunction resulting from tissue ischemia. This can make the diagnosis challenging and easily overlooked. The most commonly encountered findings include:

- Fever
  - Rigors or high fever ($>102\,°F$ argues against TTP and favors sepsis)
- Weakness (may result from fever or anemia)
- Mucosal bleeding
  - Epistaxis, gingival bleeding, hematemesis, melena
- Nausea/vomiting
- Chest pain
  - May be anginal in nature if coronary vascular occlusion present
- Dyspnea
- Ecchymosis/purpura
- Hematuria
- Abdominal pain
  - May result from gastric ulceration, pancreatitis, bowel ischemia, or perforated viscus
- Neurologic symptoms and signs (may be fluctuating)
  - Delirium/somnolence
  - Seizures
  - Focal deficits

Diagnostic Studies

Diagnosis of TTP requires a high index of suspicion and prompt hematologic laboratory evalution which should include:

- Complete blood count
  - Thrombocytopenia
  - Anemia
  - Elevated reticulocyte count
  - Leukocytosis
- Peripheral blood smear
  - Schistocytes (typically on every microscopic field) are sine qua non of TTP
  - Polychromasia
  - Paucity of platelets

- Coombs' antibody test
  - Should be negative with TTP
- Coagulation studies and associated factors
  - Normal prothombin time (PT) and partial thromboplastin time (PTT); elevation of PT or PTT supports other diagnosis such as disseminated intravascular coagulation (DIC)
- Serum chemistries
  - Elevated lactate dehydrogenase (LDH) can be very high and reflect red cell hemolysis and tissue ischemia; if LDH normal, diagnosis of TTP should be questioned
  - Increased blood urea nitrogen and creatinine if renal failure present
  - Hyperamylasemia if pancreatitis or small bowel ischemia present
- Serum level of ADAMTS-13
  - May be decreased, but lack of sensitivity and prolonged turnaround time to obtain result make assay of limited value in acute setting
- Urinalysis
  - Hematuria and proteinuria common even with normal renal function

TREATMENT

Without timely intervention, TTP from any etiology carries a high mortality rate. Therefore, a high index of suspicion is needed in any patient presenting with MAHA and thrombocytopenia, as treatment for TTP can be instituted if these two elements of the pentad are present without other explanation. Although supportive care, which often includes intensive care unit management, is important, the cornerstone of TTP management is prompt institution of therapeutic plasma exchange (TPE) via a large bore central venous catheter. The performance of TPE includes extracorporeal removal of 1-1.5 times the plasma volume and infusion of replacement fresh frozen plasma. The success of TPE may relate to removal of autoantibodies to ADAMTS-13, replacement of a vital factor with plasma infusion, or both. However, some authors question the benefit of TPE for chemotherapy-related TTP. Plasma exchange is typically performed daily until the hematocrit, platelet count and LDH stabilize. Close monitoring for complications of TPE should be performed which can include hypocalcemia from plasma infusion, catheter related thrombosis, and sepsis. Platelet transfusions are contraindicated (unless life-threatening hemorrhage is present) due to the increased risk of enhanced organ ischemia and death. Many authors recommend supplemental corticosteroids, but this may increase the risk for complications in the ill cancer patient. Refractory cases may benefit from treatment with rituximab, cyclophosphamide, or vincristine, although data is limited. Splenectomy may be useful as a last resort if other treatments prove ineffective. Finally, if the TTP was triggered by a neoplasm, treatment of the underlying process may be beneficial. Also, discontinuation of any inciting drug is vital.

Prognosis

Untreated, TTP carries a mortality rate approaching 90%, but with timely TPE mortality rates in selected patients are lower than 10%. The prognosis of TTP in the oncology population depends upon many factors including the status of the underlying malignancy, chemotherapy-induced cytopenia, and the ability to tolerate TPE. Often, TTP occurs in the terminal stages of cancer. However, if the underlying neoplasm is controlled, outcomes may be similar to patients with idiopathic TTP, although solid data are lacking in this area.

Additional Reading

Burns ER, Lou Y, Pathak A. Morphologic diagnosis of thrombotic thrombocytopenic purpura. *Am J Hematol* 2004;75:18–21.

Frangie C, LeFaucheur C, Medioni J, et al. Renal thrombotic microangiopathy caused by anti-VEGF-antibody treatment for metastatic renal cell carcinoma. *Lancet Oncol* 2007;8:177–178.

George JN. How I treat patients with thrombotic thrombocytopenic purpura-hemolytic uremic syndrome. *Blood* 2000;96:1223–1229.

George JN. Thrombotic thrombocytopenic purpura. *N Engl J Med* 2006; 354:1927–1935.

Moake JL. Thrombotic microangiopathies. *N Engl J Med* 2002;347:589–600.

Murgo AL. Thrombotic microangiopathy in the cancer patient including those induced by chemotherapeutic agents. *Semin Hematol* 1987;24:161–177.

Otrock ZK, Taher AT, Makarem JA, et al. Thrombotic thrombocytopenic purpura and bone marrow necrosis associated with disseminated gastric cancer. *Dig Dis Sci* 2007;52:1589–1591.

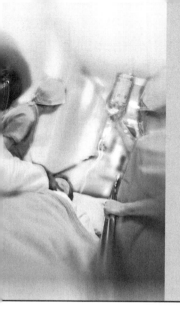

52

Heparin-Induced Thrombocytopenia

DEFINITION

Heparin-induced thrombocytopenia (HIT), an immune-mediated drug reaction resulting from IgG antibodies directed at heparin-platelet factor 4 complexes induced by exposure to heparin products, results in significant hypercoagulability and life-threatening thrombosis.

CLINICAL SETTING

The majority of cases of HIT occur in the setting of prolonged exposure to unfractionated heparin (UFH) by any route, although prior exposure may induce a rapid amnestic response and acute thrombocytopenia.

PATHOGENESIS

Unfractionated heparin is a mucopolysaccharide derived from bovine or porcine tissues with an average molecular weight of 15,000 Daltons. The mechanism of the anticoagulant effect of heparin is via an interaction with antithrombin III, which inhibits thrombin and, ultimately, fibrin clot formation. A specific pentasaccharide sequence on the heparin molecule binds to antithrombin III, conferring anticoagulant properties. Heparin products are widely utilized in clinical medicine, most often in the form of UFH or low molecular weight heparins (LMWH), which do possess cross-reactivity with heparin. The development of IgG antibodies against the heparin-platelet factor 4 (PF-4) complex may develop with subacute exposure to either intravenous or subcutaneous UFH or, less commonly, to LWMH. Antibodies can develop even in the presence of miniscule amounts of heparin exposure, such as that occurs with heparin flushes or heparin-coated vascular catheters. These antibodies typically form 5 to 10 days after exposure to heparin but may form much sooner (within hours) if the patient has had recent exposure to heparin and has circulating PF4-heparin antibodies. The PF4 epitope becomes an antigenic target when it is bound to heparin. The complex of heparin and PF4 binds to the FcγRII receptors on circulating platelets which then induces platelet activation and release of thrombogenic substances that promote thrombin generation and platelet aggregation. Thrombin formation and platelet aggregation may result in thrombosis of all sizes of veins and arteries. This can result in dysfunction and ischemia of virtually any organ system. In fact, HIT is one of the most pro-thrombotic states encountered in clinical medicine, conferring a thrombotic risk thirty-fold more than that of control populations. Thrombotic complications may occur in 30% to 50% of patients with HIT, but some authors have noted thrombosis to occur in 73% of cancer patients who develop HIT, possibly due to synergy with malignancy-induced or infection-related hypercoagulabiltiy. Thrombosis with HIT can present *de novo* as extension of an existing venous thrombosis, or as ongoing thrombosis despite anticoagulation.

Typically, platelet counts are well below 150,000 cells/mm^3 but rarely drop below 10,000 cells/mm.^{3} Occasional patients may have HIT with normal platelet counts but a drop in total count of greater than 50% of baseline levels which can make the diagnosis very difficult. Paradoxically, severe thrombocytopenia is not associated with bleeding, which should serve as a clue to HIT in patients with severe thrombocytopenia without hemorrhage. Thrombocytopenia typically recovers within 4 to 14 days after heparin cessation but the hypercoagulability remains for several weeks despite the normal platelet count. In fact, some patients with unrecognized HIT may present days to weeks later with acute thrombosis and a normal platelet count. This can lead to potentially fatal catastrophic thrombosis if heparin is administered.

Manifestations of HIT most commonly include deep venous thrombosis of the lower extremities, pulmonary embolism, or arterial limb ischemia, which often necessitates amputation. Adrenal insufficiency may result from adrenal vein thrombosis and stroke may complicate thrombosis of the dural and cerebral venous sinuses. Unusual clinical features of HIT include skin necrosis, anaphylaxis, transient amnesia with intravenous heparin, and venous gangrene of the limbs. Venous limb gangrene is important to recognize since it typically occurs when warfarin is commenced prior to recovery of the platelet count.

ETIOLOGY

The etiology of HIT in routine oncologic practice is usually limited to the following situations:

- Unfractionated heparin exposure
  - Intravenous administration for venous or arterial thrombosis
  - Subcutaneous administration for venous thrombosis prophylaxis

- ○ Heparin flushes of venous or arterial catheters
- ○ Heparin-coated vascular catheters
- Low molecular weight heparin exposure (e.g., enoxaparin, dalteparin)
  - ○ Subcutaneous, full-dose therapy to treat venous thrombosis or pulmonary embolism
  - ○ Subcutaneous, prophylactic dose

SYMPTOMS AND SIGNS

Most patients who develop antibodies are asymptomatic and do not develop specific clinical manifestations in the setting of a normal platelet count. Likewise, patients with HIT only manifesting as thrombocytopenia are asymptomatic. However, HIT with thrombosis (HITT) may present with myriad symptoms and signs, including:

- Extremity swelling
  - ○ Most common manifestation resulting from deep venous thrombosis of the lower extremity or the upper extremity if a vascular catheter present
- Dyspnea or pleurtic chest pain
  - ○ May occur with pulmonary embolism
- Angina pectoris
  - ○ May occur if coronary artery thrombosis present
- Abdominal pain
  - ○ May occur if mesenteric venous or arterial thrombosis present
- Confusion/amnesia
  - ○ May suddenly occur with intravenous heparin as amnestic response
- Hypotension
  - ○ May occur with intravenous heparin as amnestic response
  - ○ May occur if adrenal vein thrombosis and adrenal gland infarction present
- Evidence of extremity arterial ischemia
  - ○ Pain, pallor, pulselessness, parasthesis, paralysis
- Evidence of cerebral ischemia
  - ○ Focal weakness, aphasia, dysphagia

DIAGNOSTIC STUDIES

The diagnosis of HIT requires a high index of suspicion in the cancer patient since there are often many potential etiologies of thrombocytopenia in this population. Also, if the platelet count remains in the normal range despite a precipitous decline, HIT may be overlooked. The following laboratory diagnostic tests should be considered if thrombocytopenia with or without thrombosis is present and HIT is suspected:

- Enzyme-linked immunosorbent assay (ELISA)
  - ○ Widely utilized immunologic assay that detects serum IgA, IgM, and IgG antibodies

- ○ Very sensitive (>97%), less specific (74% to 86%) since detects low-titer antibodies in patients without thrombocytopenia and clinically insignificant
  - ○ Positive predictive value limited (10% to 93%) and dependent upon the pre-test probability of HIT
  - ○ Excellent negative predictive value (>95%) making a negative ELISA test helpful at excluding HIT
  - ○ ELISA may remain positive for 120 days after heparin exposure
- Functional assays
  - ○ Most common assay is the serotonin-release assay that detects antibody present only in amounts high enough to induce radiolabeled serotonin release from activated platelets
  - ○ Sensitivity of 88% to 100% and specificity of 89% to 100% but cumbersome test and not available in all laboratories

TREATMENT

If the suspicion of HIT is high, all heparin-containing compounds by any route must be discontinued. Since LMWHs are cross-reactive with PF4-heparin complexes, these drugs are contraindicated and cannot be substituted for UFH. Warfarin monotherapy is absolutely contraindicated due to the risk of skin necrosis and venous limb gangrene resulting from a decline in vitamin-K dependant endogenous anticogualation factors (e.g., protein C and S), augmenting the already thrombogenic state. In the United States, two drug classes exist for treating HIT: direct thrombin inhibitors (DTIs) and heparinoids. The heparinoids are infrequently utilized in routine practice due to their limited availability. Because of this, only DTIs will be discussed. The two most popular DTIs are lepirudin and argatroban. Lepirudin is a recombinantly synthesized analogue of the medicinal leech protein, hirudin. This agent has been shown to be effective in patients with HIT by decreasing the risk of death and new thromboembolic complications. Lepirudin is renally eliminated and must be used with caution, if at all, in the presence of moderate to severe renal dysfunction or in the elderly. Another disadvantage of lepirudin is the formation of antihirudin antibodies that enchance the anticoagulant effect and may increase the bleeding risk. Re-exposure to lepirudin may result in fatal anaphylaxis so patients should not receive this agent more than once.

Argatroban is an arginine-based synthetic DTI that has been demonstrated to decrease the risk of new thrombosis, amputation, and death in patients with HIT. Since argatroban is not renally eliminated, it can be used safely in patients with renal failure, which is common in the cancer and critally ill populations. However, lepirudin must be utililized with caution in patients with liver dysfunction due to widespread metastasis or underlying cirrhosis since it is hepatically cleared. Both lepirudin and argatroban prolong the partial thromboplastin time (PTT), which is used routinely to monitor the anticoagulant effect. The ecarin clotting time may also be used to monitor the anticoagulant effect of DTIs. Importantly, there are no antidotes for anticoagulation reversal for lepirudin or argatroban. If life-threatening hemorrhage occurs, infusion of recombinant factor VIIa could be considered. Warfarin can be safely added in low doses (5 mg or less daily) when the platelet count is in the normal range to avoid venous limb gangrene or skin necrosis. Since the DTIs prolong the prothrombin time (PT), this must be taken into account when determining when to stop these agents after commencing warfarin. The INR should be well within the therapeutic range for 2 consecutive days with overlap with the DTI for 5 days before discontinuation. Since antibodies and hypercoagulability can persist for several weeks, treatment with warfarin for several months if suggested.

PROGNOSIS

The prognosis of HIT is favorable if immediatedly recognized, all heparin compounds are discontinued and timely therapy with a DTI is instituted. If HIT is not promptly recognized and treated, patients are at risk for devastating and life-threatening complications. Some authors have found that HIT in the cancer population carries a higher risk of extremity amputation due to arterial thrombosis or venous limb gangrene and possibly death.

ADDITIONAL READING

Alving BM. How I treat heparin-induced thrombocytopenia. *Blood* 2003; 101:31–37.

Arepally GM, Ortel TL. Heparin-induced thrombocytopenia. *N Engl J Med* 2006; 355:809–817.

Hassell K. The management of patients with heparin-induced thrombocytopenia who require anticoagulant therapy. *Chest* 2005;127:S1–S8.

Opantry L, Warner MN. Risk of thrombosis in patients with malignancy and heparin-induced thrombocytopenia. *Am J Hematol* 2004;76:240–244.

Pradoni P, Falanga A, Piccioli A. Cancer, thrombosis and heparin-induced thrombocytopenia. *Thromb Res* 2007;120:S137–S140.

Warkentin TE, Kelton JG. A 14-year study of heparin-induced thrombocytopenia. *Am J Med* 1996;101:502–507.

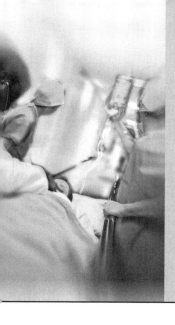

53

Hyperviscosity Syndrome

DEFINITION

Hyperviscosity syndrome (HVS) results from complications related to increased blood viscosity from markedly increased circulating cellular elements or plasma protein levels.

CLINICAL SETTING

Most cases of HVS occur in the setting of an IgM paraproteinemia (Waldenström's macroglobulinemia [WM]) or significant increases in the erythrocyte or leukocyte counts complicating a variety of hematologic diseases.

PATHOGENESIS

The viscosity of circulating whole blood is primarily determined by the level of plasma proteins and cellular elements such as erythrocytes and leukocytes. As serum viscosity increases relative to water (which has a value of 1), blood flow becomes sluggish, especially in the microvasculature. Clinical manifestations of HVS only occur when blood viscosity exceeds more than four times that of water. Dehydration with a decrease in total body water increases serum viscosity as well. The most common hematologic disease implicated in HVS is WM, a monoclonal paraproteinemia characterized by clonal overproduction of IgM. The IgM molecule is a pentamer of IgG molecules, which results in a very large macroglobulin with a molecular weight of approximately 900,000–1,000,000 kDd. This pentamer possesses a high intrinsic viscosity and is too large to traverse out of the extravascular space. The IgM paraprotein may bind water through its carbohydrate comoponents as well as "pull" extravascular fluid into the intravascular compartment further contributing to hyperviscosity. Also, immunoglobulin molecules are cationic proteins and can lower the normal repulsive forces that exist between normal erythrocytes. Patients with IgA myeloma may experience hyperviscosity due to the dimeric nature of the paraprotein, with HVS occurring in up to 25% of patients in some series. IgG myeloma is rarely (fewer than 5% of cases) associated with HVS unless the the paraprotein level is extremely elevated, although IgG subclass 3 possesses a higher intrinsic tendency to aggregate and may occasionally result in HVS.

Extreme leukocytosis (>100,000 cells/mm3) associated with acute myelogenous leukemia can result in hyperviscosity due to the hyperleukocytosis syndrome (discussed in subsequent section) which results from the immature, relatively large myeloid cells adhering to the endothelium via various integrin proteins. The vast number of blasts also increases viscosity to a degree. Significant elevations in serum hematocrit (e.g., >55% to 60%) due to myeloproliferative disorders or chronic hypoxia may occasionally cause HVS, especially in the setting of intravascular fluid depletion, co-existing hypercoagulability, or prolonged immobility.

Whatevever the etiology of HVS, the pathogenic mechanism of organ dysfunction results from sluggish blood flow within the microvasculature, leading to increased stasis and tissue ischemia. Vascular beds predisposed to HVS include the retinal, cerebral, pulmonary, coronary, and renal circulations, which can result in visual disturbance, neurologic symptoms, hypoxia, angina, and renal failure, respectively. Patients with preexisting left ventricular systolic dysfunction may experience sudden decompensation due to the elevated plasma viscosity which increases cardiac workload.

ETIOLOGY

The etiologies of HVS most commonly encountered in the oncologic population include:

- Waldenström's macroglobulinemia
- Multiple myeloma
  - Most commonly in the setting of IgA or IgG3 subtypes
- Polycythemia vera or secondary polycythemia
- Myeloproliferative disorders
  - Chronic myelogenous leukemia (CML), essential thrombocythemia
- Hyperleukocytosis syndrome complicating acute myelogenous (or much less commonly chronic) leukemia
- Cryoglobulinemia
  - Most common in setting of monoclonal cryoglobinemia associated with underlying lymphoproliferative disease
- Severe dehydration

SYMPTOMS AND SIGNS

Since HVS often presents with non-specific symptoms and signs, the diagnosis must be considered in the compatible clinical setting in patients who present with the following:

- Headache
- Epistaxis
- Visual changes or loss
- Confusion
- Seizures
- Neurologic symptoms
  - Tinnitus, vertigo, ataxia
- Dyspnea
- Anginal chest pain
- Pulmonary rales or cardiac gallop if heart failure is present
- Abnormal retinal/fundal examination
  - Dilated, sausage-like retinal veins classic finding in patients with WM
  - Retinal edema or hemorrhage
- Focal neurologic findings
  - Cerebellar signs, decreased visual acuity, paralysis

Diagnostic Studies

The diagnosis of HVS requires a high index of suspicion, supplemented by judicious use of various laboratory and imaging studies. Some of the studies include:

- Plasma viscosity
  - Measured relative to water, values exceeding 4 are associated with development of HVS
- Complete blood count
  - May reveal extreme leukocytosis in setting of acute myelogenous leukemia or CML with blast crisis
  - May reveal polycythemia in setting of myeloproliferative disorders or chronic hypoxia
- Serum protein electrophoresis and immunofixation
  - Elevation of total protein and gamma-globulin peak are characteristic of paraproteinemias (multiple myeloma or WM)
  - Immunofixation important to identify immunoglobulin type as IgM, IgA, or IgG (subtying of IgG can be considered if HVS complicates IgG myeloma)
- Janus Kinase (JAK) 2 mutation
  - Indicated if polycythemia vera or essential thrombocytosis suspected
- Serum cryoglobulins
  - Useful if monoclonal or polyclonal cryoglobulinemia is suspected
- Chest radiography
  - May resemble findings of pulmonary edema with interstitial infiltrates and small pleural effusions
- Computed tomography or magnetic resonance imaging scan of the brain
  - May reveal intracerebral hemorrhage, edema, or infarction

Treatment

Since HVS may result in critical organ ischemia and dysfunction, rapid treatment should be instituted in symptomatic patients, especially those with neurologic, cardiac, or pulmonary symptoms. General supportive measures such as crystalloid administration, oxygenation (with mechanical ventilation as necessary), hemodynamic monitoring and support, and avoidance of nephrotoxins are important. Although patients with HVS may appear to be volume overloaded clinically or radiographically, diuretics should be avoided, as decreases in intravascular water further increase plasma viscosity and may exacerbate hyperviscosity. Treatment of underlying neoplastic disorders with chemotherapy should be considered. For instance, HVS in the setting of hyperleukocytosis resulting from acute myelogenous leukemia may respond to cytoreduction with hydroxyurea prior to commencing definitive chemotherapy. Phlebotomy with saline replacement is indicated for polycythemia-related HVS. The definitive acute treatment for symptomatic or severe HVS is pheresis therapy. Patients with WM or myeloma require extracorporeal removal of serum proteins with plasmapheresis and those with hyperleukocytosis require leukopheresis to remove excess blasts. An exception is hyperleukocytosis associated with acute promyelocytic leukemia, as the coagulopathy may worsen with plasmapheresis. Cerebral ischemia related to hyperleukocytosis from acute leukemia may benefit from cranial irradiation if other measures fail.

PROGNOSIS

Prognosis of HVS is related to the timely performance of pheresis therapy and supportive care as well as the treatability of the underlying disease process. Patients with WM or multiple myeloma have a favorable prognosis with modern chemo- and immunotherapy if they recover from HVS. Acute myelogenous leukemia or blast crisis of CML have a less favorable prognosis.

ADDITIONAL READING

Blum W, Porcu P. Therapeutic apheresis in hyperleukocytosis and hyperviscosity syndrome. *Semin Thromb Hemost* 2007;33:350–354.

Crawford J, Cox EB, Cohen HJ. Evaluation of hyperviscosity in monoclonal gammopathies. *Am J Med* 1985;79:13–22.

Frewin R, Henson A, Provan D. ABC of clinical haematology: haematological emergencies. *BMJ* 1997;314:1333–1336.

Gertz MA, Kyle RA. Hyperviscosity syndrome. *J Intensive Care Med* 1995;10:128–141.

Mehta J, Singhal S. Hyperviscosity syndrome in plasma cell dyscrasias. *Semin Thromob Hemost* 2003;29:471–476.

Menke MN, Feke GT, McMeel JW, et al. Hyperviscosity-related retinopathy in Waldenstrom macroglobulinemia. *Arch Ophthalmol* 2006;124:1601–1606.

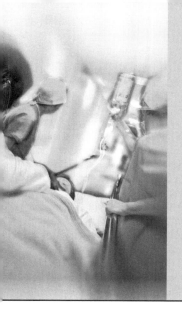

54

Hyperleuko-cytosis Syndrome

DEFINITION

Hyperleukocytosis syndrome (HLS) is a life-threatening complication of acute leukemia in which extreme leukocytosis results in symptoms of leukostasis caused by sludging of leukemic blasts within the microvascular circulation.

CLINICAL SETTING

The majority of cases of HLS occur in the setting of acute myelogenous leukemia (AML) associated with circulating leukocyte counts exceeding 100,000 cells/mm^3 with rare cases complicating acute lymphocytic leukemia (ALL) or chronic leukemias when the leukocyte count exceeds 200–400,000 cells/mm^3.

PATHOGENESIS

Acute myelogenous leukemia is the most common leukemia associated with the development of HLS due to the intrinsic properties of the leukemic blast cells. Although HLS can complicate any subtype of AML, most cases are due to acute promyelocytic leukemia (APL [M3]) and acute monocytic leukemias (M4 and M5). The pathogenesis of HLS is, in part, due to not only the increased circulating cellular mass which increases serum viscosity, but also to cellular factors that affect blast-endothelial cell interaction. This is demonstrated by the fact that patients with AML manifest symptoms of HLS with much lower total leukocyte/blast counts than patients with ALL. This may be explained by the larger cell size of myeloid blasts as well as various adhesion molecules and integrins present on the surface of myeloid blasts that result in adhesion to the microvascular endothelium. For instance, myeloid blasts may express E-selectin and vascular cell adhesion molecule-1 (VCAM-1) which induce binding to capillary endothelium within various organs.

The pathogenesis of HLS-induced organ dysfunction results from this blast-endothelial interaction resulting in leukostasis and sluggish oxygenation in various organs, most significantly the pulmonary microcirculation, brain, and kidneys. Pulmonary leukostasis interferes with gas exchange resulting in hypoxia and acute respiratory failure. Pulmonary alveolar hemorrhage is an uncommon manifestation of HLS. Cerebrovascular ischemia, infarction, or hemorrhage can occur due to occlusion of cerebral vessels. Retinal vessel involvement with resulting hemorrhage or ischemic retinal necrosis can occur. Large vessel thrombosis of the extremity vasculature can result in limb gangrene and renal vein thrombosis may cause acute renal failure. Disseminated intravascular coagulation (DIC) often complicates APL or monocytic leukemia due to release of lysosomal contents that trigger the coagulation cascade. Treatment of acute leukemias with chemotherapy may result in rapid cell lysis with release of purines, potassium, and phosphorus into the circulation resulting in tumor lysis syndrome with various complications, which are discussed in another section.

ETIOLOGY

The majority of cases of HLS complicate AML but the following other types of leukemia have been reported on occasion:

- Acute myelogenous leukemia
  - Most commonly associated with APL (M3) and monocytic (M4 and M5) subtypes
  - Presence of 11q23 abnormalities and Philadelphia (t9:22) chromosome may increase risk of HLS
- Acute lymphoblastic leukemia
  - Uncommon unless leukocyte count exceeds 250–400,000 cells/mm^3
  - Philadelphia chromosome-positive cases have higher risk
- Chronic myelogenous leukemia
  - May occur in setting of blast crisis with rapid increase in leukocyte count
- Chronic lymphocytic leukemia
  - Uncommon; mean leukocyte count of 950,000 cells/mm^3 in one study

SYMPTOMS AND SIGNS

The diagnosis of HLS is clinical and requires a high index of suspicion due to the non-specific clinical manifestations, which include:

- Fatigue
- Fever
- Blurred vision
- Headache
- Epistaxis

- Tinnitus
- Decreased hearing
- Dyspnea
- Cough
- Abdominal pain
- Priapism
- Mucosal bleeding if DIC is present
- Abnormal retinal examination
  - Hemorrhage, edema, vessel engorgement, optic disc edema
- Neurologic signs
  - Stupor, coma, focal deficits, decreased hearing acuity
- Pulmonary rales
- Acral cyanosis

DIAGNOSTIC STUDIES

Although HLS is primarily a clinical diagnosis, the following diagnostic studies are useful to confirm the diagnosis and document complications:

- Complete blood count
  - Leukocyte counts often strikingly elevated and correlate with development of HLS depending on the type of leukemia; one study revealed the following mean leukocyte counts in cases of HLS
    - AML: 303,000 cells/mm^3
    - ALL: 634,000 cells/mm^3
    - CML: 510,000 cells/mm^3
    - CLL: 950,000 cells/mm^3
  - Anemia and thrombocytopenia typical of acute leukemia
  - Spurious thrombocytosis reported by automated cell counter may occur from leukocyte fragmentation
- Peripheral blood smear
  - Reveals numerous blast cells
  - Myeloid blasts are typically larger than lymphoid blasts
- Leukocrit
  - Elevated fractional leukocyte volume may correlate with symptoms
- Plasma viscosity
  - Symptoms of hyperviscosity syndrome may develop if viscosity exceeds 4 in relation to water
- Coagulation studies
  - Elevated partial thromboplastin time (PTT) and prothrombin time (PT) and hypofibrinogenemia indicative of APL or DIC
- Computed tomography or magnetic resonance imaging of brain
  - May reveal evidence of cerebral edema, thrombosis, hemorrhage, or infarction

- Chest radiography
  - May reveal interstitial or alveolar infiltrates similar to pulmonary edema
- Serum chemistries
  - Elevations in lactate dehydrogenase (LDH) are common
  - Important to monitor for development of tumor lysis which causes hyperkalemia, hyperphosphatemia, hypocalcemia, and acute renal failure
- Uric acid
  - Often elevated due to increased cell mass and breakdown
  - May increase to very high levels with chemotherapy if tumor lysis syndrome develops
- Urinalysis
  - May reveal hematuria, proteinuria, or uric acid crystals

TREATMENT

The presence of neurologic or pulmonary symptoms in the setting of HLS constitutes a medical emergency due to the risk of cerebral hemorrhage and acute respiratory insufficiency, which are the most common causes of death. Basic supportive measures include oxygenation (and mechanical ventilation as necessary), urinary alkalinization, and vigorous hydration with crystalloid fluids. Prevention of tumor lysis syndrome with allopurinol or rasburicase should be administered to avoid urate nephropathy and acute renal failure. Transfusion of blood products should be avoided, if possible, since this may further elevate the plasma viscosity and compromise blood flow within the microcirculation. Pharmacologic cytoreduction with hydroxyurea followed by chemotherapy may be useful in cases of AML and rapid institution of all-trans retinoic acid (ATRA) and anthracycline chemotherapy should be provided for patients with APL. Patients with APL-induced DIC may require infusion of cryoprecipitate or fresh frozen plasma to reduce the risk of cerebral hemorrhage. Imatinib is indicated in patients with CML. Cranial irradiation has been utilized to treat neurologic dysfunction resulting from HLS, but this is not routinely suggested.

The most efficient and reliable modality to treat HLS is acute leukoreduction with leukapheresis. One leukapheresis treatment may decrease the circulating leukocyte count by 30% to 40%, resulting in improvement of symptoms and hematologic variables. Leukapheresis may also recruit marginated leukemic cells into the vascular space with subsequent removal. However, leukapheresis is not a definitive therapy for any leukemia and only serves as a temporizing measure to improve rheologic parameters and treat acute complications until definitive chemotherapy can be instituted.

PROGNOSIS

The development of HLS often portends a poor prognosis in patients with AML (and ALL) with early deaths typically attributable to cerebral hemorrhage or acute respiratory failure. Patients with APL have a very favorable long-term prognosis if they do not succumb during the initial presentation from coagulopathy or HLS. While leukapheresis is very useful at acute cytoreduction and resolving manifestations of HLS, no data at present demonstrate that this procedure improves overall survival or decreases mortality.

ADDITIONAL READING

Blum W, Porcu P. Therapeutic apheresis in hyperleukocytosis and hyperviscosity syndrome. *Semin Thromb Hemost* 2007;33:350–354.

Cavenagh JD, Gordon-Smith ED, Gibson FM, et al. Acute myeloid leukemia blast cells bind to human endothelium *in vitro* utilizing E-selectin and vascular adhesion molecule-1. *Br J Haematol* 1993;85:285–291.

Majhail NS, Lichtin AE. Acute leukemia with a very high leukocyte count: confronting a medical emergency. *Cleve Clin J Med* 2004;71:633–637.

Stucki A, Rivier AS, Gikic M, et al. Endothelial cell activation by myeloblasts: molecular mechanisms of leukostasis and leukemic cell dissemination. *Blood* 2001;97:2121–2129.

Tan D, Hwang W, Goh YT. Therapeutic leukapheresis in hyperleukocytotic leukemias—the experience of a tertiary institution in Singapore. *Ann Acad Med Singapore* 2005;34:229–234.

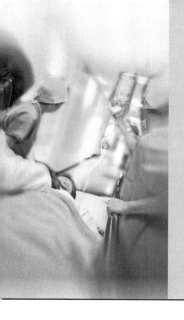

55

Retinoic Acid Syndrome

DEFINITION

The retinoic acid syndrome (RAS) develops in approximately 25% of patients from 2 to 21 days after commencing therapy for acute promyelocytic leukemia (APL) with the vitamin A analogue all-trans retinioic acid (ATRA) and is characterized by fever, weight gain, edema, and body cavity effusions.

CLINICAL SETTING

The RAS is limited to patients being treated with ATRA for APL, and most often occurs during induction therapy.

PATHOGENESIS

The pathogenesis of the RAS is very complex but basically relates to the differentiating effects of ATRA upon the neoplastic leukemic cells. The development of ATRA has transformed the therapy for APL and induces remission in more than 90% of patients when combined with anthracycline chemotherapy. ATRA is structurally related to vitamin A (a retinoid) which induces differentiation of APL into more mature neutrophils. A characteristic pathogenic feature of APL is maturation arrest of neoplastic myeloid cells at the promyelocyte stage resulting from a fusion gene formed by a chromosomal translocation between the retinoic acid receptor α (RARα) and promyelocytic leukemia (PML) genes [t(15;17)(q22;q11)], although uncommon variants do exist. This fusion protein acts as a dominant negative inhibitor of the normal RARα protein, which results in maturation arrest. Generally, leukemic APL cells manifest numerous cytoplasmic granules and Auer rods, which contain coagulation factors that result in the development of disseminated intravascular coagulation (DIC), which may result in fatal cerebral bleeding. Administration of ATRA releases the maturation arrest of cells at the promyelocyte stage so that more mature functional granulocytes form. With the administraion of ATRA there is often a significant rise in the total leukocyte count, which may result in hyperleukocytosis syndrome. The pathogenesis of the RAS syndrome continues to be elucidated, but essentially results from ATRA-induced differention changes in cytokine secretion and adhesive qualities of APL cells. Implicated cytokines involved in the pathogenesis of the RAS include interleukin (IL)-1, IL-6, IL-8, and tumor necrosis factor (TNF). The induction of matrix metalloproteinase-9 (MMP-9) may also foster tissue infiltration. *In vivo* studies have demonstrated that ATRA induces increased cell-adhesion mechanisms and the ability of the cells to transmigrate the vascular space into local tissues. Also, ATRA induces aggregation of APL cells via the expression of various integrins and intercellular adhesion molecules (ICAM). Integrins increase attachment of cells to various ICAM ligands which induce endothelial damage and allow migration of cells out of the vasculature. Autopsy studies of fatal cases of the RAS always demonstrate infiltration of various organs with maturing and mature granulocytes. These granulocytic cells release tissue-damaging chemicals and enzymes. Involved tissues often reveal cellular damage and endothelial damage that contributes to end-organ dysfunction, reminiscent of sepsis or adult respiratory distress syndrome. The end result of the RAS is endothelial disruption and a cascade of tissue events culminating in edema, hemorrhage, fibrin deposition, and respiratory failure due to granulocytic infiltration of the alveoli and interstitium. Peripheral edema and effusions involving the pericardium, pleural space, and peritoneal cavity are almost universal with the RAS and result from a capillary leak-type syndrome, similar to that which occurs with the administration of IL-2.

Common causes of morbidity and mortality in RAS include respiratory failure and pericardial tamponade from pericardial effusion. Mechanisms of respiratory failure include neutrophilic infiltration of lung interstitium and alveoli causing diffuse alveolar damage, alveolar fibrin deposition, and alveolar hemorrhage, all of which lead to hypoxemic respiratory insufficiency. Pericardial tamponade results from pericardial effusion. Acute renal failure may result not only from intravascular fluid depletion and hypotension from capillary leak, but also from renal parenchymal infiltration with maturing granulocytes. Acute febrile neutrophilic dermatosis resulting from cutaneous infiltration of granulolcytes may occur in some patients and is thought to result from elevated cytokine levels.

ETIOLOGY

The etiology of the RAS is the administration of ATRA. A similar syndrome can occur in patients treated with arsenic trioxide, but will not be discussed.

SYMPTOMS AND SIGNS

The diagnosis of the RAS is primarily clinical, based on typical symptoms and signs occurring during initiation of ATRA therapy. The most common findings include:

- Dyspnea (present in more than 80% of cases)
- Fever (present in more than 80% of cases)
- Headache
- Bone pain
- Peripheral edema
- Tachycardia
  - May result from fever, intravascular volume depletion, cytokine release, or pericardial effusion
- Hypotension
  - May result from vasodilation, intravascular volume depletion, or pericardial effusion/tamponade
- Weight gain
- Oliguria
- Ascites/abdominal distention
- Pulmonary rales or diminished breath sounds
- Scrotal ulceration
- Erythematous skin nodules (Sweet's syndrome)

DIAGNOSTIC STUDIES

As noted, the diagnosis of the RAS is clinical and typically made presumptively in patients at risk who develop dyspnea, fever, and edema after commencing ATRA therapy. However, several diagnostic studies may be helpful:

- Complete blood count
  - Leukocytosis, often extreme
- Peripheral blood smear
  - Often reveals maturing granulocytes, mature neutrophils, and APL cells
- Serum chemistries
  - May reveal elevations in lactate dehydrogenase, blood urea nitrogen, and creatinine
- Chest radiography
  - Pulmonary infiltrates or edema pattern occur in approximately 50% of patients
  - Pleural effusions
  - Enlargement of pericardial cardiac silhouette may indicate pericardial effusion
- Echocardiography
  - Useful to delineate extent of pericardial effusion and assess for tamponade physiology
- Skin biosy
  - May reveal nodular infiltration of netrophils (Sweet's Syndrome)

TREATMENT

Treatment of suspected RAS should be commenced expeditiously since treatment delay increases the risk for poor outcome. Supportive medical care including crystalloid administration, oxygenation (and mechanical ventilation as necessary), hemodynamic support, correction of coagulopathy, and electrolyte management are vital. However, the definitive treatment for the RAS is dexamethaxone, 10 mg intravenously twice daily for 3 or more days. Prophylactic dexamethaxone should be considered in patients who present with leukocytosis (e.g., >10–15,000 cells/mm^3). Temporary cessation of ATRA may be required in critically ill patients with this syndrome.

PROGNOSIS

Mortality rates for the RAS of approximately 28% to 33% were reported in early studies of ATRA for APL, with most patients succumbing to respiratory, hepatic, or renal failure. However, with prompt initiation of supportive care and dexamathasone, currently mortality rates for the RAS are approximately 5%. Some authors, however, have demonstrated reduced event-free survival and overall survival rates in APL patients who develop the RAS.

ADDITIONAL READING

Avvisati G, Tallman MS. All-trans retinoic acid syndrome in acute promyelocytic leukaemia. *Best Pract Res Clin Haematol* 2003;16:419–432.

Bi K, Jiang G. Relationship between cytokines and leukocytosis in patients with APL induced by all-trans retinoic acid or arsenic trioxide. *Cell Mol Immunol* 2006;3:421–427.

DeBotton S, Dombret H, Sanz M, et al. Incidence, clinical features, and outcome of all-trans retinoic acid syndrome in 413 cases of newly diagnosed acute promyelocytic leukemia. *Blood* 1998;92:2712–2718.

Frankel SR, Eardley A, Lauwers G, et al. The "retinoic acid syndrome" in acute promyelocytic leukemia. *Ann Intern Med* 1992;117:292–296.

Larson RS, Tallman MS. Retinoic acid syndrome: manifestations, pathogenesis, and treatment. *Best Pract Res Clin Haematol* 2003;16:453–461.

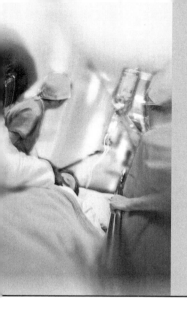

56

Acquired Hemophilia

DEFINITION

Acquired hemophilia (AH) is an uncommon, but potentially fatal, bleeding disorder resulting from the spontaneous development of inhibiting antibodies directed against blood coagulation factors, most commonly to factor VIII.

CLINICAL SETTING

Acquired antibodies to factor VIII occuring in the setting of hematologic malignancies or various solid tumors accounts for 10% of cases of AH.

PATHOGENESIS

The spontaneous development of neutralizing antibodies (also known as inhibitors) to factor VIII results in an acquired hemophilic state and may complicate various autoimmune diseases, the post-partum state, or malignant disease. These auto-antibodies inhibit the function of factor VIII in the coagulation cascade, resulting in prolongation of the partial thromboplastin time (PTT) and a bleeding diathesis. The precise mechanism of auto-antibody formation secondary to malignancy remains to be elucidated but may result from immune dysfunction caused by a T-lymphocyte response to tumor antigens. These antibodies bind to various epitopes on the factor VIII molecule and inhibit normal function. That malignant cells may be the source of auto-antibody production is supported by several reported cases of AH in the literature that resolved with eradication of the malignancy. Other potential mechanisms of auto-antibody production in the cancer population include bacteremia and various antibiotics such as penicillins. Acquired hemophilia most often manifests as spontaneous, life-threatening hemorrhage. The most common sites of hemorrhage in malignancy-associated AH are the soft tissues (not joints as with congenital hemophilia), skin, the urinary tract, and gastrointestinal tract, although any body site may experience hemorrhage. The inhibitors not only inactivate endogenous factor VIII, but also pharmacologic factor VIII which is often ineffective in standard doses.

ETIOLOGY

The development of factor VIII inhibitors and AH in the cancer population may result not only from a variety of neoplasms, but also from other mechanisms, such as:

- Solid tumors
  - Prostate cancer
  - Lung cancer
  - Pancreatic cancer
  - Colorectal cancer
  - Gastric cancer
  - Breast cancer
  - Renal cell cancer
  - Bladder cancer
  - Hepatobiliary cancer
  - Brain tumors
  - Melanoma
- Hematologic malignancies
  - Acute and chronic leukemias
  - Non-Hodgkin's lymphoma
  - Multiple myeloma
  - Myelodysplastic syndrome
  - Myelofibrosis
- Medications
  - Penicillins
  - Sulphonamides
- Infection
  - Gram-negative bacteria
  - Septic shock

SYMPTOMS AND SIGNS

The most common symptom of AH is bleeding, or ecchymosis, and may present with various symptoms and signs depending on the site of bleeding such as:

- Epistaxis
- Headache (in the setting of intracranial hemorrhage)
- Hematemesis
- Melena

- Hematochezia
- Hematuria
- Back pain (in the setting of retroperitoneal hemorrhage)
- Ecchymosis
- Soft tissue swelling
- Joint swelling/hemarthrosis (rare)

DIAGNOSTIC STUDIES

Bleeding has many potential etiologies in the cancer population so the diagnosis of AH requires a high index of suspicion. The most useful studies in the diagnosis of an acquired factor VIII inhibitor include:

- Partial thromboplastin time (PTT)
  - Prolongation of the PTT is typical and may exceed 100 seconds in some patients
- Mixing study
  - Failure to correct the PTT of the patient's plasma when normal plasma is added is consistent with presence of an inhibitor to clotting factor
    - Some cases may require incubating the sample for 2 hours since an initial correction of the PTT may reverse
- Factor VIII level
  - May be very depressed ($<1\%$) in some patients
- Factor VIII inhibitor level
  - Measured in Bethesda units (BU)

TREATMENT

Since AH may result in massive hemorrhage, prompt treatment should be instituted in any bleeding cancer patient with the typical laboratory findings of prolongation of the PTT, low factor VIII level, and increased anti-factor VIII inhibitor. Patients with a low inhibitor level (e.g., <5 BU) may be treated with high-dose recombinant factor VIII. However, patients with higher inhibitor levels require a "bypass" agent such as the prothrombin-complex concentrate known as FEIBA (Factor VIII Inhibitor Bypassing Activity). Another bypassing agent potentially useful in the setting of high inhibitor levels is recombinant factor VIIa. Treatment of the underlying malignancy with chemotherapy has been successful at eradicating inhibitors. Immunosuppressive therapy to decrease production of anti-factor VIII auto-antibodies with prednisone and cyclophosphamide are occasionally useful. Intravenous immune globulin, rituximab, and 2-chlorodeoxyadenosine have been reported by some authors to control inhibitor levels.

PROGNOSIS

Without prompt treatment, AH can result in fatal hemorrhagic shock or intracranial bleeding. With control of bleeding and inhibitor production, and if the underlying neoplasm is controlled, patients have a favorable prognosis. However, patients with acute hematologic malignancies and thrombocytopenia have a poor prognosis.

ADDITIONAL READING

De la Fourchardiere C, Flechon A, Droz JP. Coagulopathy in prostate cancer. *Neth J Med* 2003;61:347–353.

Holme PA, Brosstad F, Tjonnfjord GE. Acquired haemophilia: management of bleeds and immune therapy to eradicate autoantibodies. *Haemophilia* 2003;11:510–515.

Kreuter M, Retzlaff S, Weis UE, et al. Acquired haemophilia in a patient with Gram-negative urosepsis and bladder cancer. *Haemophilia* 2005;11:181–185.

Sallah S, Nguyen NP, Abdallah JM, et al. Acquired hemophilia in patients with hematologic malignancies. *Arch Pathol Lab Med* 2000;124:730–734.

Sallah S, Wan JY. Inhibitors against factor VIII in patients with cancer: analysis of 41 patients. *Cancer* 2001;91:1067–1074.

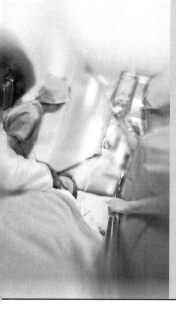

57

Acute Hemolytic Transfusion Reaction

DEFINITION

An acute hemolytic transfusion reaction (AHTR) is an uncommon, but frequently fatal, complication during or shortly following transfusion of ABO-incompatible packed red blood cells that is characterized by rapid intravascular hemolysis.

CLINICAL SETTING

Most cases of AHTR occur in the setting of a clerical error during transfusion of packed red blood cells.

PATHOGENESIS

The ABO antigen system is the most important system in erythrocyte serology and immunohematology. A simplified discussion of the ABO system will be presented. The interested reader should look to major textbooks for in-depth discussion. The ABO system consists of three allelic genes: A, B, and O. The A and B genes encode glycosyltransferase enzymes that ultimately synthesize the A and B antigens, respectively. These enzymes are responsible for the addition of single carbohydrate residues to a basic antigenic glycoprotein with a terminal L-fucose sugar present on the erythrocyte, known as the H antigen. For instance, the A gene produces N-acetyl galactosamine which, when added to the H antigen, produces blood group A. Similarly, the B gene produces D-galactose which when added to the H antigen produces blood group B. The O gene does not produce any enzyme to add carbohydrate to the H antigen. As such, blood group O is rich in H antigen but lacks A and B antigens. The A and B (as well as H) antigens are also present on most somatic cells including platelets and leukocytes. Approximately 80% of people produce these "secretor" genes and therefore these antigens are found in various body fluids and secretions such as plasma, tears, sweat, and semen. Naturally formed antibodies to the A and B antigens are present in the plasma of people whose red blood cells lack the corresponding antigen and this forms the basis of ABO-incompatible AHTR.

Naturally occurring antibodies (isoagglutinins) are present against A or B antigens. For instance, individuals with blood group A exhibit antibodies against blood group B, and vice versa. The isoagglutinin antibodies are typically IgM that activate complement upon activation. These antibodies are absent at birth, but form by 6 months of age when the immune system is exposed to exogenous ABH antigens naturally found in environmental sources such as plants, dust, and food stuffs. Antibodies are formed against the antigens that are absent within the individual. For instance, if a patient is transfused an ABO-incompatible unit of packed red blood cells, a brisk antibody response (typically IgM, but less commonly IgG) against the donor erythrocytes occurs. Less common causes of AHTR are IgG antibodies directed against other antigen systems such as Kell, Kidd, and Vel. The pathogenic features of an AHTR primarily result from IgM-induced complement mediated lysis of red cells which causes hemolysis via activation of C5-9 terminal complement component known as the membrane attack complex. A cytokine storm also occurs resulting in significant elevations of interleukin (IL)-1, IL-6, IL-8, and tumor necrosis factor (TNF) which causes many of the systemic manifestations and hemodynamic collapse associated with AHTR. Liberation of histamine, bradykinins, and vasoactive amines also contribute to the pathogenesis. Disseminated intravascular coagulation (DIC) may ensue due to formation of antigen-antibody complexes and direct activation of the clotting cascade via complement and erythrocyte damage. Massive intravascular hemolysis results in hemoglobinuria which can cause acute tubular necrosis and renal failure.

ETIOLOGY

The etiologies of AHTR are few in modern clinical practice.

- Transfusion of ABO-incompatible red blood cells
  - Most often results from clerical error resulting in transfusion of unit(s) to wrong patient
  - Mislabeling of unit during collection or storage
- Transfusion of ABO-incompatible platelets (rare)

SYMPTOMS AND SIGNS

Most cases of AHTR occur within the first several minutes of transfusion, but some patients may not experience symptoms until a few hours afterward. The most common clinical manifestations include:

- Abrupt rigors
- Fever

- Dyspnea
- Wheezing
- Chest pain
- Vomiting
- Pain at intravenous infusion site
- Flank pain
- Tachycardia
- Hypotension
- Oliguria
- Hemoglobinuria
- Jaundice

DIAGNOSTIC STUDIES

Patients suspected of experiencing an AHTR should have the transfusion immediately discontinued and the following diagnostic studies obtained:

- Complete blood count
  - Anemia and leukocytosis common
  - Thombocytopenia may indicate DIC
- Direct antiglobulin (Coombs') test on post-transfusion specimen
- Visual inspection of patient's plasma to assess for hemoglobinemia
  - Free hemoglobin imparts a pinkish tinge to plasma
- Plasma free hemoglobin
- Urine free hemoglobin
- Haptoglobin
  - Decreased from hemoglobin binding to haptoglobin
- Serum chemistries
  - May reveal elevated blood urea nitrogen and creatinine if renal failure present
  - Increased potassium may result from hemolyzed erythrocytes
  - Indirect hyperbilirubinemia
- Coagulation studies (PT/PTT, fibrinogen) if DIC suspected

TREATMENT

Cessation of infusing blood products is the first step in the treatment of an AHTR. Maintenance of adequate intravenous access for volume infusion as well as airway support and oxygenation is vital. While instituting treatment, the tubing and blood bag should be disconnected and sent to the blood bank for testing and simultaneous laboratory studies from the patient should be obtained, as noted previously. Vigourous crystalloid infusion is important to prevent hemoglobinuria-induced acute tubular necrosis. Mannitol may be useful to promote osmotic diuresis. Some patients may require hemodialysis if renal dysfunction, hyperkalemia, or metabolic acidosis is severe. Administration of vasopressors to treat hypotension and shock should be considered. Some authors recommend intravenous hydrocortisone. Transfusion of frozen plasma, platelets, and erythrocytes may be necessary to treat DIC and cytopenia.

PROGNOSIS

The prognosis of an ABO-incompatible AHTR depends somewhat on the volume of blood transfused, with mortality rates of 25% to 44% with less than or greater than 1000 milliliters of blood transfused. Cancer patients with underlying cardiopulmonary or renal disease may experience severe morbidity such as respiratory failure, shock, and renal failure and contribute to higher mortality rates.

ADDITIONAL READING

Bakdash S, Yazer MH. What every physician should know about transfusion reactions. *CMAJ* 2007;177:141–147.

Climent-Peris C, Velez-Rosario R. Immediate transfusion reactions. *P R Health Sci J* 2001;20:229–235.

Eder AF, Chambers LA. Non-infectious complications of blood transfusion. *Arch Pathol Lab Med* 2007;131:708–718.

Perrotta PL, Snyder EL. Non-infectious complications of transfusion therapy. *Blood Rev* 2001;15:69–83.

Tenorio GC, Gupte SC, Munker R. Transfusion medicine and immunohematology. In: Munker R, Hiller E, Glass J, et al., eds. *Modern Hematology: Biology and Clinical Management.* 2nd ed. Totowa, NJ: Humana Press, 2007, pp 401–432.

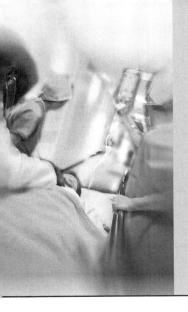

58

Bone Marrow Necrosis

DEFINITION

Bone marrow necrosis (BMN) is a clinicopathologic process characterized by necrosis of large, diffuse areas of bone marrow stroma and myeloid tissues with preservation of bone trabecular architecture.

CLINICAL SETTING

Approximately 90% of cases of BMN have been attributed to malignant disease, with the majority occurring in patients with various hematopoietic neoplasms or metastatic solid cancers.

PATHOGENESIS

The pathogenesis of BMN is not fully elucidated but failure of the bone marrow microcirculation is felt to be the key event. Briefly, the anatomy of the bone marrow consists of an arterial inflow and venous outflow interposed with a network of venous sinuses surrounding the hematopoietic environment. The venous sinuses consist of an inderdigitating network of single-layer endothelium supported by basement membrane and adventitial cells. Within this interstitium lie the fat cells and hematopoietic elements. Failure of blood inflow and oxygenation of the developing hematopoietic and stromal cells leads to cellular death and necrosis. Histologically, BMN is characterized by necrotic cellular material with indistinct cell walls, pyknotic nuclei, and eosinophilic cytoplasm as well as amorphous eosinophilic gelatinous transformation of the stroma. An important histologic hallmark of BMN is preservation of the spicular architecture in contradistinction to avascular necrosis (AVN) of bone. If necrotic bone marrow debris enters the systemic circulation, embolism to the lungs can result in severe hypoxia and acute respiratory failure.

Occlusion of the bone marrow microvasculature is felt to result in bone marrow hypoxia and release of inflammatory cytokines such as tumor necrosis factor (TNF) resulting in stromal and hematopoietic cellular damage. The majority of cases of BMN complicate hematologic neoplasms such as acute leukemia, although disseminated lymphomas and solid organ tumors have been implicated. Inflammatory damage to the endothelium by tumor cell mediated cytokines, vascular thrombi, or endothelial damage from cytotoxic chemotherapy result in vessel narrowing and occlusion with subsequent poor blood inflow. Although not a malignant disease, sickle cell anemia has been associated with BMN due to deformed, rigid erythrocytes occluding the marrow vascular network. Disseminated intravascular coagulation (DIC) resulting from malignancy or sepsis may cause BMN via fibrin plug vessel occlusion. Aggregates of disseminated carcinoma cells have been noted occluding marrow blood vessels. Rapidly replicating leukemic cells may outgrow the local blood supply and impinge upon the local vasculature resulting in occlusion. Whatever the mechanism, BMN leads to hematopoietic failure characterized by anemia, thrombocytopenia, and frequently leukopenia. Systemic symptoms may not only result from these cytopenias, but also from release of cytokines such as TNF.

ETIOLOGY

Causes of BMN within the oncology population include both malignant disease and various anti-cancer therapies, including:

- Hematopoietic malignancies
  - Acute myeloid leukemia
  - Acute lymphocytic leukemia
  - Non-Hogkin's lymphoma
  - Hodgkin's lymphoma
  - Myeloproliferative disorders
  - Myelodysplastic syndrome
  - Chronic lymphocytic leukemia
  - Hairy cell leukemia
- Metastatic solid malignancies
  - Gastric carcinoma
  - Colon carcinoma
  - Breast carcinoma
  - Ovarian carcinoma
  - Prostate carcinoma
- Chemotherapeutic agents and other anti-cancer drugs
  - Fludarabine
  - Interferon-α
  - All-trans retinoic acid (ATRA)
  - Granulocyte colony stimulating factor (G-CSF)

- Non-malignant etiologies
  - Sepsis
  - DIC
  - Starvation/malnutrition
  - Anti-phospholipid antibody syndrome

SYMPTOMS AND SIGNS

There are no pathognomonic symptoms or signs of BMN, but the following manifestations should prompt consideration of the diagnosis in any cancer patient:

- Bone pain (present in approximately 80% of patients)
  - Usually acute and severe involving the lower back in most patients
- Fever
- Fatigue
- Dyspnea
  - May result from embolization of necrotic bone marrow to the lungs resulting in acute respiratory distress syndrome

DIAGNOSTIC STUDIES

Diagnosis of BMN requires a high index of suspicion and is often overlooked in the cancer population due to non-specific symptoms and frequency of cytopenias in this population. However, the most useful studies for diagnosis include:

- Complete blood count
  - Anemia and thrombocytopenia present in more than three-fourths of patients; leukopenia less common
  - Leukoerythroblastic peripheral blood smear (e.g., the presence of circulating nucleated erythrocytes and immature leukocytes) is characteristic of BMN
  - Schistocytes
- Serum chemistries
  - Increased lactate dehydrogenase (LDH) and alkaline phosphatase common
- Magnetic resonance imaging (MRI) of bone
  - Non-invasive method for evaluating major areas of bone marrow such as the vertebrae, pelvis, and proximal long bones
  - Increased water content of bone marrow forms basis of utility of MRI in the diagnosis of BMN
  - Characteristic findings of BMN include
    - Diffuse geographic areas of central hypointensity on T2-weighted images surrounded by gadolinium-enhancing rim
- Bone marrow aspiration and biopsy
- Diagnostic study of choice for confirmation of BMN
  - Bone marrow tap may be "dry" on occasion due to coagulative necrosis of bone marrow; watery dark red or clear fluid aspirate on occasion

- ○ Aspiration findings
  - Background of diffuse amorphous eosinophilic material surrounding necrotic cellular elements
  - Necrotic cells exhibit loss of normal staining patterns with vacuolated eosinophilic cytoplasm, pyknotic nuclei, and indistinct cell membranes
- ○ Biopsy findings
  - Preservation of spicular architecture
  - Increased reticulin

TREATMENT

In addition to disease-specific therapy such as chemotherapy, the mainstay of treatment for BMN is supportive care with transfusion of blood products, antibiotics for infection, and adequate nutrition.

PROGNOSIS

The prognosis of BMN in the setting of malignancy, especially metastatic carcinoma, is poor, with some studies revealing survival times of 4 to 14 weeks. Although some patients with hematologic malignancies may recover with chemotherapy and supportive care, the median survival for this group of patients ranges between 1 and 4 months.

ADDITIONAL READING

Dunn P, Shih LY, Liaw SJ, et al. Bone marrow necrosis in 38 adult cancer patients. *J Formos Med Assoc* 1993;92:1107–1110.

Janssens AM, Offner FC, Van Hove WZ. Bone marrow necrosis. *Cancer* 2000; 88:1769–1780.

Paydas S, Ergin M, Baslamisli F, et al. Bone marrow necrosis: clinicopathologic analysis of 20 cases and review of the literature. *Am J Hematol* 2002; 70:300–305.

Ranaghan L, Morris TC, Desai ZR, et al. Bone marrow necrosis. *Am J Hematol* 1994;47:225–228.

Scudla V, Dusek J, Macak J, et al. Bone marrow necrosis in malignant diseases. A report on seven intravitally recognized cases. *Neoplasma* 1989;36:603–610.

Tang YM, Jeavons S, Stuckey S, et al. MRI features of bone marrow necrosis. *AJR* 2007;188:509–514.

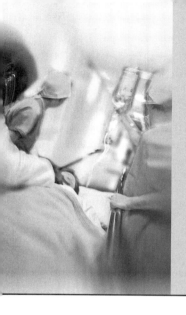

59

Transfusion-Associated Graft-Versus-Host Disease

DEFINITION

Transfusion-associated graft-versus-host disease (TA-GVHD) is an uncommon but fatal complication of blood product transfusion that results from immunocompetent donor lymphocytes attacking tissues in an immunoincompetent host who cannot destroy the donor cells.

CLINICAL SETTING

In the non-hematopoietic stem cell transplantation setting, TA-GVHD complicates transfusion of non-irradiated donor blood products to an immunosuppressed host, most commonly during induction therapy for acute leukemia.

PATHOGENESIS

Patients with profound immunodeficiency, such as that occurs with acute leukemia or prolonged chemotherapy for hematologic neoplasms, may not be able to mount an immune response against immunocompetent transfused donor T-lymphocytes. Only cellular blood products, such as packed red cells, contain sufficient numbers of viable T-lymphocytes to be capable of invoking a graft-versus-host response. Immunosuppressed cancer patients with bone marrow involvement such as acute leukemia, are especially prone to TA-GVHD as the donor T-lymphocytes engraft within the host marrow environment. Hodgkin's disease is often associated with intrinsic immune dysfunction and patients receiving chemotherapy and/or radiotherapy are especially prone to developing TA-GVHD, if unirradiated products are transfused. The recipient's bone marrow is recognized as foreign tissue to the host

T-lymphocytes which attack the hematopoietic elements resulting in bone marrow aplasia. Rarely, immunocompetent patients who receive blood transfusions from relatives develop TA-GVHD if they share HLA haplotypes. Most cases occur within 8 to 10 days following transfusion therapy, with a range of 2 to 50 days in some series. The target organs affected from TA-GVHD include tissues with large populations of lymphoid cells such as the skin, gastrointestinal tract, liver, and bone marrow. Skin involvement presents as acute desquamating rash which can affect a significant portion of the body and may behave clinically as a severe burn. Donor T-lymphocyte attack of host gastrointestinal mucosa and liver may result in severe exudative diarrhea and hepatic dysfunction, respectively. Gastrointestinal involvement with TA-GVHD may cause severe mucosal ulceration and de-epithilialization, resulting in significant losses of blood, water, and protein. Bacterial translocation across the denuded epithelium may result in sepsis. Hepatocellular dysfunction may cause severe hepatitis and subsequent impairment of protein synthesis, clotting factor formation, and drug metabolism. Destruction of small bile ducts results in jaundice and ascites. Bone marrow aplasia, similar to aplastic anemia, the hallmark feature of TA-GVHD, is recognized as foreign tissue by the donor T cells. Bone marrow failure may result in bleeding due to thrombocytopenia, severe anemia, and sepsis due to leukocyte destruction. It is the severe bone marrow aplasia that results in the almost universal mortality rate of TA-GVHD. Gamma irradiation of cellular blood products with 25–30 Gy destroys all immunocompetent lymphoid cells and should be performed before transfusion therapy in high-risk patients.

ETIOLOGY

Only cellular blood products containing sufficient numbers of immunoreactive T-lymphocytes have been implicated in TA-GVHD and include:

- Packed red blood cells
- Platelet concentrates
- Granulocyte concentrates

SYMPTOMS AND SIGNS

The diagnosis of TA-GVHD is very difficult to make and may easily be overlooked if clinicians do not appreciate this disease process or if they are unaware of recent transfusion therapy. Nonetheless, TA-GVHD should be considered in any immunosuppressed cancer patient who presents with the following:

- Fever
  - May result from infection or cytokine release
- Fatigue
- Anorexia
- Nausea/vomiting
- Diarrhea
  - May be watery or bloody and often is profuse

- Pallor
  - May result from profound anemia
- Icterus
- Desquamating rash
- Petechiae
  - May result from thrombocytopenia
- Tachycardia
- Hypotension
  - May result from diarrhea-induced volume depletion or septic shock
- Ascites
- Edema

Diagnostic Studies

Diagnosis of TA-GVHD is mainly a clinical diagnosis but the following studies may aid in diagnosis:

- Complete blood count
  - Always reveals pancytopenia
- Liver enzymes
  - Elevation of transaminases and bilirubin
- Coagulation studies
  - Increased partial thromboplastin time (PTT) and prothrombin time (PT) common
- Hepatic ultrasound
  - May reveal hepatomegaly and ascites
- Liver biopsy
  - Lymphocytic infiltration of hepatocytes, bile ducts, and portal tracts
  - Hepatocyte necrosis
- Skin biopsy
  - Lymphocytic dermal infiltration
- Gastrointestinal mucosal biopsy
  - Hallmark lesion is focal crypt cell necrosis
- Bone marrow biopsy
  - TA-GVHD is characterized by bone marrow aplasia with increased fat content and a paucity of cellular elements

Treatment

Treatment of TA-GVHD in the patient with active malignancy is especially difficult not only because of the effects of the underlying disease, but also because of the pancytopenia, profound immune suppression, and end-organ damage characteristic of this syndrome. Supportive medical care including frequent transfusion therapy, treatment of infection, correction of coagulopathy, fluid resuscitation, electrolyte repletion, and nutrition support are vital. Some authors have treated

TA-GVHD similar to aplastic anemia with agents such as corticosteroids, antithymocyte globulin, and cyclosporine with little benefit. Prevention of TA-GVHD is best prevented with gamma-irradiation of all cellular blood products prior to transfusion in at-risk patients.

PROGNOSIS

The prognosis of TA-GVHD is dismal with mortality rates exceeding 90% despite aggressive intervention.

ADDITIONAL READING

Anderson KC, Weinstein HC. Graft-versus-host disease after transfusion. *N Engl J Med* 1990;323:315.

Holland PV. Prevention of transfusion-associated graft-vs-host disease. *Arch Pathol Lab Med* 1989;113:285.

Nambiar A, Leitman S. Transfusion therapy. In: *Hematology-Oncology Therapy.* Boyiadzis MM, Lebowitz PF, Frame JN, et al., eds. New York: McGraw-Hill, 2007, pp. 607–630.

Shivdasani RA, Haluska FG, Dock NL, et al. Graft-versus-host disease associated with transfusion of blood from unrelated HLA-homozygous donors. *N Engl J Med* 1993;328:766.

Tenorio GC, Gupte SC, Munker R. Transfusion medicine and immunohematology. In: *Modern Hematology: Biology and Clinical Management.* Munker R, Hiller E, Glass J, et al., eds. Totowa, NJ: Humana Press, 2007, pp. 401–432.

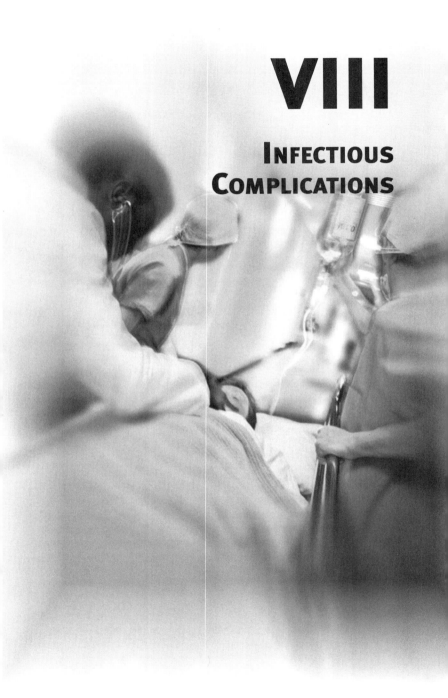

VIII

INFECTIOUS
COMPLICATIONS

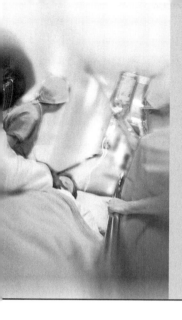

60

Overwhelming Post-Splenectomy Infection

DEFINITION

Overwhelming post-splenectomy infection (OPSI) is a devastating clinical syndrome characterized by the rapid onset of fulminant septic shock occurring months, or even years, after removal of the spleen, or less commonly, in conditions of functional asplenia.

CLINICAL SETTING

Most cases of OPSI occur within the first few years of splenectomy but it may not be until decades later and often in patients rendered disease-free following anti-cancer therapy or splenectomy for the primary condition. Uncommonly, OPSI can occur in patients with intact spleens but impaired splenic function, a condition known as "functional asplenia" which can occur in a variety of oncologic disorders.

PATHOGENESIS

The spleen is a central component of the reticuloendothelial system, where filtration and phagocytosis of bacteria in the bloodstream, removal of parasitized erythrocytes, production of antibodies, and opsonization take place. The spleen, originally described as an "organ of mystery" by Galen (130–200 AD), is the largest single aggregate of lymphoid tissue and is inserted between the arterial supply and venous return of all circulating blood. As alluded to earlier, the spleen plays an important role in host immune function but is also involved with normal erythrocyte homeostasis. For instance, senescent red blood cells are removed in the splenic cords via a process known as culling. Additionally, the spleen can remove unwanted intra-erythrocytic elements, while maintaining overall cell viability, by pitting the cells as they pass through the splenic sinuses within the slit-like fenestrations of the sinusoidal endothelium. Asplenic patients lose this pitting ability and cannot remove various intracellular constituents. Therefore, asplenic hosts typically manifest pathognomonic changes within circulating erythrocytes. Most notable among them is the Howell-Jolly body. Howell-Jolly inclusions are nuclear remnants that are normally removed but, if identified on a peripheral blood smear, are indicative of asplenia and provide a valuable clue if the presence of a spleen is unknown in the septic cancer patient. Patients with functional hyposplenism may also exhibit Howell-Jolly bodies and their presence regardless of whether anatomic or functional hyposplenism is considered to increase the risk of OPSI.

The most important role of the spleen relates to normal immune system function such as the production of opsonins which are complement proteins that adhere to circulating bacteria to enhance clearance of these bacterial-complement complexes. Opsonization is vital for adequate defense against encapsulated organisms, especially *Streptococcus pneumoniae*, the most common organism implicated associated with OPSI. In fact, asplenia renders the patient approximately 600 times more susceptible to encapsulated bacterial sepsis. Although myriad bacterial species have been implicated in OPSI, *S. pneumoniae* is clinically the most important and dangerous due to the intrinsic virulence of the organism. Decreased production of the splenic opsonin, properdin, and complement component C3 may also increase infection risk. Impaired splenic production of IgM also impairs the primary immune response to bacteremia. Combined, the loss of normal filtration, poor opsonization of bacteria, and decreased production of properdin, C3, and IgM explain the markedly increased risk of OPSI in the asplenic host, with lifetime risk exceeding 5%. However, aplenic patients with underlying hematologic malignancy have an even higher risk of OPSI and death from fulminant sepsis. Often, no primary source of infection can be ascertained, although meningitis remains a common focus, especially for *S. pneumoniae* and *N. meningitidis*. Overwhelming bacteremia causes findings typical of severe sepsis including low systemic vascular resistance, hypotension, anuria, disseminated intravascular coagulation, and occasionally, acute adrenal hemorrhage (Waterhouse-Friderichsen syndrome).

ETIOLOGY

The etiologies of asplenia in the hematology-oncology patient include surgical and functional asplenia, both of which are associated with the development of OPSI:

- Splenectomy
  - Staging for Hodgkin's disease
  - Marked splenomegaly (e.g., myelofibrosis, chronic myeloid leukemia, hairy cell leukemia)
  - Immune thrombocytopenic purpura (ITP)
  - Hereditary spherocytosis

- ○ Splenic lymphoma
- ○ Thalassemia
- Functional asplenia
  - ○ Sickle cell anemia
  - ○ Splenic lymphoma
  - ○ Hairy cell leukemia
  - ○ Amyloidosis
  - ○ Splenic irradiation
  - ○ Malignant histiocytosis
  - ○ Allogenic bone marrow transplantation/graft versus host disease
  - ○ Chemotherapy
  - ○ Corticosteroids

The bacterial etiologies of OPSI are many, with *S. pneumoniae* accounting for approximately 90% in some series. Reported etiologies, however, include:

- *S. pneumoniae* (etiology of 85% to 90% of cases)
- *Haemophilus influenzae*
- *Neisseria meningitidis*
- *Capnocytophaga canimorsus*
  - ○ Gram-negative bacterium that resides in the oral flora of dogs and, less commonly, cats that causes syndrome characterized by fulminant septic shock and *pupura fulminans* following a bite or scratch from a dog or cat
- *Staphylococcus aureus*
- *Salmonella* species
- *Pseudomonas aeruginosa*
- *Escherichia coli*
- *Klebsiella pneumoniae*
- *Pleisomonas shigelloides*
- Intra-erythrocytic parasites
  - ○ *Babesia microti* (Eastern seaboard of United States)*, B. bovis* (Europe) — Tick-borne protozoan organisms that may cause hemolytic anemia
  - ○ Malarial organisms*: Plasmodium vivax, malariae, falciparum*

SYMPTOMS AND SIGNS

The diagnosis of OPSI must be considered in any acutely ill, febrile asplenic patient, who manifests any of the following clinical manifestations, keeping in mind that non-specific symptoms are quite common:

- Fever/rigors
- Sore throat
- Headache
- Stiff neck
  - ○ Indicative of a meningeal source from infection with *S. pneumoniae* or *N. meningitidis* in adult patients

- Myalgias
- Vomiting
- Diarrhea
- Confusion
- Oliguria
- Hypotension
- Tachycardia
- Nuchal rigidity
  - May occur with a meningeal source of infection
- Petechiae/purpura
- Ecchymosis (DIC)
- Gangrene of digits (*purpura fulminans*)

DIAGNOSTIC STUDIES

Diagnosis of OPSI is primarily clinical and should be suspected in any asplenic patient who presents with an acute febrile illness, even without an apparent focus of infection. However, various diagnostic studies may be helpful in establishing the diagnosis and include:

- Peripheral blood smear
  - Howell-Jolly bodies
  - Bacteria may be visualized within granulocytes or extracellular
- Wright's or Gram stained peripheral blood buffy coat
  - Useful to identify intracellular bacteria
- Blood cultures
  - Typically positive within 24 hours, especially if *S. pneumoniae* is the etiology of OPSI
- Cultures of skin lesions
  - Petechial or purpuric lesions may reveal organisms on Gram staining and culture
- Urine pneumococcal antigen
- Lumbar puncture
  - Since meningitis is common in OPSI, cerebrospinal fluid should be obtained in most patients

TREATMENT

Treatment for suspected OPSI should not be delayed while awaiting diagnostic studies since the course is typically fulminant over a period of hours in many cases. Blood cultures should be immediately obtained while awaiting empiric antibiotics to arrive from the pharmacy. Tailoring the regimen based on the bacterial isolate can be performed when the culture data is received. Local antibiotic resistance patterns, especially to *S. pneumoniae*, should be taken into account when selecting initial therapy. Ceftriaxone or vancomycin (if the prevalence of high-level penicillin resistance to pneumococci is common) are usually appropriate empiric regimens. Additional coverage against gram-negative organisms (e.g., *P. aeruginosa*) should be considered in the appropriate clinical setting. *B. microti* is often treated with clindamycin and quinine. Antimalarial coverage should be provided in the returning asplenic traveler who has visited an endemic area. Finally, prevention of pneumococcal OPSI with the polyvalent pneumococcal vaccine is suggested in patients about to undergo, or who have recently had, a splenectomy. Other suggested immunization strategies include the *H. influenza* type B and the meningococcal vaccines, which should be optimally administered at least 14 days before an elective splenectomy. Consideration should be given for provision of oral antibiotics to be taken by the patient at the onset of febrile illness if there is the potential for delay in seeking medical care and for a medic alert bracelet indicating the presence of asplenia.

PROGNOSIS

Prognosis of OPSI in the patient with hematologic malignancy is quite poor, and is higher than patients who are asplenic from benign or traumatic etiologies. Mortality rates of up to 70% have been reported, with 68% of deaths occurring within 4 hours and 80% within 24 hours.

ADDITIONAL READING

Brigden ML, Pattullo AL. Prevention and management of overwhelming post-splenectomy infection—an update. *Crit Care Med* 1999;27:836–842.

Brown EJ, Hosea SW, Frank MM. The role of the spleen in experimental pneumococcal bacteremia. *J Clin Invest* 1981;67:975–982.

Ndon JA. Capnocytophaga canimorsus septicemia caused by a dog bite in a hairy cell leukemia patient. *J Clin Microbiol* 1992;30:211–213.

Sumaraju V, Smith LG, Smith SM. Infectious complications in asplenic hosts. *Infect Dis Clin N Am* 2001;15:551–565.

Waghorn DJ. Overwhelming infection in asplenic patients: current best practice preventive measures are not being followed. *J Clin Pathol* 2001; 54:214–218.

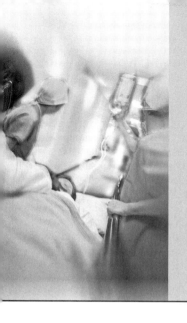

61

Disseminated Candidiasis

Definition

Disseminated candidiasis (DC) is a life-threatening infection characterized by bloodstream and tissue invasion with various *Candida* species and often results in death due to sepsis and multiple organ dysfunction.

Clinical Setting

Most cases of DC occur in patients with hematologic malignancies who have undergone cytotoxic chemotherapy resulting in prolonged and deep neutropenia and have received broad-spectrum antimicrobial therapy.

Pathogenesis

Candida albicans causes approximately 40% to 50% of cases of DC, but other species are increasing in frequency due to the common administration of broad-spectrum antibiotics and antifungal drugs. *Candida glabrata* and *C. parapsilosis* are the most common non-*albicans* species causing DC, but other isolates include *C. lusitaniae, C. tropicalis, C. krusei, C. rugosa,* and, *C. guilliermondii.* All *Candida* species are commensals of healthy humans, but can be pathogenic in various circumstances, especially malignancy. These organisms can be isolated from areas with a warm and moist environment such as the mouth, gastrointestinal tract, and vagina. *Candida* grows on basic culture media as budding cells but in tissue, both yeast forms and pseudohyphae are present. An exception is *C. glabrata* which forms no true hyphae or pseudohyphae. *Candida albicans* is well-known for forming germ tubes in serum, a useful test for identification in the microbiology laboratory.

Candida species can become virulent in the setting of immunosuppression and mucosal disruption, which are frequently encountered in the oncology population, especially those patients with hematologic malignancies undergoing stem cell transplantation or induction chemotherapy. Colonization of various sites is present in most patients who eventually develop DC, usually in the setting of broad-spectrum antibacterial drugs which allows for yeast overgrowth. *Candida* may enter the bloodstream through central venous catheters, disrupted oral or intestinal mucosa from cytotoxic chemotherapy, abdominal surgery, uretheral catheterization, or from maceration or disruption of the skin. *Candida* can evade host immune defenses and antifungal therapy due to their ability to produce a biofilm on venous catheters or tissue. Once within the bloodstream, sepsis syndrome with hemodynamic instability and multiple organ dysfunction commonly occurs, which may result in rapid death. *Candida albicans*, as well as other species, has a propensity to seed various sites such as the skin, eyes, liver, kidneys, and lungs. Invasion of small dermal vessels can result in characteristic tender, erythematous nodules in patients with acute leukemia. *Candida* may involve the retinal vessels and vitreous humor resulting in blindness. A condition known as hepatosplenic candidiasis characteristically occurs in patients who have recently undergone induction chemotherapy and manifests shortly after neutrophil recovery. The hepatic parenchyma becomes seeded via the portal venous system as *Candida* organisms translocate across denuded intestinal mucosa. Hematogenous invasion of the kidneys can result in pyelonephritis and papillary necrosis and lung involvement may manifest as pulmonary nodules and infiltrates.

ETIOLOGY

The etiologies and risk factors for DC in the cancer patient include:

- Cytotoxic chemotherapy
  - Induction chemotherapy with cytosine arabinoside
  - Hematopoietic stem cell transplantation with high-dose chemotherapy and graft-versus-host disease
- Hematologic malignancy
  - Acute myelogenous leukemia with prolonged, deep neutropenia
- Mucositis
  - Oral or gastrointestinal mucosal disruption from chemotherapy
- Broad-spectrum antibiotics
- Fluconazole prophlyaxis
  - May increase risk of DC due to *C. glabrata* and *C. krusei*
- Corticosteroids
- Central venous catheters
- Acute renal failure
- Total parenteral nutrition
- Intensive care unit admission
- Prolonged hospitalization

- Diabetes mellitus/hyperglycemia
- Perforated colon cancer
- Recent gastrointestinal surgery

Symptoms and Signs

Patients with DC often have similar symptoms to patients with bacterial sepsis or focal bacterial infections. However, *Candida* species have a propensity to seed particular organs, which may aid in diagnosis in the proper setting. The clinician should consider DC in any cancer patient who develops any of the following, especially in the recovery phase of neutropenia—a time in which DC is especially prone to manifest:

- Fever
- Rigors
- Delirium
- Visual changes/loss
  - May result from *Candida* invasion of the retina, vitreous humor, or anterior chamber
- Painful oral lesions
  - Often a feature in patients with neutropenia and recent administration of chemotherapy that serves as a portal of entry for bloodstream invasion
- Cough
  - Pneumonia is a rare complication of DC
- Diarrhea
  - Often a feature of gastrointestinal mucositis in patients with neutropenia and recent administration of chemotherapy that serves as a portal of entry for bloodstream invasion
- Abdominal pain
  - Right upper quadrant pain occurring during the period of neutrophil recovery is suggestive of hepatosplenic cadidiasis
  - *Candida* peritonitis is a rare complication of colonic perforation from chemotherapy associated mucositis
- Flank pain or renal colic
  - Involvement of the renal parenchyma can result in pyelonephritis or renal papillary necrosis which can present as flank pain and renal colic, respectively
- Painful skin lesions
  - Typically small (0.5–1.0 cm) and can involve any area of the body
- Hypotension
  - Common feature of septic shock due to DC
- Tachycardia
- Abnormal ophthalmoscopic examination
  - Retinal findings include bilateral whitish exudates
  - Retinal detachment may be noted

- Vitreous humor may be cloudy if endophthalmitis occurs
- Hypopyon may occur on rare occasion if infection spreads to anterior chamber
- Erythematous, tender skin nodules that may undergo necrosis
  - Vascular invasion by *Candida* species can result in skin lesions with a necrotic center
- Erythema surrounding venous catheter
- Cardiac murmur
  - Suggestive of hematogenous seeding of the aortic or mitral valves
- Abdominal tenderness
  - Right upper quadrant tenderness suggestive of hepatosplenic candidiasis or rarely, candidal cholecystitis
- Flank tenderness
  - Suggestive of *Candida* pyelonephritis

DIAGNOSTIC STUDIES

Diagnosis of DC requires a high index of suspicion and should be considered in any cancer patient, especially those with hematologic malignancies and neutropenia, who develop evidence of sepsis or unexplained organ dysfunction. Since DC is often overlooked and not discovered until autopsy, the following studies should be considered in at-risk patients:

- Blood cultures
  - Routine blood culture media often positive for *C. albicans* and other species but blood cultures may be negative even in setting of fulminant DC or organ infection
  - Positive germ tube test provides preliminary evidence that isolated species is *C. albicans*
- Urine culture
  - Although urine is frequently colonized in the presence of an indwelling catheter, growth of *Candida* may indicate pyelonephritis and cystitis
- Culture of central venous catheter tip
- Chest radiography
  - *Candida* pneumonia is rare and typically occurs in the setting of severe neutropenia and DC
  - Acute respiratory distress syndrome (ARDS) may complicate septic shock due to DC and manifest as diffuse pulmonary infiltrates
- Computed tomography of the abdomen
  - May reveal low density lesions characterstic of hepatosplenic *candidiasis*
  - Renal abscess, pyelonephritis, or hydroureter from renal papillary necrosis are occasional complications of DC
- Complete blood count
  - Severe neutropenia very common

- Liver function tests
  - Increased alkaline phosphatase characteristic of hepatosplenic candidiasis
- Skin biopsy
  - May reveal candidal organisms, vascular occlusion, and tissue necrosis
- Organ biopsy and culture
  - Biopsy via computed tomographic guidance of the liver and kidney may be useful to assess for hepatosplenic *candidiasis* or pyelonephritis

TREATMENT

Prompt institution of appropriate antifungal therapy, removal of infected central venous catheters or other prosthetic foci, and treatment of the underlying malignant condition are the cornerstones of managing DC. Patients with septic shock due to DC typically require critical care intervention including mechanical ventilation and vasopressors. Recovery of the neutrophil population is important, but ongoing cytoxic chemotherapy or residual leukemia may inhibit marrow recovery. The three classes of antifungal drugs with activity against *Candida* species include the azoles (e.g., fluconazole, voriconazole, posaconazole), the polyenes (e.g., amphotericin B deoxycholate and lipid-based amphotericin formulations), and the echinocandins (e.g., caspofungin, micafungin, anidulafungin). Fluconazole-resistant *C. albicans* and *C. glabrata* isolates are increasing due to the increased use of fluconazole for antifungal prophylaxis in patients with hematologic malignancies. Additionally, some species such as *C. krusei* are intrinsically resistant to fluconazole, which is an important consideration when choosing empiric therapy for suspected DC. Voriconazole is a newer azole with extended antifungal spectrum against most *Candida* species, including *C. krusei*, and is a viable empiric treatment option in patients with suspected DC. Amphotericin B is the historic fungicidal agent of choice for DC. The deoxycholate form is often poorly tolerated by the ill cancer patient due to adverse effects such as rigors, renal failure, anemia, and electrolyte depletion. The lipid-formulated derivatives of amphotericin are better tolerated and retain excellent anti-*candida* activity against the majority of clinically encountered species, with the exception of the intrinsically polyene-resistant *C. lusitaniae*. The echinocandins are increasingly utilized for DC due to excellent susceptibility and side-effect profiles. One major study showed that caspofungin is equivalent to amphotericin B for invasive *candidiasis* with candidemia and is better tolerated. Empiric therapy for the neutropenic or hemodynamically unstable patient with suspected DC should consist of either an amphotericin B formulation, an echinocandin, or voriconazole. Some authors recommend use of a -cidal agent such as amphotericin B or an echinocandin in this situation. Combination therapy with amphotericin and an azole can be considered in critically ill patients with a deep seated focus or poor response to monotherapy. Treatment should continue for at least 14 days after the last positive blood culture and all signs and symptoms of infection have resolved.

PROGNOSIS

The prognosis of DC in patients with acute leukemia or recent stem cell transplantation is high, with crude mortality rates approaching 40%. Failure to recover an adequate neutrophil count or the development of multiple organ dysfunction syndrome is associated with almost universal mortality. The importance of prompt antifungal drug administration cannot be overstated in the cancer population as mortality rates are decreased threefold if treatment is instituted within 12 hours.

ADDITIONAL READING

DiNubile MJ, Hille D, Sable CA, et al. Invasive candidiasis in cancer patients: observations from a randomized clinical trial. *J Infect* 2005;50:443–449.

Megalakaki C, Perlorentzou S, Dadakaridou M, et al. Candidemia in patients with acute leukemia. *J BUON* 2006;11:191–195.

Mora-Duarte J, Betts R, Rotstein C, et al. Comparison of caspofungin and amphotericin B for invasive candidiasis. *N Engl J Med* 2002;347:2020–2029.

Patterson TF. Advances and challenges in management of invasive mycoses. *Lancet* 2005;366:1013–1025.

Spellberg B, Ibrahim AS, Edwards JE, et al. Mice with disseminated candidiasis die of progressive sepsis. *Clin Infect Dis* 2005;192:336–343.

Spellberg BJ, Filler SG, Edwards JE. Current treatment strategies for disseminated candidiasis. *Clin Infect Dis* 2006;42:244–251.

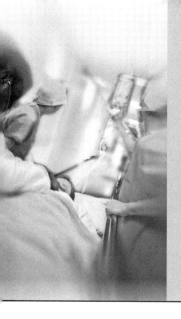

62

Rhinocerebral Mucormycosis

DEFINITION

Rhinocerebral mucormycosis (RCM) is a rapidly progressive, and often fatal, necrotizing vascular infection involving organisms from the *Zygomycetes* class that most often affects the nasal sinuses, resulting in rapid tissue necrosis and secondary brain invasion.

CLINICAL SETTING

The vast majority of cases of RCM occur in immunosuppressed patients with uncontrolled diabetes mellitus, hematologic malignancies, or those who have received aggressive cytotoxic chemotherapy with prolonged neutropenia.

PATHOGENESIS

Mucormycosis is a term referring to infection caused by various members of the *Mucoraceae* family. Although the taxonomy of this group of fungal organisms is complex, the most commonly isolated organisms causing human infections include species of *Rhizopus, Rhizomucor, Cunninghamella, Absidia,* and *Saksenaea*. The most commonly isolated organisms responsible for mucormycosis infections in adults are from the genus *Rhizopus*. Mucormycosis can affect various organs including the paranasal sinuses, tracheobronchial-pulmonary tissues, and the gastrointestinal tract. The most common form of infection resulting from this group of organisms is RCM, which most often occurs in immunosuppressed patients, such as patients with hematologic malignancies with prolonged neutropenia and chemotherapy-induced mucositis and immune dysfunction. Hyperglycemia and metabolic acidosis from poorly controlled diabetes mellitus also increases the risk of infection. Prolonged iron-chelation therapy with deferoxamine in patients who undergo chronic transfusion therapy increases the risk of RCM since this agent chelates iron into a form that the organisms can utilize.

Rhizopus and other organisms that cause mucormycosis are environmentally ubiquitous, thriving on decaying vegetation, soil, feces, and high-sugar content foodstuffs. Infection is typically acquired by inhalation of spores, which are often present in the ambient air. Histologically, *Rhizopus* and other closely related organisms are characterized by broad, aseptate hyphae with right-angle branching. Growth of tissue specimens on media is difficult but resembles mold colonies when incubated at room temperature. These organisms are intrinsically angiotropic, leading to vascular thrombosis and tissue necrosis, which is the hallmark of RCM and infections at other sites. Histopathologic specimens may reveal not only intravascular thrombosis teeming with organisms, but also destruction of the arterial wall and vasa vasorum, which can result in hemorrhage from vascular rupture. Typically, RCM commences within the paranasal sinuses leading to ischemic necrosis of the mucosa, followed by invasion and destruction of the hard palate and skull, with secondary invasion of the brain tissue. However, RCM may involve many sites within the skull, upper respiratory tract and brain, leading to various manifestations including proptosis, blindness, seizures, stroke, or coma. Post-mortem pathologic findings in patients with RCM include large hemorrhagic cavities within the fronatal or temporal lobes, sinus destruction, and mastoid bone involvement. Since RCM spreads by rapid vascular invasion and advancing tissue necrosis, curative treatment is often elusive, especially in the later stages of disease.

ETIOLOGY

The underlying etiologic disease processes that predispose to RCM in the cancer population include:

- Hematologic malignancies
  - Acute myelogenous leukemia, especially during induction therapy
  - Hairy cell leukemia
  - Myelodysplastic syndrome
  - Non-Hodgkin's and Hodgkin's lymphoma
- Bone marrow transplantation
- Chemotherapy
  - Prolonged neutropenia, tissue breakdown, immunosuppression, and mucositis related to chemotherapy increase the risk
- Corticosteroids
- Chronic iron-chelating therapy
  - Utilized in setting of chronic transfusion therapy such as with myelodysplastic syndrome
- Poorly controlled diabetes mellitus
- Metabolic acidosis

As noted, the taxonomic organization of mucormycosis is complex, however, the clinician should have a basic knowledge of the etiologic agents responsible for RCM. Species of the following organisms are some of the most frequently isolated from clinical samples of patients with RCM:

- *Rhizopus*
- *Rhizomucor*
- *Cunninghamella*
- *Absidia*
- *Mucor*
- *Saksenaea*

Symptoms and Signs

Since RCM is a rapidly progressing infection with a high mortality rate, a high index of suspicion is needed to diagnose the condition before extensive tissue destruction takes place. Unfortunately, early symptoms and signs are often non-specific, and only after signficiant tissue necrosis occurs, do the classic findings of eschar formation within the nasal cavity become evident. Nonetheless, the clinician should consider RCM in any at-risk cancer patient who develops any of the following:

- Fever
- Nasal obstruction
- Sinus, periorbital, or facial pain
- Bloody, thin nasal discharge
- Maxillary tooth pain
- Otalgia
- Diplopia
- Confusion
  - Indicative of cerebral involvement
- Seizures
  - Indicative of cerebral involvment
- Facial swelling
- Black eschar within nasal cavity or on hard palate
  - A black, necrotic eschar is the classic finding of RCM, but at this stage significant tissue destruction has occurred
- Proptosis
  - May indicate orbital involvement
- Chemosis
- Focal neurologic signs
  - May result from focal areas of brain necrosis or hemorrhage or from ischemic infarction from blood vessel invasion and thrombosis
  - Cranial nerve dysfunction may occur with cavernous sinus thrombosis
- Coma
  - Very poor prognostic sign which is typically a terminal finding in patients with frontal lobe involvement

DIAGNOSTIC STUDIES

Diagnosis of RCM requires a very high index of suspicion and remains, for the most part, a clinical diagnosis. However, several diagnostic studies may be useful to delineate the extent of tissue involvement or prognosis. They are:

- Computed tomography of the head with attention to the sinuses (ethmoidal, maxillary, sphenoidal, and frontal), orbital area, and brain
  - Typical findings of RCM include sinus opacification, bone destruction, soft tissue swelling, and, if brain involvement is present, cerebral infarction, hemorrhage, or edema
- Computed tomographic angiogram or magnetic resonance angiogram
  - May reveal arterial occlusion or aneurysm formation if arterial invasion is present
- Tissue biopsy of involved sites such as the sinuses, hard palate, or bone
  - Classic histologic appearance of mucormycosis includes ribbon-like non-septate, broad hyphae with right-angle branching
  - Necrosis and hemorrhage are common findings in involved tissue
  - Vascular thrombosis and arterial wall invasion with organisms may be noted
- Culture of involved tissue
  - Plating material onto Sabouraud media often reveals rapid growth of mold colonies

TREATMENT

Although timely antifungal chemotherapy is important in the therapy of RCM, the crux of treatment is immediate, aggressive surgical debridement of all involved tissue. Radical debridement of necrotic and threatened tissue may require disfiguring surgery, involving radical facial reconstruction, if the patient survives. Eradication of the underlying malignancy, correction of neutropenia, hyperglycemia, and metabolic acidosis are important supportive measures. Amphotericin B is the historical antifungal agent of choice for RCM, but is associated with significant toxicity such as anemia, rigors, electrolyte depletion, and renal dysfunction. Liposomal amphotericin B has been successfully utilized and is better tolerated with less renal toxicity. The newer systemic antifungals voriconazole and caspofungin are not active against mucormycosis and should not be utilized if RCM is suspected. Posaconazole, a newer azole administered as an oral elixir, has demonstrated *in vitro* activity although clinical trials are lacking.

PROGNOSIS

The prognosis of RCM is generally poor, especially if the diagnosis is delayed and debridement is suboptimal. Patients with hematologic malignancies, hematopoietic stem cell transplantation, and prolonged neutropenia, have an especially poor prognosis with mortality rates of approximately 70%. Invasion of the cerebral tissue with subsequent hemorrhagic necrosis is almost uniformly fatal.

ADDITIONAL READING

Blair SL, Schwarz RE. Critical care of patients with cancer: surgical considerations. *Crit Care Clin* 2001;17:721–739.

Georgala A, Vekemans M, Husson M, et al. Zygomycosis in the immunocompromised patient: a case report. *Acta Biomed* 2006;77:S2:5–9.

Lerchenmuller C, Goner M, Buchner T, et al. Rhinocerebral zygomycosis in a patient with acute lymphoblastic leukemia. *Ann Oncol* 2001;12:415–419.

Pagano L, Offidani M, Fianchi L, et al. Mucormycosis in hematologic patients. *Haematologica* 2004;89:207–214.

Paterson PJ, Marshall SR, Shaw B, et al. Fatal invasive cerebral *Absidia corymbifera* infection following bone marrow transplantation. *Bone Marrow Transplantation* 2000;26:701–703.

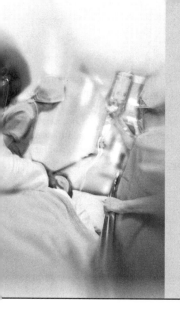

63

Acute Infectious Meningitis

DEFINITION

Acute infectious meningitis (AIM) refers to acute meningeal inflammation resulting from infection with various bacterial or, less often, fungal organisms.

CLINICAL SETTING

Some authors have reported that as many as one in six cases of central nervous system infections occur in patients with malignancy, with AIM occurring most commonly in brain tumor patients who have undergone craniotomy or in patients undergoing aggressive therapy for hematologic malignancy.

PATHOGENESIS

This discussion will primarily focus on acute bacterial meningitis in the cancer patient, although fungal meningitis will be briefly discussed. The most common etiologies of community-acquired AIM are *Streptococcus pneumoniae, Neisseria meningititis*, and *Haemophilus influenzae*. However, the responsible organisms in the cancer population are quite different, and depend upon the various predisposing factors that are present within this population. Although myriad infecting agents can cause AIM in the cancer patient, *Staphylococcus aureus, S. pneumoniae,* and *Listeria monocytogenes* are responsible for more than one-half of the cases of malignancy-associated AIM. Meningitis due to the skin commensals *S. aureus* and *S. epidermidis* most commonly occurs following craniotomy for a primary or metastatic brain tumor. Encapsulated bacteria such as *S. pneumoniae* is quite common in patients with impaired humoral defenses, such as those with multiple myeloma or chronic lymphocytic leukemia. Solid tumors and hematopoietic malignancies, as well as chemotherapy, increase the risk of infection with *L. monocytogenes*. The underlying immunologic deficit due to the type of malignancy or treatment is important in the pathogenesis of AIM. For instance, neutrophil dysfunction or neutropenia increases the risk of bacterial infections, especially in the setting of hematologic malignancy. Any focus of bacterial infection in the setting of prolonged and deep neutropenia may result in bacteremia (prolonged or transient) with subsequent seeding of the meninges. Impairment of cell mediated immunity and T-cell function are risk factors for a wide variety of nervous system infections, including AIM. For instance, patients receiving corticosteroid therapy or those with Hodgkin's disease are prone to infections with *L. monocytogenes* and *Cryptococcus neoformans*. Splenectomy predisposes to pneumococcal meningitis.

As noted, the meninges may become seeded with bacteria through hematogenous spread, or by direct extension from a contiguous source such as a surgical incision, a ventriculoperitoneal catheter, lumbar puncture, sinusitis, epidural abscess, or craniofacial osteomyelitis. Bacteria within the cerebrospinal fluid (CSF) replicate in rapid fashion due to the paucity of immune defenses. Normal CSF contains very few phagocytic neutrophils and only small amounts of complement and immunoglobulins, which results in poor opsonization of bacteria. Regardless of how bacteria (or less commonly, fungi) reach the subarachnoid space, proliferation elicits an inflammatory response of the vasculature, meninges, and the parenchyma leading to increased levels of cytokines such as interleukin (IL)-1, IL-6, and tumor necrosis factor (TNF). Studies of patients with community acquired meningitis have shown that the levels of inflammatory cytokines directly correlate with the severity of symptoms and risk of a poor outcome. The majority of neurologic complications of AIM result from this inflammatory response to the organism. Increased permeability of the blood brain barrier from IL-1 and TNF leads to vasogenic edema with leakage of leukocytes and proteins into the subarachnoid space. This can overwhelm absorptive mechanisms and result in communicating hydrocephalus and interstitial cerebral edema. Neutrophil breakdown with release of cytotoxic enzymes can lead to cytoxic edema and cell necrosis. As a consequence of these mechanisms and disruption of normal cerebral vascular autoregulation, a cycle of cerebral edema with fatal brain herniation may ensue. Cerebral infarction may occur from inflammatory or infectious occlusion of arteries (*endarteritis obliterans*) within the brain parenchyma which may result in extensive tissue necrosis. Basilar meningeal involvement may also result in cranial nerve dysfunction. Diffuse cortical inflammation may result in refractory seizures or coma. Other pathogenic events occurring during the course of AIM include hyponatremia from the syndrome of inappropriate anti-diuretic hormone (SIADH) release or cerebral salt-wasting syndrome, multiorgan dysfunction syndrome, respiratory failure, and cerebral venous sinus thrombosis.

ETIOLOGY

Cancer patients are at risk for AIM from a variety of infectious organisms, most often bacteria. Opportunistic pathogens are occasionally implicated in patients with prolonged and profound immunosuppression as may be the case with acute leukemia and hematopoietic stem cell transplantation. Some of the most commonly reported etiologies of AIM include:

- *S. pneumoniae*
  - Patients with humoral deficiency or hypogammaglobulinemia such as chronic lymphocytic leukemia or multiple myeloma are especially prone to invasive pneumococcal infection
- *S. aureus*
  - Most often occurs in setting of prior craniotomy or placement of an intraventricular catheter or ventriculoperitoneal shunt
- *S. epidermidis*
  - Typically complicates placement of an intraventricular catheter or ventriculoperitoneal shunt
- *L. monocytogenes*
- *Propionibacterium acnes*
  - Skin commensal that may cause meningitis following craniotomy or intraventricular device
- *H. influenzae*
- *Pseudomonas aeruginosa*
  - Common cause of post-neurosurgical meningitis
- Other Gram-negative bacilli (*Escherichia coli, Enterobacter, Klebsiella, Proteus* species)
- *Aspergillus* species
  - Most commonly occurs in setting of deep and prolonged neutropenia associated with induction chemotherapy or hematopoietic stem cell transplantation for acute leukemia
- *Cryptococcus neoformans*
- *Candida* species
  - Typically occurs in the setting of prolonged neutropenia, broad-spectrum antimicrobial use, or total parenteral nutrition

SYMPTOMS AND SIGNS

Although AIM in the cancer patient can present in a classic fashion with sudden headache, fever, and neck stiffness, symptoms in this patient population may be more subtle due to multiple comorbidities, use of corticosteroids and analgesia, and the presence of underlying cognitive function. Therefore, the clinician should consider AIM if any of the following symptoms and signs are present:

- Headache
- Fever

- Neck pain/stiffness
- Photophobia
- Nausea/vomiting
- Confusion
- Seizures
  - Focal seizures usually indicative of focal areas of arterial ischemia, hemorrhage, or necrosis
  - Generalized seizures may complicate cerebral edema, infarction, hyponatremia, or secondary to antibiotics (e.g., quinolones, high-dose penicillin, carbapenems)
- Tachycardia
- Hypertension and bradycardia (Cushing reflex)
  - Indicative of severe cerebral edema and impending brain herniation
- Papilledema
  - Indicative of increased intracranial pressure
- Nuchal rigidity
- Kernig's sign
- Brudzinski's sign
- Focal neurologic deficits (cranial nerve paralysis or focal extremity weakness)
  - Indicative of focal area of infarction/necrosis secondary to *endarteritis obliterans*, vascular thrombosis, or brain abscess
- Coma
  - May result from cerebral edema, brain herniation, or status epilepticus

DIAGNOSTIC STUDIES

As a general rule, diagnostic studies should not delay definitive therapy, since many studies have shown higher morbidity and mortality rates associated with delayed antibiotic therapy in patients with acute community acquired meningitis. However, patients with underlying malignancy often have other causes for fever, headache, confusion, and neurologic deficits such as metastasis, metabolic derangements, radiation toxicity, and chemotherapy effects. Additional diagnostic testing is frequently performed in this population including:

- Lumbar puncture (LP)
  - Gold standard diagnostic test of choice; common findings include:
    - Increased total leukocyte and neutrophil count (> 10–100 cells/mm^3)
      - May not be elevated in setting of severe neutropenia
    - Mononuclear pleocytosis
      - May be present with early bacterial meningitis, fungal meningitis, viral infections, or neoplastic meningitis
    - Decreased glucose (< 40 mg/dl)
    - Increased protein (> 45 mg/dl)
    - Increased opening pressure (> 180 mmH$_2$0)
    - Positive Gram stain (in approximately 50% to 60%)

- Positive CSF culture (in approximately 80%, but may be lower in the setting of recent antibiotic use or slow-growing organisms)
  - Latex agglutination testing helpful if *S. pneumoniae* is suspected but overall sensitivity and specificity in the cancer population is limited
  - Positive limulus lysate test which detects Gram-negative endotoxin in approximately 75% of patients with Gram-negative AIM
  - India ink preparation or cryptococcal antigen assay if *C. neoformans* is suspected
  - Immunocompromised and cancer patients have a higher risk of an underlying mass lesion which may increase the risk of cerebral herniation with LP
    - LP should not be performed until imaging of the central nervous system is carried out to exclude a space-occupying lesion in patients presenting with seizures, focal neurologic findings, papilledema, known solid tumor with propensity for brain metastasis, or concern about a focal infectious process such as toxoplasmosis
- Computed tomography (CT) or magnetic resonance imaging (MRI) of the brain
  - CT is useful to detect acute hemorrhage, edema, bone destruction, or midline shift; less sensitive than MRI for detecting cerebral mass lesions
- Blood cultures
  - Should be obtained immediately (before LP) and before antibiotic therapy

TREATMENT

Since treatment delay increases the risk of adverse outcome, patients with suspected acute bacterial meningitis should be administered antibiotics before cerebral imaging if an LP needs to be deferred until a space-occupying lesion is excluded. Empiric antibiotic therapy is based upon the organism(s) most likely to cause AIM in the specific clinical situation with the guiding principle of utilizing bactericidal antibiotics for prolonged time periods. For instance, patients with humoral immunodeficiency (e.g., CLL, myeloma) should be administered agents active against *S. pneumoniae* such as ceftriaxone and vancomycin. The regimen can be modified based on culture and susceptibility data. Empiric therapy for post-neurosurgical meningitis includes vancomycin to cover *S. aureus* and *S. epidermidis* and an antipseudomonal agent such as cefepime or imipenem. Patients with risk factors for *L. monocytogenes* such as old age or cell mediated immunity defects should receive ampicillin and gentamicin. Antibiotic regimens should subsequently be tailored to culture results. Meningitis due to fungal organisms requires amphotericin B and, occasionally, flucytosine. Supportive care including hemodynamic monitoring, seizure control, respiratory support, nutritional support, electrolyte and glucose management, venous thromboembolism prophylaxis, and gastritis prophylaxis are important adjuncts. Patients with impending herniation may require placement of an intraventricular pressure monitor, but underlying coagulopathy, thrombocytopenia, and neutropenia make this a risky procedure in the cancer population.

PROGNOSIS

Mortality rates for community-acquired meningitis range from 19% to 37% with as many as 30% of survivors experiencing chronic neurologic dysfunction such as hearing loss or focal deficits. Although precise outcome data in the oncology population with AIM are limited, mortality rates of 60% have been reported in immunocompromised patients with a central nervous system infection. Patients with hematologic malignancy and recent stem cell transplantation with prolonged neutropenia have a very high mortality.

ADDITIONAL READING

Beaman MH, Wesselingh SL. Acute community-acquired meningitis and encephalitis. *Med J Aust* 2002;176:389–396.

Mylonakis E, Hohmann EL, Calderwood SB. Central nervous system infection with *Listeria monocytogenes*: 33 years experience at a general hospital and review of 776 episodes from the literature. *Medicine (Baltimore)* 1998;77:313–336.

Pruitt AA. Nervous system infections in patients with cancer. *Neurol Clin N Am* 2003;21:193–219.

Roos KL, Tyler KL. Meningitis, encephalitis, brain abscess, and empyema. In: Harrison's *Principles of Internal Medicine.* 16th ed. Kasper DL, Fauci AS, Longo DL, et al., eds. New York: McGraw-Hill, 2005, pp 2471–2490.

Van de Beek D, de Gans J, Tunkel AR, et al. Community-acquired bacterial meningitis in adults. *N Engl J Med* 2006;354:44–53.

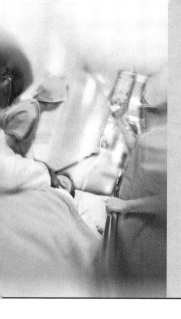

64

Infectious Encephalitis

DEFINITION

Infectious encephalitis (IE) refers to infection of the brain parenchyma, and occasionally meninges (meningoencephalitis), spinal cord (encephalomyelitis), or nerve roots (encephalomyeloradiculitis), resulting in central nervous system dysfunction.

CLINICAL SETTING

Excluding endemic and epidemic viral etiologies, IE in the oncology population is typically caused by a limited number of organisms. IE occurs most often in the setting of impaired cell-mediated immunity such as that occurs with lymphoreticular neoplasms or chronic corticosteroid use.

PATHOGENESIS

Viruses and certain protozoal organisms cause most cases of malignancy-associated IE; seasonal and geographic viral encephalitis will not be discussed. As with infectious meningitis, the immune status of the host plays a primary role in the susceptibility of IE. For instance, patients with impaired T-lymphocyte function due to Hodgkin's lymphoma, hematopoietic stem cell transplantation, and chronic corticosteroid or immunosuppressive therapy, have an increased risk for viral IE with cytomegalovirus (CMV), varicella zoster virus (VZV), and herpes simplex viruses (HSV). Cytotoxic chemotherapy and cranial irradiation for solid neoplasms have been associated with HSV infections. Encephalitis due to the feline protozoan *Toxoplasma gondii* may complicate chronic steroid use, human immunodeficiency virus (HIV)-associated malignancy, or hematopoietic stem cell transplantation. Human herpes virus (HHV)-6 encephalitis seems to be a unique pathogen implicated in causing IE of the temporal lobes in patients who have undergone stem cell transplantation. This syndrome may resemble reactivation HSV encephalitis, which possesses tropism for the temporal lobes and endothelium, resulting in inflammatory hemorrhagic necrosis of the brain parenchyma. Temporal lobe involvement by any organism may induce behavioral changes and seizures. Varicella zoster virus (VZV) has been implicated in causing acute inflammatory necrotizing encephalitis in cancer patients. Patients with humoral deficiency due to chronic lymphocytic leukemia, multiple myeloma, or splenectomy may develop IE due to echoviruses. Immunocompromised patients should be cautioned against working in outdoor soil since contamination with the raccoon pinworm *Baylisascaris procyonis* may cause encephalitis. West Nile encephalitis may be of concern in the cancer patient who receives multiple blood transfusions as this agent has been shown to be transmitted by various blood products. The West Nile virus can involve not only the brain but also the anterior horn cells resulting in a paralytic syndrome. Profound immunosuppression can result in progressive multifocal leukoencephalopathy (PML) due to the JC virus. Reactivation of VZV may cause encephalitis through two pathogenic mechanisms. Large vessel granulomatous angiitis and encephalitis may follow a recent outbreak of zoster involving the trigeminal distribution. Small vessel diffuse vasculitis and encephalitis typically follows an episode of zoster involving any dermatome, although some patients may not have a history of a rash.

Regardless of the etiology and mode of acquisition, IE typically causes cerebral dysfunction with the clinical manifestations varying depending upon predominant sites of involvement. Cortical inflammation and edema can produce delirium, somnolence, disruptive behavior, focal deficits, or seizure activity. As noted, HSV IE has a predilection for inciting an inflammatory response with hemorrhagic necrosis, typically involving the temporal lobes. Ongoing cerebral edema may result in increased intracranial pressure and cerebral herniation syndromes. Involvement of the hypothalamus may produce the syndrome of inappropriate diuretic hormone (SIADH) release.

ETIOLOGY

The etiology of IE in an indivual cancer patient varies somewhat depending on the underlying malignancy and treatment modalities. Keep in mind that, overall, HSV is the most common etiology of IE in this population. However, other etiologies should be considered in the immunosuppressed host which includes:

- HSV 1 or 2
  - HSV 1 most common form of sporadic IE
- VZV
- HHV-6
  - May resemble HSV IE in patients who have undergone hematopoietic stem cell transplantation
- Cytomegalovirus

- Encephalitis may co-exist with retinitis
- Epstein-Barr virus
- West Nile virus
  - May complicate blood product transfusion in endemic areas during the summer or fall months
- Echovirus
  - May occur in patients with CLL or myeloma
- Influenza A or B virus
- JC virus
- *Toxoplasma gondii*
- *Mycoplasma pneumoniae*

SYMPTOMS AND SIGNS

The hallmark of IE is abnormal cerebral cortex function, most often manifested by behavioral abnormalities. However, since cancer patients often manifest non-specific clinical findings, the diagnosis should be entertained with any combination of the following:

- Headache
- Fever
- Vomiting
- Confusion/behavioral changes
- Poor memory
- Aphasia
- Weakness
- Seizures
- Tachycardia or bradycardia
  - May result from autonomic dysfunction if temporal lobe or hypothalamic involvement is present
- Somnulence
- Hyperreflexia
- Ataxia
- Focal weakness in setting of encephalomyeloradiculitis
- Coma

DIAGNOSTIC STUDIES

Although the diagnosis of IE is often made clinically, diagnostic studies are necessary to confirm suspected cases, ascertain specific infectious etiologies, and assess for complications. The most widely utilized diagnostic studies for IE in the cancer population include:

- Magnetic resonance imaging (MRI) of the brain
  - MRI with gadolinium enhancement is the imaging study of choice, especially when HSV is suspected. Typical findings of HSV IE include enhancement, necrosis, or hemorrhage of the temporal lobe(s)

- Cerebrospinal fluid (CSF) analysis
  - CSF findings of IE most often include lymphocytic pleocytosis and elevated protein with normal glucose concentration
  - Red blood cells in the CSF may indicate HSV infection due to the hemorrhagic nature of this infection
  - Polymerase chain reaction (PCR) is the diagnostic study of choice for HSV (over 95% sensitive and specific) but is also available for CMV, VZV, EBV, enteroviruses, HHV-6, JC virus, and toxoplasmosis
- Viral serologies
  - IgM serologies most helpful in acute setting and available for most implicated viruses, including West Nile
- Electroencephalogram (EEG)
  - Although non-specific slowing of background activity is common with any type of encephalitis, patients with HSV IE may manifest characteristic findings such as lateralizing periodic sharp waves and slow wave patterns
- Cerebral angiogram
  - Rarely necessary but may be indicated in diagnostically uncertain situations to exclude vasculitis due to VZV or paraneoplastic etiology
- Brain/meningeal biopsy
  - Although imaging studies and PCR analysis of CSF lead to a diagnosis in many patients, indications for brain/meningeal biopsy include
    - Uncertainty between IE and neoplastic involvement
    - Progression of abnormalities on MRI with treatment
    - Concern for vasculitis in setting of VZV infection

TREATMENT

In addition to meticulous supportive care and correction of cytopenias, effective specific therapy for IE remains limited to a few pathogens. Most importantly, patients with suspected HSV IE should be immediately treated with intravenous acyclovir while awaiting CSF PCR results. If HSV infection is confirmed, treatment should be continued for at least 14 days. Acyclovir is also indicated for VZV encephalitis. Ganciclovir is indicated for CMV IE. Foscarnet has been used with limited success in cases of HHV-6 IE. There is no effective antiviral agent to treat JC virus. Toxoplasmosis is often treated with pyrimethamine and sulfadiazine.

PROGNOSIS

The prognosis of IE in patients with malignancy depends upon many factors including the status and stage of the underlying neoplasm, the degree of immunosuppression, and presence of organ dysfunction. The most important prognostic factor in patients with encephalitis due to HSV is the level of consciousness upon initiation of treatment. Regardless of the etiology of IE, cancer patients with refractory seizures, coma, focal deficitis, or ongoing cerebral edema have a very high mortality.

ADDITIONAL READING

Beaman MH, Wesselingh SL. Acute community-acquired meningitis and encephalitis. *Med J Aust* 2002;176:389–396.

Hirai R, Mitsuyoshi A, Shoji H, et al. Herpes simplex encephalitis presenting with bilateral hippocampal lesions on magnetic resonance imaging, simultaneously complicated by small cell lung carcinoma. *Intern Med* 2005;44:1006–1008.

Pruitt AA. Nervous system infections in patients with cancer. *Neurol Clin N Am* 2003;21:193–219.

Schmutzhard E. Viral infections of the CNS with special emphasis on herpes simplex infections. *J Neurol* 2001;248:469–477.

Whitley RJ. Herpes simplex encephalitis: adolescents and adults. *Antiviral Res* 2006;71:141–148.

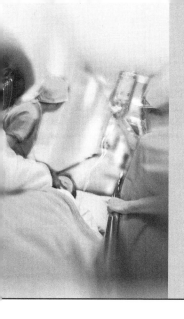

65

Perirectal Abscess

DEFINITION

Perirectal abscess (PRA) is an infection of the lower rectum and perianal area that often results from occlusion and infection of mucosal glands within the anal crypts.

CLINICAL SETTING

Within the oncology population, patients with acute myelogenous leukemia (AML) are the most vulnerable to developing PRA (2% to 8%) as a result of neutropenia, neutrophil dysfunction, and chemotherapy-induced mucositis. Patients with solid tumors undergoing chemotherapy are also at risk.

PATHOGENESIS

The pathogenesis of PRA is multifactorial with immunosuppression playing the primary role in commencement and spread of infection. Underlying benign anorectal disorders such as hemorrhoids and anal fissures increase the risk of developing PRA. Patients with AML may manifest a PRA at initial presentation as a result of profound neutropenia and granulocyte dysfunction, which often occurs following minor epithelial trauma. Diarrhea due to neutropenic enteritis or chemotherapy may lead to mucosal ulceration with subsequent bacterial invasion. Patients undergoing cytotoxic chemotherapy, especially for small cell lung carcinoma, may also develop PRA. Leukemic infiltration of perianal epithelium or rectal mucosa may facilitate infection as well. Occlusion of the mucosal glands within the anal crypts with denuded epithelium and fecal material results in rapid bacterial growth, most often with anaerobes and Gram-negative bacilli. Due to the paucity of neutrophils, infection can subsequently spread rapidly to the ischiorectal fossa, supralevator space, and the perineum, occasionally resulting in Fournier's gangrene. Translocation of bacteria into the bloodstream results in sepsis and, occasionally, multiple organ dysfunction syndrome (MODS). Positive blood cultures are present in approximately 20% to 25% of cases. Underlying immunosuppresion due to hematologic malignancy or chemotherapy increases the risk for rapid tissue destruction that may result in uncontrollable sepsis and death. The vast majority of cases of PRA are polymicrobial in nature containing anaerobic and Gram-negative bacteria. *Bacteroides fragilis* and *Eschercia coli* are the most common isolates, although most cultures yield several bacterial species.

ETIOLOGY

The most frequently isolated bacterial species from PRA include:

- *Bacteroides fragilis*
- *Clostridium perfringens*
- *Escherichia coli*
- *Klebsiella pneumoniae*
- *Proteus mirabilis*
- *Enterobacter cloacae*
- *Pseudomonas aeruginosa*
- *Enterococcus faecalis, E. faecium*
- *Staphylococcus aureus*
- *Streptococcus* species

SYMPTOMS AND SIGNS

Although the most common symptoms of PRA are perianal pain and fever, patients may present with other clinical manifestations, which may be atypical in the setting of neutropenia, including:

- Perianal pain (present in approximately 70% of patients)
- Fever
- Diarrhea
- Rectal bleeding
- Tenesmus
- Perianal erythema and/or induration
  - Patients with neutropenia may exhibit only erythema and induration without fluctuance. With neutrophil recovery, fluctuance and spontaneous drainage may occur
- Perianal ulceration/purulent discharge
- Midline anal fissure
  - An anal fissure involving the midline has been noted in association with acute leukemia

- Perianal tenderness
  - Clinical dictum usually states that a rectal examination should be avoided in neutropenic patients to avoid invoking bacteremia; however, studies are not conclusive regarding this, with some revealing no increased risk of rectal examination in this setting
- Perianal or perineal crepitus
  - May occur due to infection with anaerobes, especially with gas-forming Clostridial species such as *C. septicum*, *C. welchii*, or *C. perfringens*
- Perineal or scrotal swelling
  - May occur if Fournier's gangrene complicates PRA

Diagnostic Studies

Diagnosis of PRA in the cancer patient requires a high index of suspicion, especially in the setting of neutropenia since fluctuance may be absent. Patients with febrile neutropenia, especially due to AML or small cell lung cancer, should have a perianal examination; however, helpful diagnostic studies may include:

- Complete blood count
  - Neutropenia or agranulocytosis common
  - Thrombocytopenia common in settting of AML or chemotherapy
  - Circulating leukemic blasts may be present
- Blood cultures
  - Positive in approximately 20% to 25% of cases
- Culture of purulent material
- Perianal skin biopsy
  - May be useful if leukemic infiltration of perianal area is suspected, but may be hazardous in setting of neutropenia and/or thrombocytopenia
- Computed tomography
  - May be helpful to visualize abscess, fistula, or soft tissue gas
  - May reveal concurrent neutropenic enterocolitis/typhlitis in setting of AML and neutropenia

Treatment

Treatment of PRA requires a high index of suspicion with prompt administration of broad-spectrum antibiotics. Agents with activity against Gram-negative bacilli (including *P. aeruginosa*), *S. aureus*, streptococci, enterococci, and anaerobes are imperative; such agents include piperacillin-tazobactam, ticarcillin-clavulanic acid, or the combination of a quinolone or extended-spectrum cephalosporin and metronidazole. Vancomycin should be considered if cultures reveal evidence of resistant staphylococci or enterococci. If fluctuance is present, surgical consultation and incision and drainage should be considered. However, most patients with profound neutropenia manifest induration which may be treated initially with conservative measures such as warm compresses, sitz baths, stool softeners, analgesics, and antibiotics. Profuse diarrhea may require treatment to limit fecal contamination and decrease perianal trauma. Granulocyte stimulating factor (G-CSF) can be considered, although data regarding effect on outcome are unclear. If abscess formation becomes evident with neutrophil recovery, spontaneous drainage may occur, but surgical drainage should be considered if ongoing sepsis is present. If a perirectal fistula occurs, surgical repair is indicated upon hematologic remission. Severe cases with ongoing sepsis may require diverting colostomy. Fortunately, most patients respond to conservative measures. Some authors recommend perianal radiation therapy if leukemic infiltration is documented, although chemotherapy is typically commenced first.

PROGNOSIS

Most patients respond to conservative measures and do not require surgical intervention, although as many as 40% of patients with PRA required drainage in some series. Mortality rates for PRA are 10% to 30%, with higher mortality rates in the leukemic population.

ADDITIONAL READING

Diehl KM, Chang AE. Acute abdomen, bowel obstruction, and fistula. In: Abeloff MD, Armitage JO, Niederhuber JE, et al., eds. *Clinical Oncology*, 3rd ed. Philadelphia: Elsevier Churchill Livingstone, 2004, pp 1025–1045.

Earle MF, Fossieck BE, Cohen MH, et al. Perirectal infections in patients with small cell lung cancer. *JAMA* 1981;246:2464–2466.

Grewal H, Guillem JG, Quan SHQ, et al. Anorectal disease in neutropenic leukemic patients. *Dis Colon Rectum* 1994;37:1095–1099.

North JH, Weber TK, Rodriguez-Bigas MA, et al. The management of infectious and noninfectious anorectal complications in patients with leukemia. *J Am Coll Surg* 1996;183:322–328.

Quadri TL, Brown AE. Infectious complications in the critically ill patient with cancer. *Semin Oncol* 2000;27:335–346.

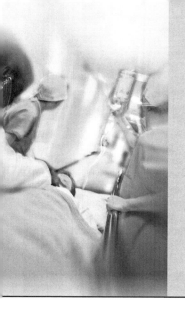

66

Ecthyma Gangrenosum

DEFINITION

Ecthyma gangrenosum (EG) is a distinct infectious syndrome characterized by invasive necrotic skin ulcerations resulting from vascular involvement with a variety of organisms, most commonly *Pseudomonas aeruginosa*.

CLINICAL SETTING

The majority of cases of EG occur in the setting of profound neutropenia and immunosuppression, most commonly due to acute leukemia.

PATHOGENESIS

Although EG may result from many infectious organisms, it most commonly complicates local or systemic infection with *P. aeruginosa*. Immunosuppression from hematologic, or, less commonly, solid malignancies, chemotherapy, hypogammaglobulinemia, neutropenia, or corticosteroid use are key factors in the development of EG. The two primary mechanisms involved in the pathogenesis of EG are bacteremia with secondary hematogenous skin involvement (the classic form) and direct skin inoculation at the site of a vascular catheter, biopsy, scratch, or surgical incision. The localized form is typically not associated with bacteremia if treated promptly and has a more favorable prognosis than the bacteremic form of EG. This discussion will primarily focus on the virulent bacteremic form of EG.

Pseudomonas aeruginosa is a ubiquitous Gram-negative opportunistic pathogen normally isolated from water, soil, and damp hospital surfaces. Patients with prolonged hospitalization, broad-spectrum antibiotic use, and severe illness commonly become colonized with this organism. In the setting of prolonged neutropenia, hematologic malignancy, or cytotoxic chemotherapy, fulminant bacteremia may ensue from intestinal translocation, intravascular catheters, or urinary catheters. Classic EG results when bacteria lodge within dermal blood vessels, causing an infectious vasculitis and secondary thrombosis, which eventually leads to tissue necrosis. Tissue necrosis is characterized phenotypically as the classic purple or black central eschar. The perivascular area and surrounding tissue teem with organisms that multiply rapidly. The vasculitis is hemorrhagic in nature. Bacterial collagenases and elastases destroy the elastic lamina of the vascular wall and surrounding tissue, allowing rapid tissue spread of infection and ongoing sepsis. Tissue cultures and biopsies almost always yield the responsible organism, *P. aeruginosa*, although a variety of bacteria and fungal organisms are responsible for EG in some cases. Leukopenia and hypogammaglobulinemia inhibit the host's ability to control the infection. The buttocks, perineum, and proximal limbs are most frequently affected, but any site can be involved and multiple lesions are not uncommon. The most common cause of death in patients with EG is typically septic shock and multiple organ dysfunction from uncontrolled bacteremia.

ETIOLOGY

Many organisms have been reported to cause EG, including:

- *P. aeruginosa*
- *Klebsiella pneumoniae, K. oxytoca*
- *Escherichia coli*
- *Serratia marcescens*
- *Stenotrophomonas maltophilia*
- *Citrobacter freundii*
- *Morganella morganii*
- *Aeromonas hydrophila*
- *Staphylococcus aureus*
- *Fusarium solani*
- *Aspergillus fumigatus*
- *Candida albicans*
- *Rhizopus* species
- *Exserohilum* species
- Herpes simplex virus

SYMPTOMS AND SIGNS

Since a variety of skin lesions can occur in the critically ill oncology population, a high index of suspicion is necessary to diagnose EG, which should be considered if any of the following are present:

- Fever
- Tachycardia

- Hypotension
- Painless erythematous macule with pale surrounding halo (initial lesion)
- Progression (usually within 24 hours) to painful, dark red-purple well-demarcated nodules
- Blue-black centrally necrotic and tender ulceration occasionally surrounded by erythematous halo (this is the classic lesion of EG)
- Purulent discharge with crust
- Hemorrhagic bullae

DIAGNOSTIC STUDIES

Diagnosis of EG is primarily clinical based on the appropriate setting such as neutropenia following induction chemotherapy for acute leukemia, and the rapid development of a characterstic skin lesion(s). However, useful diagnostic adjuncts include:

- Blood cultures
  - Almost universally positive in classic form of pseudomonal EG
- Gram stain and culture of aspirate or discharge from lesion
  - Gram-negative bacilli on Gram stain with growth of *P. aeruginosa* or other organisms
- Biopsy
  - Typical findings include tissue necrosis, hemorrhage, small vessel thrombosis, vasculitis, and perivascular infiltration with numerous organisms
  - Hyphae noted with fungal EG
- Computed tomography, especially if large lesion or perineal involvement

TREATMENT

Treatment of EG should be instituted immediately, without waiting for histologic or culture data. Since bacteremia with *P. aeruginosa* is present with most cases of classic EG, antipseudomonal antibiotic therapy with two agents should be commenced. For example, an antipseudomonal penicillin or cephalosporin in combination with an aminoglycoside, aztreonam, or quinolone. Surgical debridement may be necessary in cases of rapid tissue necrosis and multiple surgeries are occasionally needed. Supportive care with attention to nutrition, correction of neutropenia, and eradication of the underlying malignancy (usually acute leukemia) is also important.

PROGNOSIS

The prognosis of EG in patients with acute leukemia and prolonged neutropenia is poor, especially if restoration of the neutrophil count is prolonged or if the underlying leukemic process does not respond to treatment. Overwhelming sepsis with multiple organ dysfunction syndrome is an ominous sign with a very high mortality in the oncology patient with EG, especially if mechanical ventilation or vasopressor use is required.

Additional Reading

Chan YH, Chong CY, Puthucheary J, Loh TF. Ecthyma gangrenosum: a manifestation of *Pseudomonas* sepsis in three paediatric patients. *Singapore Med J* 2006;47:1080–1083.

Downey DM, O'Bryan MC, Burdette SD, et al. Ecthyma gangrenosum in a patient with toxic epidermal necrolysis. *J Burn Care Res* 2007;28:198–202.

Fast M, Woerner S, Bowman W, et al. Ecthyma gangrenosum. *Can Med Assoc J* 1979;120:332–334.

Jones SG, Olver WJ, Boswell TC, et al. Ecthyma gangrenosum. *Eur J Haematol* 2002;69:324.

Levy I, Steiin J, Ashkenazi S, et al. Ecthyma gangrenosum caused by disseminated *Exserohilum* in a child with leukemia: a case report and review of the literature. *Pediatr Dermatol* 2003;20:495–497.

Reich HL, Fadeyi DW, Naik NS, et al. Nonpseudomonal ecthyma gangrenosum. *Am Acad Dermatol* 2004;50:S114–S117.

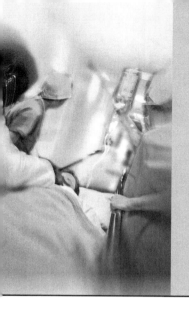

67

Vibrio vulnificus Sepsis

DEFINITION

Vibrio vulnificus sepsis is an uncommon, but highly lethal, infection characterized by the rapid development of necrotizing bullous skin lesions and septic shock following ingestion of raw shellfish or soft tissue inoculation acquired while cleaning seafood or bathing in warm seawater.

CLINICAL SETTING

The vast majority of cases of *Vibrio vulnificus* sepsis occur in the setting of underlying cirrhotic liver disease, malignancy, cytotoxic chemotherapy, or high-dose corticosteroids.

PATHOGENESIS

Vibrio vulnificus is a motile, curved, halophilic (salt-requiring), Gram-negative bacteria commonly isolated in warm seawater worldwide, but most commonly in the Gulf of Mexico and Hawaii. The organism has also been isolated in the marine waters off the coast of Cape Cod, and even within lakewater in New Mexico, Oklahoma, and Utah. The organism especially thrives in the southern United States during the months of March through November, the time period when most infections occur. Most severe human infections follow ingestion of raw or undercooked shellfish, especially oysters and crabs, or through exposure of a superficial wound with seawater or drippings from uncooked, raw seafood. The focus of this discussion will pertain to primary bacteremia obtained via ingestion of undercooked seafood, since aggressive soft tissue infections may occur in normal hosts, but virtually all cases of primary bacteremia occur only in patients with severe underlying illness, such as cancer.

Cirrhosis is the most well-known predisposing condition for *V. vulnificus* infection. Impaired reticuloendothelial function and elevated ferritin contribute to the pathogenesis, since iron is vital for growth of *V. vulnificus*. The organism is able to extract iron from hemoglobin as a nutrient source. In fact, iron overload from thalassemias, hemolytic anemias, chronic transfusion therapy for myelodysplastic syndromes, and hereditary hemochromotosis, all increase the risk of primary bacteremia and sepsis with this organism. Hypogammaglobulinemia (as can occur in nephrotic syndrome, chronic lymphocytic leukemia and multiple myeloma) increases the risk of sepsis due to decreased IgG levels which are important for host control of this organism. Neutropenia resulting from chemotherapy or acute myeloid leukemia increases the risk of *V. vulnificus* sepsis since neutropenia impairs phagocytic clearance of the bacteria. Poor opsonization, due to reticuloendothelial system dysfunction present in various hematopoietic neoplasms, as well as splenectomy, contributes to the poor immune response in the cancer population.

Several properties of *V. vulnificus* contribute to the virulence of the organism. The major determinant of virulence is the presence of a polysaccharide capsule which impairs phagocytosis and serum killing, and directly stimulates release of inflammatory cytokines such as interleukin (IL)-1, IL-6, and tumor necrosis factor (TNF). The hallmark of *V. vulnificus* sepsis is treatment-refractory hypotension, which likely results from cytokine and bradykinin generation. Another hallmark of *V. vulnificus* sepsis is the rapid development of hemorrhagic bullae and skin necrosis. Elaboration of extracellular toxins as well as elastase, collagenase, and phospholipase invoke vascular and dermal injury resulting in bullae formation and cutaneous necrosis. Necrotizing vasculitis has been reported from direct bacterial invasion of vascular endothelium, which may contribute to necrosis of skin, subcutaneous tissues, and muscle. Death occurs from refractory septic shock and multiple organ dysfunction syndrome.

ETIOLOGY

Vibrio vulnificus sepsis most commonly occurs in immunocompromised hosts following ingestion of, or, uncommonly, exposure of damaged skin to the following marine organisms:

- Raw oysters (cause majority of cases)
  - Virtually all oysters and 10% of crabs harvested from the Chesapeake Bay during summer months contain *V. vulnificus*
  - Very commonly isolated from shellfish along the southern Gulf states from March through November
- Raw or undercooked crabs
- Contaminated seawater contacting food during preparation

- Shrimp
- Mackerel
- Tilapia (reported to cause necrotizing skin infection and septic shock after skin puncture by a fin during cleaning)

SYMPTOMS AND SIGNS

The diagnosis of *V. vulnificus* sepsis requires a high index of suspicion, but should be considered in any cancer patient presenting with fever and hemorrhagic or bullous skin lesions, especially involving the lower extremities, which is the most frequent site of cutaneous involvement. Reported symptoms and signs of this infectious syndrome include:

- Fever/rigors
  - Typically abrupt onset
- Nausea/vomiting
- Diarrhea
- Confusion
- Lower extremity pain
  - May predate onset of skin lesions by several days
- Tachycardia
- Hypotension
- Skin changes
  - Erythematous, cellulitis-like lesions initially involving the legs
  - Hemorrhagic, bullous skin lesions are the classic finding and may evolve and spread over hours
  - Cutaneous necrosis

DIAGNOSTIC STUDIES

Diagnosis of *V. vulnificus* sepsis is primarily clinical since the rapid onset of high fever, hemorrhagic bullous skin lesions, and shock in the setting of seafood exposure in a compromised host is nearly pathognomonic. As such, recognition of this syndrome by all clinicians involved with the care of cancer patients is vital. However, useful diagnostic adjuncts include:

- Blood cultures
  - Positive in majority of cases of primary bacteremia
  - Prompt review of the initial Gram-stain specimen obtained from blood culture bottles with identification of curvilinear, Gram-negative bacilli useful for facilitating diagnosis
- Aspirate and culture of bullae
- Biopsy of cutaneous lesion
  - May reveal organisms within tissue, thrombotic occlusion of small blood vessels, necrotizing vasculitis, and hemorrhagic tissue necrosis

- Complete blood count
  - Leukopenia more common than leukocytosis
  - Thrombocytopenia common
  - Schistocytes and reticulocytes may indicate disseminated intravascular co-agulation (DIC), which is very common
- Coagulation studies
  - Typically reveal changes of DIC
- Electrocardiogram
  - Heart block has been rarely reported
- Chest radiography
  - Commonly reveals diffuse bilateral pulmonary infiltrates compatible with acute respiratory distress syndrome (ARDS)

TREATMENT

Prompt institution of appropriate antibiotics is imperative in any suspected case of *V. vulnificus* sepsis. Tetracyclines are the agents of choice and should be provided intravenously at maximally tolerated doses. Cefotaxime and ciprofloxacin are reasonable alternatives. Aggressive debridement of devitalized and necrotic tissue is important; some patients may require limb amputation to control infection. Aggressive critical care support with intravenous volume resuscitation, vasopressors, and mechaninal ventilation are important treatment adjuncts. No randomized trials exist regarding administration of intravenous immunoglobulin infusion, but this could be considered in patients with underlying lymphoid malignancies or multiple myeloma.

Of vital importance, is prevention of *V. vulnificus* sepsis in patients undergoing cytotoxic chemotherapy or with liver metastases, CLL, myeloma, hypogammaglobulinemia, splenectomy, or iron overload states. Patients with any of these risk factors should be cautioned against consumption of raw or undercooked seafood in any form. Additionally, these patients should wear gloves if involved with seafood or shellfish preparation and avoid seawater contact with broken skin.

PROGNOSIS

The fatality rate of *V. vulnificus* sepsis is approximately 50% in most series. Patients presenting with hypotension have a mortality rate approaching 100%. Reported mortality rates are lower, but still approximately 33%, in patients who receive antibiotic within 24 hours of onset of the illness.

ADDITIONAL READING

Barton JC, Ratard RC. *Vibrio vulnificus* bacteremia associated with chronic lymphocytic leukemia, hypogammaglobulinemia, and hepatic cirrhosis: relation to host and exposure factors in 252 *V. vulnificus* infections reported in Louisiana. *Am J Med Sci* 2006;332:216–220.

Bonner JR, Coker AS, Berryman CR, et al. The spectrum of vibrio infection in a gulf coast community. *Ann Intern Med* 1983;99:464–469.

Ikeda T, Kanehara S, Ohtani T, et al. Endotoxin shock due to *Vibrio vulnificus* infection. *Eur J Dermatol* 2006;16:423–427.

Koenig KL, Mueller J, Rose T. *Vibrio vulnificus:* hazard on the half shell. *West J Med* 1991;155:400–403.

Neill MA, Carpenter CCJ. Other pathogenic vibrios. In: Mandell, Douglas, and Bennett's *Principles and Practice of Infectious Diseases.* 6th ed. Mandell GL, Bennett JE, Dolin R, eds. Philadelphia: Elsevier Churchill Livingstone, 2005, pp. 2544–2548.

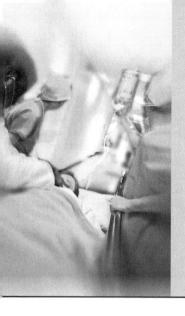

68

Clostridium septicum Spontaneous Myonecrosis

DEFINITION

Spontaneous myonecrosis is a rapidly progressive and highly fatal necrotizing infection of skeletal muscle that results from bacteremia with the anaerobic bacillus, *Clostridium septicum*.

CLINICAL SETTING

Spontaneous necrosis of skeletal muscle and sepsis due to *C. septicum* most often occurs in the setting of known or occult malignant disease, most commonly colorectal carcinoma or acute leukemia.

PATHOGENESIS

Clostridium septicum is a Gram-positive, gas-producing, obligate anaerobic bacillus that, unlike other clostridial species, has a propensity to invade and necrose normal skeletal muscle tissue resulting in spontaneous (atraumatic) myonecrosis and gas gangrene. Myonecrosis can occur in sites distant from the initial portal of entry. The ability of this organism to invade normal tissue results from the production of various toxic enzymes such as hyalouronidase, deoxyribonuclease, and various hemolysins. The most well-described exotoxins produced by *C. septicum* include α, β, γ, and δ. The α-toxin possesses lecithinase activity that can cause breakdown of the cell membranes of circulating erythrocytes and skeletal muscle, resulting in massive intravascular hemolysis and myonecrosis, respectively. The β-toxin induces transmural necrosis of the bowel wall, facilitating invasion of the adjacent tissue and subsequent metastatic infection. *Clostridium septicum* is a rare constituent of normal colonic flora, but frequently colonizes patients with colorectal carcinoma or enteritis of any cause, such as that due to chemotherapy or leukemia (e.g., neutropenic enterocolitis). The presence of a colorectal neoplasm may induce an acidic and hypoxic mileau favoring overgrowth of *C. septicum*. Subsequent ulceration of tumor or bowel mucosa from any cause likely results in bacterial translocation, resulting in bacteremia and subsequent metastatic seeding of distant skeletal muscle culminating in myonecrosis. Rare cases of *C. septicum* myonecrosis resulting from endometrial and gallbladder carcinoma have been reported.

Once *C. septicum* lodges in skeletal muscle, most often the limb or trunk musculature, the organism propogates in rapid fashion resulting in local edema, hemorrhage, gas formation, and tissue necrosis. Rhabdomyolysis can result in myoglobinuric acute renal failure. Curiously, pathologic specimens reveal a paucity of neutrophilic inflammation—a phenomenon resulting from enzymatic dissolution of leukocytes and inflammatory cells. Necrotic muscle contains abundant Gram-positive bacilli and cystic spaces that result from gas production within myocytes. Death results from refractory septic shock with multiple organ dysfunction syndrome.

Etiology

Approximately 80% of patients who develop *C. septicum* myonecrosis have an underlying malignant disease, most commonly colorectal carcinoma or acute leukemia, which account for approximately three-fourths of all cases. Myonecrosis may be the initial manifestation of occult malignancy in some patients, especially those with colon carcinoma. The most commonly reported etiologies in the oncology population include:

- Colon or rectal carcinoma
- Acute myelogenous or lymphocytic leukemia
- Large granular lymphocytic leukemia
- Gallbladder carcinoma
- Endometrial carcinoma
- Ovarian carcinoma
- Prostate carcinoma
- Neutropenic enterocolitis/typhlitis
- Chemotherapy-associated gastrointestinal ulceration (etoposide, cytarabine, anthracyclines)

Symptoms and Signs

Spontaneous myonecrosis due to *C. septicum* may present with abdominal pain in the patient with neutropenic colitis or with severe extremity pain in the patient with known or an occult visceral, especially colon, cancer. Clinical manifestations that should prompt the clinician to consider this diagnosis include:

- Fever
- Extremity pain
  - May be excruciating with absence of cutaneous findings in early stage of illness: "pain out of proportion to physical findings"

- Malaise
- Nausea/vomiting
- Abdominal pain
  - Typically severe, generalized, and progressive if a perforated colon cancer or severe enterocolitis in the setting of chemotherapy or neutropenia due to leukemia is present
- Diarrhea
- Tachycardia
- Hypotension, often refractory to treatment
- Delirium
- Abdominal tenderness
  - Generalized tenderness and peritoneal signs typically indicate perforation of a colorectal tumor or transmural necrosis of the intestinal wall in the setting of neutropenic enterocolitis
- Extremity tenderness and swelling
  - Findings of compartment syndrome may be present in some patients: massive edema, loss of distal motor function, and parasthesia
- Skin discoloration
  - Begins with area of erythema with rapid expansion and development (within hours) of bullae and purple skin discoloration
- Crepitus
  - Hallmark finding indicative of gas formation within soft tissue and muscle

DIAGNOSTIC STUDIES

Diagnosis of *C. septicum* myonecrosis requires a very high index of suspicion since treatment delay is associated with a poor response to even the most aggressive therapy. The diagnosis may be made clinically in patients who present with sudden onset of fever, excruciating extremity and/or muscle pain, and rapid evolution of skin changes and crepitus, whether or not there is a history of malignancy. However, useful diagnostic adjuncts include:

- Aspiration of bullous skin lesion for Gram stain and culture
  - Thin, grayish-colored fluid (resembling dirty dishwater) with a foul smell
  - Gram stain reveals plump Gram-positive bacilli with absence of leukocytes (a valuable clue to the diagnosis)
  - *C. septicum* colonies on solid agar resemble a "medusa head," which provides a valuable clue to the diagnosis
- Blood cultures
  - May become positive within hours on anaerobic media due to the presence of overwhelming bacteremia
- Biopsy of involved skin, subcutaneous tissue, and muscle—may not be an option in cases of rapidly progressive septic shock
  - Typical histologic findings include abundant organisms, a lack of neutrophilic and inflammatory cell infiltrate, and necrotic myocytes with vaculozation from intramuscular gas formation

- Plain radiography of involved extremity
  - May reveal soft tissue gas
- Computed tomography
  - More sensitive at detecting soft tissue gas within muscle groups as well as edema and necrotic tissue
  - In cases of bowel involvement typical findings include wall thickening and edema, *pneumatosis intestinalis*, ascites, and, in cases of a colonic malignancy, a localized-phlegmatous mass
- Serum chemistries
  - Elevated creatine phosphokinase (CPK) due to myonecrosis; may be extremely elevated leading to acute renal failure
  - Elevated lactate dehydrogenase (LDH) may result from muscle necrosis, end-organ ischemia resulting from hypotension and shock, or intravascular hemolysis
- Complete blood count and peripheral blood smear
  - Leukocytosis, leukopenia, and thrombocytopenia common
  - May reveal leukemic blasts in cases related to neutropenic enterocolitis
  - Severe anemia may occur if α-toxin mediated intravascular hemolysis or disseminated intravascular coagulation (DIC) is present
    - Spherocytes on blood smear indicative of α-toxin-induced hemolysis
    - Schistocytes on blood smear indicative of DIC
- Coagulation studies
  - Findings of DIC are common such as prolonged clotting times and hypofibrinogenemia

TREATMENT

Prompt treatment of suspected *C. septicum* myonecrosis is mandatory and must be instituted before culture and imaging data are available since treatment delay is closely correlated with a poor outcome. The antibiotic of choice is intravenous penicillin G in high-dose (e.g., 18–24 million units daily in divided doses). Alternatives for the penicillin-intolerant patient include metronidazole, imipenem, and clindamycin. Some authors recommend routine administration of clindamycin which may decrease bacterial protein synthesis and subsequent toxin production. The cornerstone of effective therapy for myonecrosis is timely surgical debridment with wide excision of all involved muscle tissue. Amputation may be necessary. Compartment syndrome requires immediate fasciotomy. Daily surgery to assess for ongoing muscle necrosis and serial debridement is often necessary. Patients with necrotic bowel or perforated colon carcinoma and uterine carcinoma require colectomy or hysterectomy, respectively. Hyperbaric oxygen is recommended by some authors. Supportive critical care measures including aggressive volume resuscitation, vasopressors, and mechanical ventilation are necessary in most patients.

Prognosis

Even with prompt, aggressive medical and surgical therapy, mortality rates for *C. septicum* myonecrosis range from 30% to 75% in some series. Treatment delay of greater than 12 hours of presentation has been associated with mortality rates of nearly 100% in some studies. Most patients die on the first day of illness. Survivors without prior diagnosis of malignancy require a colonoscopy to exclude colorectal carcinoma, due to the close association with spontaneous clostridial myonecrosis. Search for other malignancies should be considered depending on the clinical scenario.

Additional Reading

Chew SSB, Lubowski DZ. *Clostridium septicum* and malignancy. *ANZ J Surg* 2001;71:647–649.

Katlic MR, Derkac WM, Coleman WS. *Clostridium septicum* infection and malignancy. *Ann Surg* 1981;193:361–364.

Kornbluth AA, Danzig JB, Bernstein LH. *Clostridium septicum* infection and associated malignancy. Report of two cases and review of the literature. *Medicine* (Baltimore) 1989;68:30–37.

Lorimer JW, Eidus LB. Invasive *Clostridium septicum* infection in association with colorectal carcinoma. *Can J Surg* 1994;37:245–249.

Pelletier JPR, Plumbley JA, Rouse EA, et al. The role of *Clostridium septicum* in paraneoplastic sepsis. *Arch Pathol Lab Med* 2000;124:353–356.

Stevens DL, Musher DM, Watson DA, et al. Spontaneous, non-traumatic gangrene due to *Clostridium septicum*. *Rev Infect Dis* 1990;12:286–296.

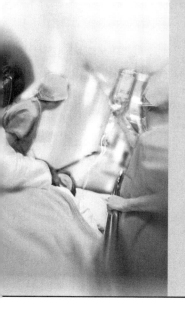

69

Streptococcus bovis Endocarditis

DEFINITION

Endocarditis is an infection of the endothelial surface of the cardiac valves, most often the aortic and mitral, that may result in valvular destruction, heart failure, and death. *Streptococcus bovis* is an occasional etiology of endocarditis, which has important diagnostic and long-term treatment implications due to a close association with occult malignancy.

CLINICAL SETTING

Over 50% of patients with *S. bovis* endocarditis are found to harbor an occult colon carcinoma, which is often diagnosed only after *S. bovis* bacteremia is identified. Occasionally, other visceral neoplasms can result in *S. bovis* bacteremia.

PATHOGENESIS

Streptococcus bovis is a normal commensal of the human gastrointestinal tract. This organism is a member of the Lancefield group D streptococci which also includes the genus, *Enterococcus*. Since diagnostic and treatment approaches differ between treatment of *Enterococcus* species and *S. bovis*, accurate microbiological differentiation is vital. The group D organisms are identified by the ability to grow in 40% bile and to hydrolyze esculin. However, the enterococci grow in 6.5% sodium chloride whereas *S. bovis* is salt-sensitive and does not grow in a salt-laden environment. Biochemical evidence of starch hemolysis by *S. bovis* is another reliable method of differentiation from enterococci. In addition, *S. bovis* is 10 to 5000 times more susceptible to penicillin G than are the enterococci, which are frequently penicillin-resistant.

Several studies have demonstrated that the fecal flora of patients with colorectal carcinoma is altered, providing a growth advantage for *S. bovis*, possibly due to tumoral-related metabolic changes in the luminal mileau. Whatever the mechanism, *S. bovis* likely gains access to the bloodstream via translocation through friable tumoral mucosa. The organism typically adheres to abnormal valves affected by pathologic calcification, mitral valve prolapse, or rheumatic valvular disease. Endocarditis due to *S. bovis* is typically subacute in nature, resulting in prolonged systemic symptoms such as fever, weight loss, and myalgia which result from circulating cytokines. Immune complex phenomena may result in glomerulonephritis, hematuria, or joint effusions. If left untreated, large vegetations may form, disrupting coaptation of the valves and leading to eventual valvular incompetence and heart failure. Embolization of vegetations may result in stroke, mesenteric infarction, coronary artery occlusion and myocardial infarction, or lower extremity ischemia. Other streptococci such as *S. sanguis* and group G streptococci have been reported in association with colorectal tumors, probably by a similar mechanism, although the association with underlying neoplasia is not as robust.

Etiology

Most cases of malignancy-related *S. bovis* endocarditis occur in association with the following conditions:

- Colorectal carcinoma
  - Cecal involvement most common site in some series
- Esophageal carcinoma
- Hepatobiliary carcinomas
- Colonic polyps
- Colonoscopic biopsy

Symptoms and Signs

Endocarditis resulting from *S. bovis* presents with symptoms similar to subacute bacterial endocarditis from other bacteria, although patients with underlying colon cancer may manifest findings related to their neoplasm. Common manifestations include:

- Fever
- Weight loss
- Malaise
- Anorexia
- Night sweats
- Arthralgias/myalgias
- Back pain
- Hematuria

- Abdominal pain
  - May be associated with large colonic malignancy
  - Sudden severe pain may indicate embolic occlusion of mesenteric arterial vasculature with vegetation
- Chest pain/angina
  - May indicate embolic occlusion of coronary artery with vegetation
- Hemoccult-positive stool
- Mass lesion on rectal examination if distal cancer is present
- Heart murmur
  - Aortic and mitral regurgitant murmurs most common
- Physical findings of microembolic phenomena or circulating immune complexes
  - Subconjunctival petchiae, retinal hemorrhages, painful acral nodules (Osler's nodes), painless palmar/plantar macules (Janeway lesions), or splinter hemorrhages involving nail beds

DIAGNOSTIC STUDIES

The diagnosis of endocarditis in the cancer patient requires a very high index of suspicion due to the non-specific symptoms and signs. Definitive diagnosis requires additional diagnostic studies which include:

- Blood cultures
  - Often, the diagnosis of *S. bovis* endocarditis is made after blood cultures yield the organism
- Echocardiogram
  - Transesophageal echocardiography (TEE) is superior to transthoracic echocardiography (sensitivity and specificity exceed 90%) at detecting typical findings of endocarditis such as:
    - Vegetations, valvular insufficiency, myocardial abscess, aortic root abscess
- Electrocardiogram
  - May reveal heart block if the conduction system is involved by abscess formation
- Erythrocyte sedimention rate (ESR)
  - Although not specific, most patients with deep seated infection have an elevated ESR
- Complete blood count
  - Thrombocytosis, anemia, and leukocytosis common findings with bacterial endocarditis
  - Hypochromic, microcytic anemia may be present due to occult blood loss from colonic malignancy
- Gastrointestinal endoscopy
  - Colonoscopy is recommended in any patient with *S. bovis* isolated from a blood culture if no prior history of malignancy is present

o Esophagogastroduodenoscopy should be considered if the colonoscopy is normal

TREATMENT

Treatment of *S. bovis* endocarditis consists of prolonged intravenous administration of bactericidal antibiotics. Penicillin G is the drug of first choice since the organism is exquisitely sensitive to this agent with typical MICs ranging from 0.01-0.12 $\mu g/ml$. Penicillin alone for 4 weeks is adequate therapy for most patients. Ampicillin is an effective alternative if high-dose penicillin G is unavailable. Alternative antibiotics for the penicillin-allergic patient include vancomycin and clindamycin. Most patients have a favorable response to antibiotic therapy, but valve repair or replacement may be indicated if there is refractory congestive heart failure, more than one significant embolic episode, very large vegetation, uncontrolled bacteremia with failure to sterilize blood cultures, severe mitral or aortic regurgitation, and valvular or myocardial abscess. If colon carcinoma is present, standard surgical resection and chemotherapy should be applied once the patient is treated adequately for endocarditis.

PROGNOSIS

The prognosis of *S. bovis* endocarditis is favorable if antibiotic therapy is instituted prior to valvular destruction. The long-term prognosis primarily depends upon the stage of the underlying neoplasm and response to treatment.

ADDITIONAL READING

Burns CA McCaughey M, Lauter CB. The association of *Streptococcus bovis* fecal carriage and colon neoplasia: Possible relationship with polyps and their premalignant potential. *Am J Gastroenterol* 1985;80:42-46.

Klein RS, Recco RA, Catalano MT, et al. Association of *Streptococcus bovis* with carcinoma of the colon. *N Engl J Med* 1977;297:800-802.

Klein RS, Catalano MT, Edberg SC, et al. *Streptococcus bovis* septicemia and carcinoma of the colon. *Ann Intern Med* 1979;91:560-562.

Reynolds JG, Silva E, McCormack WM. Association of *Streptococcus bovis* bacteremia with bowel disease. *J Clin Microbiol* 1983;17:696-697.

Wantanakunakorn C. *Streptococcus bovis* endocarditis. *Am J Med* 1974;56:256-260.

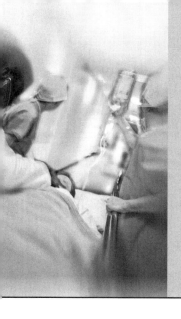

70

Transfusion Transmitted Bacteremia

DEFINITION

Transfusion transmitted bacteremia (TTB) is a relatively uncommon, but often fatal, etiology of sepsis that results from transfusion of various blood products utilized in various clinical settings.

CLINICAL SETTING

Although TTB has been reported following transfusion of red blood cells and plasma products, the majority of cases follow transfusion of platelet concentrates, which are commonly administered to patients with acute leukemia and chemotherapy-associated thrombocytopenia.

PATHOGENESIS

Rates of bacterial contamination of blood products have remained relatively stable over the last decade, in comparison to the drastic decline in the risk of transmission of various viral pathogens such as hepatitis C or the human immunodeficiency virus (HIV). In fact, bacterial contamination of blood products is the most common infectious risk posed by transfusion therapy and the second most common cause of transfusion-related mortality, second only to clerical errors. The contamination of various blood components varies with a rate of 1 per 1,000–3,000 of random donor and single donor platelets. The risk of sepsis is 1 in 25,000 units of platelets transfused. The risk for TTB from red blood cell transfusion is many-fold lower, with sepsis occurring in 1 in 250,000 units of red cells transfused. However, many cases of TTB may go unnoticed since fever during or following a transfusion may be attributed to a non-hemolytic transfusion reaction or to an infection at another site.

Bacterial contamination of blood products can occur by a variety of mechanisms. During blood donation, bacterial flora residing on the donor's skin may be introduced into the collection device since no method of skin cleansing is able to eradicate 100% of bacteria. As the needle is inserted into the donor vein, a skin plug may be forced into the needle and subsequently into the collection bag; bacteria residing on the skin and within sweat glands (most commonly *Staphylococci*) may subsequently grow and contaminate the collected blood. Red blood cell concentrates are an uncommon cause of TTB since these products are refrigerated at 4°C, a process that inhibits growth of most bacterial species. An exception to this, however, is the Gram-negative, iron-loving organism *Yersinia enterocolitica*, which is able to grow at a low temperature (psychrophilic). *Y. enterocolitica* is provided an ideal iron-rich, cold environment during the storage of packed red blood cells. *Yersinia enterocolitica* occasionally causes inflammatory colitis and mesenteric adenitis. Patients with subclinical or recent infection with this organism may be bacteremic and transmit the bacteria during blood donation. Other psychrophilic bacteria that may cause TTB with red cell transfusion include *Pseudomonas* species and *Serratia liquefaciens*. Since fresh frozen plasma (FFP) and cryoprecipitate are stored frozen, bacterial contamination is rarely associated with these products.

However, rare cases of TTB due to *Pseudomonas aeruginosa* and *Burkholderia cepacia* have been cultured from FFP and cryoprecipitate that have been thawed in contaminated water baths. A rare cause of TTB is contamination of blood collection bags or tubing; *Serratia marcescens* bacteremia has occurred in this setting.

Host factors that increase the risk of clinically significant sepsis following a contaminated transfusion include chemotherapy or corticosteroid use, prolonged neutropenia, solid tumors, hematopoietic malignancy, hypogammaglobulinemia, and malnutrition. However, otherwise healthy individuals have experienced fatal sepsis when transfused products laden with large amounts of endotoxin-releasing Gram-negative bacteria. Gram-negative organisms are most often implicated in the development of fatal septic shock, which likely results from endotoxin production and a subsequent cytokine storm culminating in multiple organ dysfunction syndrome.

ETIOLOGY

The bacterial etiology of TTB largely depends upon whether platelets or red blood cells are transfused, since these products are stored at different temperatures. The most commonly reported organisms include:

- Platelet transfusions
  - *Staphylococcus epidermidis, S. aureus*: accounts for 47% of cases
  - *Streptococci*
  - *Bacillus cereus*
  - *Clostridium perfringens*

- *Propionibacterium acnes*
- *Salmonella* species
- *Klebsiella* species
- *Serratia marcescens, S. liquifaciens*
- *Acinetobacter* species
- *Enterobacter* species
- *Y. enterocolitica*
- Red blood cell transfusions
  - *Y. enterocolitica*
  - *S. marcescens, S. liquifaciens*
  - *Enterobacter*
  - *Acinetobacter*
  - *Pseudomonas*
  - *E. coli*
  - *S. epidermidis, S. aureus*
  - *Enterococcus faecalis*
  - *B. cereus*

SYMPTOMS AND SIGNS

Most patients who develop TTB manifest symptoms during the transfusion or within 2 hours of completion. Symptoms and signs may be attributed to a transfusion reaction or another infection, which may lead to underdiagnosis. The clinician should consider TTB if any of the following are present:

- Fever/rigors (typically abrupt during transfusion)
- Diaphoresis
- Vomiting
- Confusion
- Oliguria
- Bleeding (in cases of disseminated intravascular coagulation [DIC])
- Tachycardia
- Tachypnea
- Hypotension

DIAGNOSTIC STUDIES

Diagnosis of TTB is primarily clinical and requires a very high index of suspicion. However, useful laboratory studies to aid in diagnosis and management include:

- Blood cultures
  - Should be obtained immediately, prior to antibiotic administration
- Culture of donor blood product
  - Transfusion should be stopped and any blood product in the line or bag should be sent to the laboratory for culture and identification of the organism

- Complete blood count and blood smear examination
  - May reveal leukocytosis or thrombocytopenia which are common findings with sepsis
  - Examination of the peripheral blood smear is useful to assess for morphologic changes consistent with intravascular hemolysis or DIC
- Coagulation studies
  - May reveal evidence of DIC

TREATMENT

Differentiating TTB from an acute hemolytic transfusion reaction (AHTR) may be difficult, but abrupt rigors and high fever with hypotension and absence of hemolysis should suggest TTB. Antibiotic therapy should be commenced immediately after blood cultures are obtained. Since Gram-positive organisms are commonly associated with platelet transfusions, initial coverage should be adequate against these organisms. Vancomycin is a reasonable empiric choice. Gram-negative bacteria, however, are associated with a more fulminant septic course and initial antibiotic therapy should provide coverage against enteric Gram-negative bacilli as well as *Pseudomonas* and *Serratia* species. Patients who develop symptoms of TTB during a red blood cell transfusion should receive an antibiotic active against *Y. enterocolitica*, such as a quinolone. Supportive care including fluid resuscitation, vasopressors, mechanical ventilation, and treatment of DIC is often necessary.

PROGNOSIS

Prognosis of TTB depends upon many factors including the bacterial inoculum, bacterial species, and the immune status of the host. Cancer patients with prolonged neutropenia and hematologic malignancies have a dismal prognosis if septic shock requires the use of mechanical ventilation or vasopressors. The mortality rate of *Y. enterocolitica* TTB is 50%. Outcomes may be worse if TTB is not recognized and treated promptly. Therefore, judicious use of empiric antibiotics may be warranted in any patient with possible TTB until culture data is available.

ADDITIONAL READING

Brecher ME, Hay SN. Bacterial contamination of blood components. *Clin Microbiol Rev* 2005;18:195–204.

Dodd RY. Bacterial contamination and transfusion safety: experience in the United States. *Transfus Clin Biol* 2003;10:6–9.

Gottlieb T. Hazards of bacterial contamination of blood products. *Anaesth Intensive Care* 1993;21:20–23.

Hoelen DWM, Tjan DHT, Schouten MA, et al. Severe *Yersinia enterocolitica* sepsis after blood transfusion. *Neth J Med* 2007;65:301–303.

Morel P, Herve P. Detection of bacterial contamination of platelet concentrates. International forum 6. *Vox Sang* 2003;85:230–232.

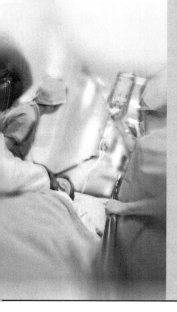

71

Pneumocystis jiroveci (carinii) Pneumonia

DEFINITION

Pneumocystis pneumonia (PCP) is a life-threatening opportunistic pulmonary infection caused by the ascomycetous fungi, *Pneumocystis jiroveci* (formerly *carinii*).

CLINICAL SETTING

Pneumonia due to *P. jiroveci* is a well-recognized complication in patients infected with the human immunodeficiency virus (HIV) but may also occur in patients with cancer, most commonly those with hematologic malignancies or receiving chronic corticosteroid therapy for malignant brain tumors.

PATHOGENESIS

Pneumocystis jiroveci is a ubiquitous fungal organism known for its inability to be propogated in any available culture medium. Person-to-person or environmental transmission is believed to be the likely mode of acquisition of infection, although some authors suggest that reactivation of dormant organisms is responsible. Most people have been exposed by early childhood without sequelae. The organism is dimorphic, existing both as trophic (1–4 μm diameter) and cystic (8 μm diameter) forms. The cyst typically contains up to eight trophic forms, which are dispersed upon cyst rupture. *Pneumocystis* exhibits pulmonary tropism, where it thrives within the alveolar spaces, without invasion unless the host is severely immunocompromised. This is a rare occurrence. The pathogenesis of PCP infection is complex, but an immunogenic surface glycoprotein termed glycoprotein A plays a key role in the attachment of the organism to host cells. The cyst wall of *Pneumocystis* consists of a variety of compoentents including beta-1, 3-glucan, chitins, and melanins which contribute to cell wall stability and evoking an inflammatory response within the lungs. The trophic forms adhere to the alveolar epithelium which subsequently activates signaling pathways within the organism culminating in increased reproduction and proliferation. The host inflammatory response to PCP results in local inflammation and pulmonary tissue damage which is in part responsible for the severe hypoxemia and respiratory failure that often complicates PCP. Vigorous subpleural inflammation can result in pneumothorax. Death due to PCP more closely correlates with the severity of lung damage than the fungal burden.

Cancer patients with severe immunosuppression involving T-lymphocytes are especially vulnerable to infection with PCP. Neutropenic patients do not exhibit a significant predisposition to PCP. The activity of CD4+ lymphocytes is the key defense against PCP, with risk of infection especially high with CD4+ counts of less than 200 cells/mm^3. CD4+ cells function as memory cells that play an important role in the recruitment of monocytes and macrophages which is to ingest and kill the organism. Recruited macrophages secrete tumor necrosis factor (TNF), interleukin-1, superoxides, and reactive nitrogen species that are vital for host defense against *Pneumocystis*. Patients with various lymphoid malignancies may manifest T-lymphocyte depletion or dysfunction thereby increasing risk of PCP. Chemotherapy and stem cell transplantation also may induce lymphopenia. Glucocorticoids are lympholytic and also increase the risk of PCP, especially in patients with lymphoma and malignant brain tumors who receive long-term therapy to control edema. Macrophage dysfunction is common in patients with hematologic malignancies which contribute to poor clearance of the organism.

Etiology

Most cases of PCP affecting cancer patients occur in the setting of chemotherapy, chronic corticosteroid administration, or hematologic malignancy. The most frequently reported underlying etiologies in the cancer population include:

- Non-Hodgkin's lymphoma
- Chronic lymphocytic leukemia
- Hodgkin's lymphoma
- Acute myelogenous or lymphoblastic leukemia
- Multiple myeloma
- Waldenström's macroglobulinemia
- Myelodysplastic syndrome
- Chronic myelogenous leukemia
- Hematopoietic stem cell transplantation
- Chemotherapy
- Corticosteroids
  - Typically when administered for malignant brain tumors and lymphoma

Symptoms and Signs

Patients with PCP may exhibit various symptoms and signs that are similar to other processes common in the oncology setting, with the most commonly reported including:

- Fever
- Dyspnea
- Non-productive cough
- Pleuritic chest pain
  - May be indicative of pneumothorax
- Tachypnea
- Tachycardia
- Rales (normal ausculatory findings are more common)

Diagnostic Studies

Diagnosis of PCP in the cancer patient requires a high index of suspicion, with the following studies most useful for diagnosis:

- Chest radiography
  - Classic finding is bilateral perihilar infiltrates in an interstitial or alveolar pattern, although nodular densities or unilateral lung infiltrates may occur
  - Pneumothorax and pleural effusion occasionally
- Computed tomography
  - More sensitive at detecting infiltrates; may be "ground glass" in nature
- Arterial blood gas
  - Hypoxia and respiratory alkalosis
- Serum lactate dehydrogenase (LDH)
  - Although not specific for PCP, LDH is often elevated which serves as a negative prognostic sign
- Complete blood count
  - Leukopenia and lymphopenia (notably CD4+ lymphopenia)
- Sputum collection (expectorated or induced with hypertonic saline) or bronchoalveolar lavage
  - Silver stains reveal characteristic trophic forms of *P. jiroveci*

Treatment

Treatment for suspected PCP in the ill cancer patient should not be delayed while awaiting sputum or bronchoalveolar specimen stains. Supportive medical care including oxygenation, mechanical ventilation, and treatment of cytopenias is paramount. The antibiotic of choice is intravenous trimethoprim-sulfamethoxazole. Inhaled pentamidine is an alternative for the sulfa-allergic patient. Corticosteroids have been shown to be beneficial if hypoxia is present by decreasing the inflammatory response in the lung.

Prognosis

If PCP is diagnosed and treated in a timely fashion, prognosis is favorable. However, uncontrolled malignancy, refractory leukopenia, and prolonged respiratory failure are associated with a high mortality rate, especially in the setting of hematologic malignancy.

Additional Reading

Bollee G, Sarfati C, Thiery G, et al. Clinical picture of *Pneumocystis jiroveci* pneumonia in cancer patients. *Chest* 2007;132:1305–1310.

Roblot F, LeMoal G, Godet C, et al. *Pneumocystis carinii* pneumonia in patients with hematologic malignancies: a descriptive study. *J Infect* 2003;47:19–27.

Thomas CF, Limper AH. Pneumocystis pneumonia. *N Engl J Med* 2004;350: 2487–2498.

Torres HA, Chemaly RF, Storey R, et al. Influence of type of cancer and hematopoietic stem cell transplantation on clinical presentation of *Pneumocystis jiroveci* pneumonia in cancer patients. *Eur J Clin Microbiol Infect Dis* 2006;25: 382–388.

Vehnuizen AC, Hustinx WNM, van Houte AJ, et al. Three cases of *Pneumocystis jiroveci* pneumonia (PCP) during first-line treatment with rituximab in combination with CHOP-14 for aggressive B-cell non-Hodgkin's lymphoma. *Eur J Haematol* 2007;80:275–276.

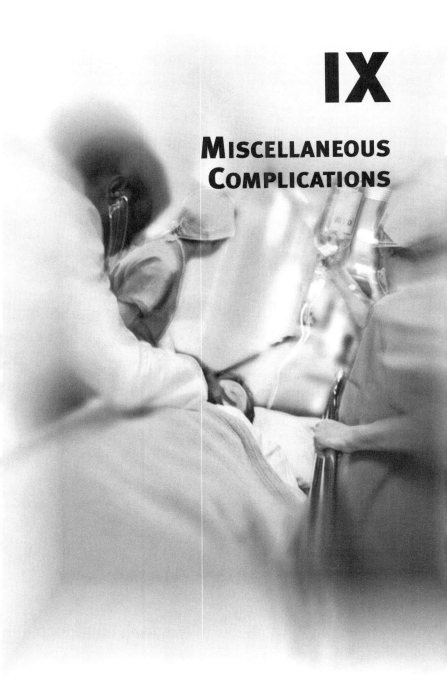

IX

MISCELLANEOUS COMPLICATIONS

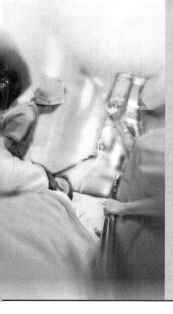

72. Hypersensitivity Reactions to Anti-Cancer Drugs

DEFINITION

Hypersensitivity reactions (HSRs) are defined as systemic reactions ranging from mild skin flushing to anaphylactic shock and typically occur during or shortly after infusion of certain chemotherapeutic drugs or monoclonal antibodies.

CLINICAL SETTING

Although there are exceptions, the majority of HSRs associated with platinum compounds occur after multiple previous cycles. In contrast, those associated with taxanes and monoclonal antibodies generally occur during the first few minutes of the first or second exposure.

PATHOGENESIS

The pathogenesis of HSRs may be either IgE-mediated (as in the case of platinum HSRs) or secondary to chemotherapy drugs, metabolites, or the diluent vehicles (as is the case with taxanes and monoclonal antibodies). An IgE mediated HSR, also known as a type I allergic reaction, is the proposed pathogenic mechanism for those reactions complicating platinum analogues, most commonly carboplatin and oxaliplatin, etoposide, and L-asparaginase, a bacterial derived protease utilized in the treatment of acute lymphocytic leukemia. Type I HSRs occur when mast cells sensitized to a specific antigen (e.g., platinum salt) are re-exposed to the antigen in the presence of the specific IgE antibodies that cause mast cells and basophils to release various mediators such as histamine, bradykinins, and leukotrienes that induce vasodilation, capillary leak, tissue edema, and smooth muscle contraction.

Vasodilatation and capillary leak-induced edema can lead to laryngeal swelling and acute airway obstruction which is a leading cause of death with HSRs. Cardiovascular collapse manifested as treatment-refractory hypotension is mediated by vasotoxic mast cell and basophil mediators such as histamine, leukotrienes, prostaglandins, and bradykinins. Type I HSRs, due to the aforementioned drugs, typically occur after several cycles of the implicated agent since it takes multiple exposures to develop IgE antibodies. Hypersensitivity to platinum compounds is a well-established phenomena and has been noted in refinery workers after prolonged inhalation of complex platinum salts. With regards to carboplatinum, a mean of eight cycles are typically administered prior to the development of HSRs, which occurs in as many as 27% patients treated with more than seven cycles of this agent. Intraperitoneal and intravesical administration of platinums may also induce HSRs in some patients.

Anaphylactoid reactions are so named due to having similar clinical manifestations as type I HSRs (e.g., urticaria, pruritis, bronchospasm, hypotension) but are not IgE mediated. Anaphylactoid reactions result from drug or vehicle-stimulated release of histamine and vasoactive mediators from mast cells. Taxane-mediated HSRs are of this type and in 95% of all reactions, occur during the first or second exposure to the drug, with the majority of cases occurring minutes into the infusion. Paclitaxel, a derivative of the yew plant, is water insoluble, and is diluted in a castor-oil compound known as Cremophor, has been shown to directly induce histamine release and hypotension in dogs. Similarly, docetaxel frequently causes HSRs, possibly mediated by the drug itself of its vehicle, polysorbate 80. Chimeric monoclonal antibodies (e.g., rituximab, cetuximab) may also induce severe infusional HSRs, due to a mechanism similar to the taxanes. Moderately severe infusion reactions manifested as bronchospasm and hypotension occur most commonly during the first infusion (77% with rituximab and 90% with cetuximab), which mandates prophylactic measures, which will be discussed below.

ETIOLOGY

Although HSRs have been reported in association with nearly all chemotherapeutic agents, most clinically significant reactions occur with the following cytotoxic agents and monoclonal antibodies:

- Platinum analogues
  - Cisplatinum, carboplatinum, oxaliplatin
- Taxanes
  - Paclitaxel, docetaxel
- Epipodophyllotoxins
  - Etoposide, teniposide
- L-asparaginase
  - *Escherichia coli* derived form most commonly implicated
- Monoclonal antibodies
  - Rituximab, traztuzumab, cetuximab, bevacizumab, alemtuzumab

Symptoms and Signs

Since most HSRs occur during or shortly after drug infusion, the clinician should consider the diagnosis if any of the following symptoms, alone or in combination, occur with any anti-cancer agent, but especially with those discussed in the previous section:

- Flushing
- Pruritis
- Fever or rigors
- Diaphoresis
- Apprehension/sense of impending doom
- Headache
- Dizziness
- Syncope
- Dyspnea
- Wheezing
- Stridor
- Chest discomfort
- Tongue swelling
- Diarrhea
- Abdominal pain
- Tumor pain
- Tachycardia
- Hypotension
- Conjunctival injection
- Erythematous rash or urticaria
- Angioedema

Diagnostic Studies

Diagnosis of HSRs to chemotherapy and monoclonal antibodies is typically a clinical diagnosis and made on the basis of the previously mentioned symptoms and signs in the proper clinical setting. Skin testing has been advocated by some authors to document true allergic reactions, but that discussion is beyond the scope of this text. In cases of severe HSRs or anaphylactic reactions, helpful studies to guide management include:

- Electrocardiogram
  - Typically reveals sinus tachycardia, but in patients with underlying cardiac disease, ischemic changes may be noted
- Chest radiography
  - May reveal acute non-cardiogenic pulmonary edema in rare cases
- Arterial blood gas
  - Respiratory alkalosis due to hyperventilation and hypoxia due to bronchospasm may be noted

○ Ominous findings include respiratory or metabolic acidosis which may complicate hemodynamic collapse

TREATMENT

Prevention of HSRs, especially with taxane therapy, involves prophylactic administration of corticosteroids and diphenhydramine. Minor HSRs consisting of pruritis or rash may resolve with interruption of the infusion or administration of an antihistamine, such as diphenhydramine. More severe HSRs manifested as urticaria, wheezing, dyspnea, or hypotension, typically require cessation of the implicated drug and administration of crystalloid fluids, corticosteroids, diphenhydramine, and H2-antagonists, such as cimetidine. Cases of suspected anaphylaxis require immediate subcutaneous injection of an epinephrine solution. If hypotension persists, dopamine or norepinephrine infusion may be necessary. Supportive care including airway control, oxygen, inhaled bronchodilators, and fluid management are important treatment adjuncts. Laryngeal edema may require urgent endotracheal intubation, or rarely, tracheostomy or cricothryoidotomy to establish a patent airway.

PROGNOSIS

The majority of cases of HSRs can be managed expectantly with temporary cessation of the implicated drug, gradual increase in the infusion rate, and pretreatment of subsequent cycles with corticosteroids, diphenhydramine, and H2-antagonists, especially prior to taxane and monoclonal antibody administration. Type 1 HSRs due to platinum analogues may require choosing an alternative cytotoxic agent, or if the platinum drug is deemed vital, using aggressive premedication with a crash cart at the bedside or attempting desensitization, although this is not without risk. Patients with acute lymphocytic leukemia who require L-asparaginase can be administered *Erwinia carotovora*-derived asparaginase or polyethylene glycol (PEG)-mediated asparaginase with frequent success. Death, although rare, can occur with severe HSRs not treated in an expedient manner.

ADDITIONAL READING

Lenz HJ. Management and preparedness for infusion and hypersensitivity reactions. *Oncologist* 2007;12:601–609.

Marinella MA. Bilateral conjunctivitis associated with rituximab. *Ann Pharmacother* 2007;41:1318.

Siu SWK, Chan RTT, Au GHK. Hypersensitivity reactions to oxaliplatin: experience in a single institute. *Ann Oncol* 2006;17:259–261.

Thomas RR, Quinn MG, Schuler B, et al. Hypersensitivity and idiosyncratic reactions to oxaliplatin. *Cancer* 2003;97:2301–2307.

Zanotti KM, Markman M. Prevention and management of antineoplastic-induced hypersensitivity reactions. *Drug Safety* 2001;24:767–779.

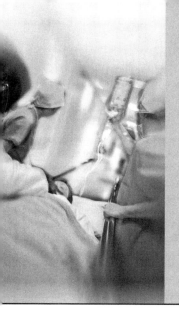

73

Chemotherapy Extravasation

DEFINITION

Chemotherapy extravasation (CE) is the escape of a cytotoxic chemotherapeutic agent out of the vein and into the surrounding tissue that may result in tissue necrosis.

CLINICAL SETTING

Most cases of CE occur during or shortly after administration of tissue vesicants, most commonly anthracyclines or vinca alkaloids, with an incidence of 0.1% to 6.5%.

PATHOGENESIS

Many cases of CE injury occur in patients with fragile or sclerosed veins or chronic lymphedema, which are more common in the elderly and patients treated with prior infusion therapy. The dorsum of the hand is especially vulnerable to extravasation injury due to the paucity of subcutaneous tissue. Although CE tissue necrosis has been associated with implanted central venous ports, most cases complicate extravasation through a peripheral venous catheter. Extravasation of chemotherapeutic agents may only cause minimal symptoms or irreversible tissue necrosis necessitating multiple reconstructive surgical procedures. The toxic effect on tissue depends upon the chemical nature of the extravasated drug. Cytotoxic agents are characterized as irritants or vesicants, depending on the degree of tissue injury they invoke. Irritant drugs typically cause a self-limited local inflammatory reaction manifested as local swelling, erythema, and pain. Local phlebitis may also occur. Long-term sequelae from irritant extravasation are rare. Examples of commonly administered irritant chemotherapeutic agents include carboplatin, cisplatin, oxaliplatin, cytarabine, and gemcitabine.

Vesicant drugs are those agents capable of inducing blister formation followed by significant tissue injury and irreversible necrosis. Tissue injury induced by vesicants may occur by several mechanisms. Anthracyclines, the most widely recognized class of vesicants, are absorbed onto the surface of local cells with subsequent entry into the nucleus causing DNA damage and cell death. After the involved cell dies, the drug is released into the surrounding tissues (a phenomenon known as endocytolysis) resulting in a cycle of further tissue injury and necrosis. Local vascular injury can result in cutaneous thrombosis, further contributing to tissue necrosis. Some drugs, notably doxorubicin, may be detected in the extravasated area for weeks to months, which is likely explained by ongoing endocytolysis. Indolent areas of cutaneous ulceration may ensue, but typically are non-healing due to lack of granulation tissue formation and poor peripheral re-epithelialization, due to fibroblast and epidermal cell injury, respectively. Other vesicants such as the vinca alkaloids and epipodophyllotoxins induce tissue injury via the lipophilic solvents utilized in commercial drug formulations. Injury from these drug classes is less severe than that due to anthracyclines since DNA damage does not occur. Taxanes may also act as tissue vesicants possibly due to microtubular dysfunction, but the tissue injury is typically much less severe than that seen with anthracylcines and vinca alkaloids.

ETIOLOGY

From a clinical standpoint, the agents implicated in CE can be characterized as irritants or vesicants.

- Irritants
  - Alkylating agents
    - Dacarbazine, carboplatin, cisplatin, cyclophosphamide, ifosfamide, oxaliplatin, thiotepa, melphalan
  - Antimetabolites
    - Cytarabine, 5-fluorouracil, gemcitabine, fludarabine, methotrexate
  - Miscellaneous agents
    - Etoposide, irinotecan, bleomycin, docetaxel, paclitaxel
- Vesicants
  - Anthracyclines
    - Doxorubicin, daunorubicin, idarubicin, epirubicin
  - Nitrogen mustard
  - Mitomycin-C
  - Vinca alkaloids
    - Vincristine, vinblastine, vinorelbine
  - Taxanes (usually cause irritant type injury, but may act as vesicant)
    - Docetaxel, paclitaxel

Symptoms and Signs

Any symptom involving the catheter site or extremity should be considered potentially related to extravasation injury. The most common clinical manifestations include:

- Intense pain around intravenous line or port site
  - Pain may be incapacitating, especially after doxorubicin extravasation
- Burning sensation
- Erythema
  - Typically occurs shortly after extravasation, but may be delayed by 1-2 hours
- Blister formation
  - Characteristic of vesicant injury from necrosis of basal layers of epidermis
- Extremity swelling
  - Typically involves distal forearm and dorsum of the hand
- Induration
  - Occurs after hours to days as tissue damage involves subcutaneous tissues
- Skin sloughing and ulceration
  - Typically complicates vesicant extravasation
- Soft tissue necrosis
  - Most commonly occurs after doxorubicin extravasation
  - Characterized by deep ulceration with eschar formation

Diagnostic Studies

The diagnosis of CE is made clinically, and is based on compatible symptoms during or shortly after intravenous administration of an implicated chemotherapeutic drug. In cases of suspected deep tissue injury, the following studies may help aid in management:

- Computed tomography or magnetic resonance imaging
  - May delineate extent of soft tissue, tendon, or vascular involvement and aid in surgical debridement plans
- Electromyography (EMG)
  - May be helpful in cases of chronic neurologic symptoms following vesicant extravasation
- Creatine phophokinase level if significant muscle necrosis is suspected

Treatment

Prevention of CE is of paramount importance, especially in the setting of anthracycline administration, and requires meticulous nursing care before, during, and after chemotherapy infusion. If possible, an implanted central venous port should be inserted into patients who require several cycles of potent vesicants such as anthracyclines. If a peripheral vein is utilized to infuse vesicant chemotherapy, the following principles should be followed:

- Avoid infusion into an extremity that has been venipunctured proximal to the infusion site in the preceding 48 hours
- Do not infuse with a butterfly needle
- Avoid infusion into an extremity affected by lymphedema, the dorsum of the hand, or over a joint
- The venous catheter should have blood aspirated to ensure brisk venous flow
- The catheter should be flushed before and after drug infusion

Treatment of vesicant CE requires prompt identification and management. In cases of peripheral CE, the infusion must be stopped and aspiration through the venous cannula should be attempted prior to catheter or needle removal. If a known antidote for the extravasated drug is available, a portion should be infused through the intravenous catheter and a portion subcutaneously infiltrated into the involved area. Specific antidotes for CE include dimethyl sulfoxide (DMSO) for anthracycline and mitomycin C; hyaluronidase for vinca alkaloids, epipodophyllotoxins, and paclitaxel; and sodium thiosulfate for nitrogen mustard and cisplatin. Hyaluronidase is an enzyme that enhances absorption of the extravasant whereas sodium thiosulfate provides an alternative alkylation target by forming non-toxic renally eliminated thioesters. Topical or subcutaneous DMSO acts as a free radical scavenger which has been shown to decrease soft tissue necrosis in animal and clinical studies. Pressure should not be applied to the involved area, since this may spread the agent into surrounding tissues. Application of cool compresses may decrease tissue injury in cases of anthracycline CE whereas warm compresses may benefit cases of vinca alkaloid CE. Surgical consultation should be obtained in cases of vesicant extravasation if debridement is necessary; skin grafting may be necessary in severe cases.

PROGNOSIS

Most cases of vesicant CE have a favorable prognosis if recognized in an expedient fashion. If CE is not recognized or treatment is delayed, necrosis may require extensive tissue resection and, rarely, amputation.

ADDITIONAL READING

Albanell J, Baselga J. Systemic therapy emergencies. *Semin Oncol* 2000;27: 347–361.

Berghammer P, Pohnl R, Baur M, et al. Docetaxel extravasation. *Support Care Cancer* 2001;9:131–134.

Krimsky WS, Behrens RJ, Kerkvliet GJ. Oncologic emergencies for the internist. *Cleve Clin J Med* 2002;69:209–222.

Lebredo L, Barrie R, Woltering EA. DMSO protects against adriamycin-induced tissue necrosis. *J Surg Res* 1992;53:62–65.

Schrijvers DL. Extravasation: a dreaded complication of chemotherapy. *Ann Oncol* 2003;16Siii:26–30.

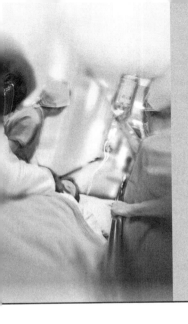

74

Neuroleptic Malignant Syndrome

DEFINITION

Neuroleptic malignant syndrome (NMS) is a life-threatening complication of various psychotropic medications characterized by hyperthermia, autonomic instability, and extrapyramidal symptoms.

CLINICAL SETTING

Cancer patients, especially in the palliative setting, are at significant risk of developing NMS when administered neuroleptic medications and dopamine antagonists utilized for symptom control of advanced malignancy.

PATHOGENESIS

Temperature homeostasis is regulated by complex centrally and peripherally-mediated control systems that maintain normal body temperature within a relatively constant range. Normal body temperature exhibits diurnal variation, with a nadir in the morning and peak values in late afternoon. Readings can vary by 1–3 °F in normal individuals. The central area responsible for temperature regulation is located in the preoptic nucleus of the anterior hypothalamus. When core body temperature increases, this area activates efferent nerve fibers to induce cutaneous vasodilation and sweating. Vasodilation dissipates body heat by convection and sweating enhances heat loss by evaporation. In contrast, if body core or skin temperature declines (as in shock states or environmental exposure), heat is conserved by cutaneous vasoconstriction and decreased sweating, which decreases heat loss from convection and evaporation, respectively. The body can only generate heat *de novo* by increased skeletal muscle contraction and tone or overt shivering—both of which are involuntary and depend on integration between the central and somatic nervous systems.

Fever is the most common disorder of temperature regulation and results when the hypothalamic set point is disrupted by inflammatory and infectious conditions that alter cytokine mileau. Hyperthermia results when peripheral temperature-regulating mechanisms are unable to maintain normal heat dissipation to maintain a body temperature that matches the hypothalamic set point, which is normal. Hyperthermia has many etiologies which include heat stroke, malignant hyperthermia of anesthesia, hormonal hyperthermia, and drug-induced hyperthermia from illicit or prescribed medications. Many medications utilized in the palliation of cancer symptoms can cause NMS. Furthermore, patients with advanced malignancy are at risk of developing NMS due to the presence of acute illness, dehydration, malnutrion, fatigue, mineral imbalance, and polypharmacy. All are factors that may increase susceptibility in the setting of psychotropic drug administration. The pathogenesis of NMS most likely results from drug-induced blockade of central dopaminergic receptors in the corpus striatum. This causes increased skeletal muscle spasticity, thereby generating excessive heat production. Impaired hypothalamic thermoregulation and autonomic dysfunction also impair heat dissipation, culminating in hyperthermia.

Hyperthemia affects homeostasis in many ways and adversely impairs various organ systems. As body temperature increases, basal metabolic rate and oxygen consumption rise. Increases in heart rate with rising body temperature may not be tolerated in patients with underlying cardiovascular disease and may induce myocardial ischemia, arrhythmias, hypotension, and acute heart failure. Neurologic damage from severe hyperthermia may induce delirium, stupor, seizures, or coma. Altered mental status often leads to aspiration and acute hypoxemic respiratory failure. Elevated body temperature can lead to dehydration via increased insensible water losses. Metabolic derangements complicating hyperthermia include metabolic acidosis, hyperkalemia, hypernatremia, and hypoglycemia. Rhabdomyolysis is a hallmark manifestation of NMS and results from extreme muscle rigidity. Increased myoglobin often leads to acute tubular necrosis and renal failure.

ETIOLOGY

The majority of NMS cases are associated with psychotropic medications and occur within 30 days of instituting therapy. The most commonly implicated drugs in the cancer population are utilized for treatment of nausea, vomiting, and terminal delirium and include:

- Butyrophenones
  - Haloperidol (most common agent responsible for NMS)
- Phenothiazines
  - Promethazine
  - Chlorpromazine

- ○ Prochlorperazine
- ○ Triethylperazine
- Metoclopramide
- Fentanyl— is known to induce muscular rigidity syndrome and has rarely been implicated in NMS

SYMPTOMS AND SIGNS

Since patients with NMS are often confused and may not be able to provide an adequate history, the following manifestations should prompt consideration of the diagnosis:

- Delirium
- Coma
- Diaphoresis
- Oliguria
- Incontinence
- Hyperthemia
- Tachycardia
- Hypertension—often labile
- Warm, dry skin
- Tremor
- Myoclonus
- Dystonia
- Dysarthria
- Muscular rigidity
  - ○ Generalized "lead pipe" rigidity is characteristic of NMS

DIAGNOSTIC STUDIES

The diagnosis of NMS is primarily clinical, but several laboratory studies may aid not only in diagnosis, but also in clinical management:

- Creatine phosphokinase
  - ○ Rhabdomyolysis universal
- Serum chemistries
  - ○ Hyperkalemia, hyperphosphatemia, and hypocalcemia frequently complicate rhabdomyolysis
  - ○ Hypernatremia occurs in setting of dehydration and increased insensible water loss
  - ○ Hypoglycemia
  - ○ Elevated urea nitrogen and creatinine indicate acute renal failure
- Complete blood count
  - ○ Leukocytosis and thrombocytopenia
- Arterial blood gases
  - ○ Respiratory acidosis and hypoxemia common and may aid in guiding decision for intubation
  - ○ Metabolic acidosis common

- Coagulation studies
  - May reveal evidence of disseminated intravascular coagulation (DIC)
- Urinalysis/microscopy
  - Dipstick analysis testing is positive for blood, but without red cells on microscopy and is indicative of myoglobinuria
  - Muddy-brown granular casts indicate myoglobinuric acute-tubular necrosis
- Urine myoglobin
- Electrocardiogram
  - Often reveals sinus tachycardia; hyperkalemia and hypocalcemia secondary to rhabdomyolysis may result in peaked T waves and QT interval prolongation, respectively

TREATMENT

Since body temperature can reach life-threatening levels (105°F), suspected cases of NMS should be immediately treated. Discontinuation of the inciting drug is mandatory. Supportive measures such as endotracheal intubation for airway protection, hydration to replace insensible fluid loss, and electrolyte management are vital. Rhabdomyolysis requires aggressive hydration and urinary alkalinization to prevent myoglobin-induced renal failure. Cooling measures such as cool water sprays, fans, and ice-packing the groin and axillae may be useful. Antipyretics such as acetaminophen or non-steroidal drugs are ineffective since the hypothalamic set point is normal. Benzodiazepines may aid in muscle relaxation. Dantrolene, a non-specific muscle relaxing agent, or bromocriptine have been utilized successfully in management of NMS.

PROGNOSIS

Morbidity from NMS often results from rhabdomyolysis-induced acute renal failure, respiratory failure, seizures, and autonomic instability. Mortality rates are approximately 10% to 20% in most studies. However, despite lack of large series, the cancer population may have higher mortality rates due to the presence of complex comorbidities.

ADDITIONAL READING

Garrido SM, Chauncey TR. Neuroleptic malignant syndrome following autologous peripheral blood stem cell transplantation. *Bone Marrow Transplant* 1998; 21:427–428.

Kawanishi C, Onishi H, Kato D, et al. Neuroleptic malignant syndrome in cancer treatment. *Palliat Support Care* 2005;3:51–53.

Morita T, Shishido H, Tei Y, et al. Neuroleptic malignant syndrome after haloperidol and fentanyl infusion in a patient with cancer with severe mineral imbalance. *J Palliat Med* 2004;7:861–864.

O'Neill WM. The neuroleptic malignant syndrome. *Clin Oncol* (R Coll Radiol) 1990;2:241–242.

Simon HB. Hyperthermia. *N Engl J Med* 1993;329:483–487.

Tanaka K, Akechi T, Yamazaki M, et al. Neuroleptic malignant syndrome during haloperidol treatment in a cancer patient. *Support Care Cancer* 1998;6:536–538.

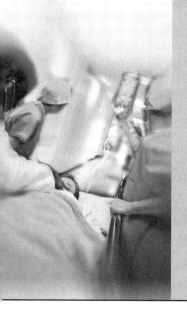

75

Acquired Methemo-globinemia

DEFINITION

Methemoglobinemia results from pathologic accumulation of methemoglobin, an oxidized (ferric, Fe^{+3}) form of hemoglobin that is unable to bind to oxygen, resulting in cyanosis despite normal PO2.

CLINICAL SETTING

Although uncommon, methemoglobinemia may occur in the cancer population following administration of various oxidant-type drugs, most often topical benzocaine anesthesia.

PATHOGENESIS

Methemoglobin is a normal byproduct of intracellular erythrocyte metabolism resulting from the oxidation of hemoglobin iron from the reduced ferrous (Fe^{+2}) state to the oxidized ferric (Fe^{+3}) state. Methemoglobin is normally maintained in the physiologic range of 1% by nicotinamide adenine dinucleotide phosphate (NADPH) and cytochrome-b5-methemoglobin reductase. However, with elevated levels, especially exceeding 25%, increased oxidized ferric iron within the hemoglobin molecule is unable to carry oxygen, which results in cyanosis from impaired tissue oxygen delivery. Also, oxygen affinity for the residual ferrous hemoglobin is increased, which shifts the oxygen dissociation curve leftward, impairing oxygen release to tissues. Methemoglobin exhibits a different spectrum of light absorption than hemoglobin (631 nm vs. 660 nm) which explains the inability of traditional transcutaneous pulse oximetry to detect methemoglobin.

In fact, despite normal PO_2, pulse-oximeter readings reveal very low saturation values. To detect methemoglobin, which exihibits a light absorption spectrum similar to carboxyhemoglobin, a co-oximetry device must be utilized, which can also provide a methemoglobin level. Routine blood gas analysis discloses a normal PO_2, which in the setting of clinical cyanosis, is highly suggestive of methemoglobinemia. Elevated plasma methemoglobin changes the color of blood to a chocolate-brown hue.

Acquired methemoglobinemia typically results from oxidizing drugs such as sulfa compounds, nitrates, topical anesthetics such as benzocaine, and rarely, alkylating agents. These drugs induce formation of ferric iron, resulting in methemoglobinemia. Depletion of the erythrocyte antioxidant glutathione and NADPH are implicated mechanisms. Reduction of the reducing ability of cytochrome-b5-methemoglobin reductase also plays a role. Congenital reductions of these enzymes systems may predispose patients to methemoglobinemia when oxidant drugs are administered.

ETIOLOGY

Although congenital enzyme deficiencies and multiple drugs have been implicated, etiologies specific to the cancer patient include:

- Topical mucosal benzocaine or cetacaine spray
  - Most common etiology in hospitalized population
  - Topical spray widely utilized for oropharyngeal anesthesia preceding esophagogastroduodenoscopy (EGD), bronchoscopy, endoscopic retrograde pancreatography (ERCP), transesophageal echocardiography (TEE), and endotracheal intubation
- Sulfa-containing antibiotics
- Dapsone
  - Occasionally administered following stem cell transplantation
- Metoclopramide
  - Frequently utilized for anti-emetic or promotility effects
- Rasburicase
  - Utilized for treatment of tumor lysis syndrome and severe hyperuricemia
  - Induces formation of hydrogen peroxide which induces oxidative stress and methemoglobin formation
- Chemotherapy
  - Cyclophosphamide
  - Ifosfamide

SYMPTOMS AND SIGNS

Symptoms of methemoglobinemia may be absent or minimal with serum levels of <25%; however, the majority of patients with levels >25% to 50% display clinical manifestations, which include:

- Dyspnea
  - Often out of proportion to co-oximetry findings of normal PO_2 and oxygen saturation
- Cyanosis
  - Often central in nature involving lips and oral mucosa
- Headache
- Confusion
- Lethargy
- Palpitations
- Anxiety
- Tachycardia
- Tachypnea
- Hypotension
- Coma
- Seizures

DIAGNOSTIC STUDIES

Diagnosis of acquired methemoglobinemia in the cancer patient should be suspected if acute cyanosis, decreased oxygen saturation levels, or both occur in the setting of no obvious pulmonary cause. Helpful diagnostic tests include:

- Arterial blood gas by co-oximetry, which has ability to detect wave lengths of methemoglobin and carboxyhemoglobin
  - "Chocolate-brown" color of arterial blood is virtually pathognomonic in the correct setting
  - Preserved PO_2 level and normal oxygen saturation
  - Elevated methemoglobin level
- Chest radiography
  - Helpful to exclude other causes of hypoxia; if normal and patient is cyanotic, very suggestive of methemoglobinemia

TREATMENT

Recognition of methemoglobinemia requires a high index of suspicion since low oxygen saturation levels and cyanosis have many causes in the critically ill cancer patient. Discontinuation of the offending drug is imperative. Intravenous methylene blue is the drug of choice and has a rapid onset. Some patients may require a second or multiple doses. Methylene blue accelerates the reduction of circulating methemoglobin by NADPH methemoglobin reductase. Patients with glucose-6-phosphate dehydrogenase deficiency have low endogenous NADPH levels and may develop acute intravascular hemolysis when administered methylene blue. Ascorbic acid is recommended in this situation.

PROGNOSIS

With rapid recognition and institution of therapy, most patients recover and have a favorable prognosis. However, methemoglobin levels above 50% may be fatal.

ADDITIONAL READING

Allen TL, Jolley SJ. Iatrogenic methemoglobinemia from benzocaine spray in trauma. *Am J Emerg Med* 2004;22:226.

Hadjiliadis D, Govert JA. Methemoglobinemia after infusion of ifosfamide chemotherapy. *Chest* 2000;118:1208–1210.

Kizer N, Martinez E, Powell M. Report of two cases of rasburicase-induced methemoglobinemia. *Leuk Lymphoma* 2006;47:2648–2650.

Marinella MA. When brown and blue make red: a case of acquired methemoglobinemia. *Heart Lung* 2006;35:205–206.

Shehadeh N, Dansey R, Seen S, et al. Cyclophosphamide-induced methemoglobinemia. *Bone Marrow Transplant* 2003;32:1109–1110.

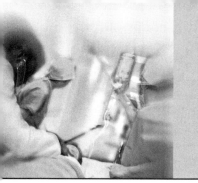

Index

U

V